Hospital Medicine Cardiology Cases

2024

First Edition

Rafael Zioni, MD

Senior Fellow
Emergency Department
Laniado Hospital
Israel

Self Publishers Worldwide
Seattle San Francisco New York
London Paris Rome Beijing Barcelona

Preface

"Hospital Medicine Cardiology Cases" is an intricate scholarly resource meticulously structured to provide an in-depth exploration of fundamental cardiology topics crucial for internal medicine practitioners and students aspiring to acquire profound knowledge in cardiology. Aligned with the ABIM exam blueprint for hospital and internal medicine, this book focuses on premier clinical cases in cardiology drawn from the latest research, aiming to furnish readers with a comprehensive grasp of essential cardiology principles. Each case within the text mirrors the ABIM exam format and is accompanied by detailed responses to enrich understanding. The primary objective of this book is to offer readers a comprehensive and current perspective on key cardiology subjects relevant to internal medicine practice and academic study. It is expertly designed to incorporate leading clinical cases sourced from up-to-date references, each presented in the ABIM exam style with thorough explanations. Additionally, the book features summarizing tables and figures to enhance learning and facilitate quick reference for readers.

Table of Contents

1 HYPERTENSION

1.1 Initial Hypertension Management: Lifestyle Changes vs Medication

Case 1

A 53-year-old man with a body mass index (BMI) of 32 presents to the clinic for a routine check-up. He has no complaints and is currently not on any medications. His blood pressure is 152/96 mmHg on two separate occasions. He reports a dietary intake high in salt and consumes alcohol occasionally, with about three drinks per week. He smokes half a pack of cigarettes per day and exercises infrequently. His father had a stroke at the age of 60, and his mother has been treated for hypertension. Laboratory tests reveal a fasting blood glucose of 110 mg/dL, HDL cholesterol of 35 mg/dL, triglycerides of 200 mg/dL, and a normal complete blood count and renal function. His serum potassium is 3.5 mEq/L.
Which of the following is the most appropriate initial step in the management of this patient's hypertension?

- A. Start a thiazide diuretic.
- B. Recommend lifestyle modifications including dietary changes, exercise, and smoking cessation.
- C. Prescribe a beta-blocker.
- D. Initiate treatment with an angiotensin-converting enzyme (ACE) inhibitor.

The correct answer is B. Recommend lifestyle modifications including dietary changes, exercise, and smoking cessation. This patient has newly diagnosed primary essential hypertension. Before initiating pharmacotherapy, it is important to address modifiable risk factors. Lifestyle modifications are the first-line treatment for patients with stage 1 hypertension and no evidence of target organ damage or cardiovascular disease. These modifications include dietary changes such as reducing salt intake, increasing potassium intake, and moderating alcohol consumption; promoting regular aerobic exercise; and smoking cessation. These changes can lead to significant reductions in blood pressure and may eliminate the need for medication in some individuals. Additionally, this patient's metabolic risk factors (elevated BMI, borderline impaired fasting glucose, low HDL, and elevated triglycerides) suggest the presence of metabolic syndrome, which further underscores the importance of lifestyle interventions. Option A is incorrect because while thiazide diuretics are a common choice for the pharmacological treatment of hypertension, the initial approach should focus on non-pharmacological interventions, especially in the absence of compelling indications for immediate drug therapy. Option C is incorrect because beta-blockers are not typically the first-line agents for the treatment of primary hypertension unless there are other indications such as heart failure or post-myocardial infarction. Option D is incorrect because ACE inhibitors are a good choice for hypertension, particularly in patients with diabetes or chronic kidney disease, but again, the initial step should be lifestyle modifications before starting pharmacotherapy in this patient.

"Essential hypertension" refers to the combination of inherited and environmental factors that contribute to the elevation of blood pressure in hypertensive patients. This particular ailment impacts an estimated 95% of individuals who have hypertension. It is uncommon for this condition to manifest prior to the age of 20; the average age of onset is between 25 and 50 years. Extensive research has been conducted on the various pathways that contribute to hypertension. These pathways encompass the overactivation of the renin-angiotensin-aldosterone and sympathetic nervous systems (RAAS), a compromised relationship between pressure and natriuresis, variations in cardiovascular and renal development, and elevated intracellular sodium and calcium levels.

Obesity, sleep apnea, excessive salt consumption, extensive alcohol use, smoking, polycythemia, nonsteroidal anti-inflammatory drug (NSAID) therapy, and low potassium levels are all causal elements. An increase in sympathetic outflow, an activation of the renin-angiotensin system, and an elevation in cardiac output are all associated with obesity. Modest blood pressure reduction results from weight loss accomplished via lifestyle modifications. In contrast, bariatric surgery substantially improves blood pressure and induces substantial weight loss in the vast majority of patients. Hypertension does indeed resolve entirely in 20 to 40% of instances.

Blood pressure has been observed to decrease in patients with sleep apnea who are treated with continuous positive airway pressure (CPAP). Certain individuals may experience an increase in blood pressure in response to increased salt consumption; therefore, patients with hypertension are advised to limit their sodium intake. Blood pressure may also be elevated as a result of excessive alcohol consumption, possibly due to an increase in plasma catecholamines. Patients who engage in binge drinking or consistently consume more than 40 g of ethanol (equivalent to two beverages) per day may develop hypertension. Blood pressure can be elevated as a result of cigarette smoking, as plasma norepinephrine levels increase. While there may be some uncertainty regarding the long-term effects of smoking on blood pressure, it is generally accepted that both smoking and excessive blood pressure contribute to an increased risk of cardiovascular disease. Variable relationships exist between exercise and hypertension. The implementation of aerobic exercise has been observed to decrease blood pressure in sedentary individuals. Nevertheless, the effect of more vigorous physical activity on blood pressure is comparatively diminished in individuals who engage in regular physical activity. A definitive correlation between stress and hypertension has yet to be established. Primary, drug-induced, or reduced plasma volume polycythemia all have the potential to increase blood viscosity and, consequently, blood pressure.

NSAIDs are typically associated with a blood pressure increase of 5 mm Hg. It is recommended that individuals with borderline or elevated blood pressure refrain from using these medications. A reduced consumption of potassium may lead to elevated blood pressure in certain patients. A recommended daily consumption is ninety millimoles. Metabolic syndrome, a collection of irregularities including adiposity of the upper body, insulin resistance, and elevated triglyceride levels, is associated with an increased risk of developing hypertension and adverse outcomes.

Filippone EJ et al. Controversies in Hypertension I: the optimal assessment of blood pressure load and implications for treatment. Am J Med. 2022;135:1043. [PMID: 35636476]

Case Note

The 53-year-old man in this case presents with new primary essential hypertension and metabolic risk factors indicative of metabolic syndrome. The most appropriate initial step in managing his hypertension is to recommend lifestyle modifications, including dietary changes, exercise, and smoking cessation. Lifestyle modifications can lead to significant reductions in blood pressure and may, in some cases, eliminate the need for medication. In tackling these modifiable risk factors, there's a potential for improved overall health and prevention of diseases linked with his metabolic syndrome. This plan should be the initial approach before considering pharmacological interventions.

1.2 Hypokalemia and Hypertension in a Young Woman: A Diagnostic Conundrum

Case 2

A 27-year-old woman presents to your clinic with a blood pressure of 158/100 mmHg, measured on three separate occasions. She has no significant past medical history and takes no medications. She does not smoke, drinks alcohol socially, and leads an active lifestyle. Her physical examination is unremarkable except for mild muscle weakness. Her father was diagnosed with hypertension in his early 30s. Laboratory tests reveal serum potassium of 2.9 mEq/L, bicarbonate of 32 mEq/L, plasma renin activity is low, and plasma aldosterone concentration is elevated. She denies the use of licorice-containing products. An abdominal ultrasound shows no abnormalities of the adrenal glands.
Which of the following is the most appropriate next step in the management of this patient's hypertension?

- A. Start treatment with an angiotensin-converting enzyme (ACE) inhibitor.
- B. Perform genetic testing for Liddle syndrome.
- C. Begin spironolactone therapy.
- D. Obtain a computed tomography (CT) scan of the abdomen to evaluate for an adrenal tumor.

The correct answer is C. Begin spironolactone therapy. This patient's clinical presentation is suggestive of a mineralocorticoid excess state, given the hypertension, hypokalemia, metabolic alkalosis, low renin, and high aldosterone levels. The absence of adrenal gland abnormalities on ultrasound makes a primary adrenal tumor less likely. The patient's clinical picture is consistent with primary hyperaldosteronism, possibly due to an inherited form such as glucocorticoid-remediable aldosteronism (GRA) or another form of familial hyperaldosteronism. Spironolactone, a mineralocorticoid receptor antagonist, is an appropriate treatment to block the effects of aldosterone and is likely to improve both her blood pressure and hypokalemia. Option A is incorrect because while ACE inhibitors are a common treatment for essential hypertension, they are not the first-line treatment for suspected primary hyperaldosteronism, which is suggested by the patient's low potassium and metabolic alkalosis. Option B is incorrect because genetic testing for Liddle syndrome, an autosomal dominant condition characterized by hypertension, hypokalemic alkalosis, low renin, and low aldosterone levels, is not consistent with the patient's elevated aldosterone levels. Liddle syndrome would present with low aldosterone due to volume expansion. Option D is incorrect because the patient's ultrasound did not show any adrenal abnormalities, making an adrenal tumor less likely. The patient's young age and familial history suggest that hyperaldosteronism may have a genetic basis rather than an adrenal tumor. Accurately measuring plasma potassium levels is crucial in hypertensive patients. While hypokalemia was once the primary indicator of hyperaldosteronism, now only 37% of affected individuals present with it - 50% have an aldosterone-producing adenoma, and 17% have adrenal hyperplasia. A frequent finding is a high serum bicarbonate level, indicating metabolic alkalosis. It is essential to consider testing for primary aldosteronism in hypertensive patients exhibiting any of the following:

1. Recurrent sustained high blood pressure
2. Resistance to three antihypertensive medications, including a diuretic
3. Well-controlled blood pressure requiring $\geq$4 medications
4. Hypokalemia unrelated to diuretics
5. Personal or family history of stroke or early-onset hypertension (<40 years)
6. Immediate family member with primary aldosteronism
7. Adrenal mass
8. Low lithium levels

Before testing, patients should correct any hypokalemia, consume a high-sodium diet ($>$ 6 g/day), and ideally discontinue oral estrogens/contraceptives, clonidine, ACE inhibitors, ARBs, beta-blockers, diuretics, and NSAIDs for $\geq$ 2 weeks. Approved medications include extended-release verapamil, hydralazine, terazosin, and doxazosin. Blood should be drawn after the patient has been awake and seated for 15–60 minutes, ideally between 8–10 am. Using a syringe and needle (not a vacutainer) and avoiding fist-clenching is recommended. Plasma potassium measurement is preferred over serum if unexpected hyperkalemia occurs, as hypokalemia can suppress aldosterone.

In primary aldosteronism, plasma renin activity (PRA) is typically under or 1.0 ng/mL/hr, and serum aldosterone is above 15 ng/dL (420 pmol/L). An aldosterone/PRA ratio < 24 rules out primary aldosteronism, while ratios of 30–64 are concerning, and > 64 support the diagnosis. Confirmatory testing includes a 24-hour urine for aldosterone, cortisol, and creatinine in an acidified container. Primary aldosteronism is confirmed with 93% specificity if urinary aldosterone exceeds 12 mcg/24 hr (33 nmol/24 hr), especially with suggestive clinical/biochemical findings. Genetic testing is advised for patients diagnosed with primary aldosteronism by age 20 or with a family history of the condition or early stroke (< 40 years) to identify familial corticosteroid-remediable aldosteronisms.

Byrd JB et al. Primary aldosteronism. Circulation. 2018;138:823. [PMID: 30359120]

1.3 Resistant Hypertension and Suspected Renal Artery Stenosis

Case 3

A 55-year-old man with a history of smoking and peripheral arterial disease presents with a 6-month history of difficult-to-control hypertension. Despite being on a regimen of amlodipine, hydrochlorothiazide, and atenolol, his blood pressure remains at 162/98 mmHg. He reports no history of renal disease, and his baseline serum creatinine has been stable at 1.2 mg/dL. On physical examination, you note diminished femoral pulses and an abdominal bruit. His laboratory tests show no electrolyte abnormalities, and his renal function is unchanged. You suspect renal artery stenosis.
Which of the following is the most appropriate next step in the evaluation of this patient?

- A. Start treatment with an angiotensin receptor blocker (ARB).
- B. Obtain a duplex ultrasound of the renal arteries.
- C. Perform a renal biopsy.
- D. Initiate a trial of a direct renin inhibitor.

The correct answer is B. Obtain a duplex ultrasound of the renal arteries. This patient has several clinical features that raise suspicion for renal artery stenosis, including resistant hypertension, a history of atherosclerotic disease (peripheral arterial disease), and an abdominal bruit. Duplex ultrasound of the renal arteries is a non-invasive test that can assess for the presence of renal artery stenosis, especially in patients with atherosclerotic disease. It is an appropriate initial imaging modality given its safety profile, lack of nephrotoxic contrast, and cost-effectiveness. Option A is incorrect because while ARBs can be used to treat hypertension, they can potentially worsen renal function in cases of bilateral renal artery stenosis or stenosis in a solitary kidney by reducing glomerular filtration pressure. Furthermore, the diagnosis should be confirmed before considering changes to antihypertensive therapy that specifically target the renin-angiotensin system. Option C is incorrect because there is no indication for a renal biopsy in this scenario. Renal biopsy is an invasive procedure and is typically reserved for cases where there is suspicion of intrinsic renal parenchymal disease, which is not suggested here. Option D is incorrect because, similar to ARBs, direct renin inhibitors can also worsen renal function in the setting of renal artery stenosis. Additionally, the diagnosis should be confirmed before considering this class of medication. Renal artery stenosis, a narrowing of the arteries supplying blood to the kidneys, is present in 1–2% of individuals with hypertension. The primary cause is atherosclerosis, but fibromuscular dysplasia should be considered in women under 50 years of age.

The decreased renal perfusion pressure leads to an excess release of renin, resulting in hypertension in patients with either a solitary kidney or bilateral renal artery lesions. Renal vascular hypertension should be suspected in the following circumstances:

- Onset of hypertension before age 20 or after age 50
- Resistant hypertension despite three or more antihypertensive medications
- Presence of epigastric or renal artery bruits (abnormal vascular sounds)

- Atherosclerotic disease of the aorta or peripheral arteries (15–25% of patients with symptomatic lower limb atherosclerotic vascular disease have concurrent renal artery stenosis)
- Abrupt increase (more than 25%) in serum creatinine levels after initiating angiotensin-converting enzyme (ACE) inhibitors
- Episodes of pulmonary edema associated with sudden surges in blood pressure

In these circumstances, further evaluation for renal artery stenosis may be warranted, as prompt diagnosis and management can help preserve renal function and potentially improve blood pressure control. Diagnostic modalities include renal artery duplex ultrasonography, computed tomographic angiography, or magnetic resonance angiography, followed by confirmatory renal angiography if indicated.

Early recognition and appropriate management of renal artery stenosis are crucial in preventing complications such as progressive renal impairment, resistant hypertension, and recurrent episodes of pulmonary edema or flash pulmonary edema.

Herrmann SM et al. Renovascular hypertension. Endocrinol Metab Clin North Am. 2019;48:765. [PMID: 31655775]

1.4 Hypertension Management in an Obese Black Man with DM and CKD

Case 4

A 60-year-old Black man with a history of type 2 diabetes and chronic kidney disease stage 3 presents with a blood pressure of 162/98 mmHg. He is currently not on any antihypertensive medications. His physical examination is notable for obesity with a BMI of 34 and no additional abnormal findings. His laboratory tests show a serum creatinine of 1.8 mg/dL, a potassium level of 4.5 mEq/L, and a urine albumin-to-creatinine ratio of 300 mg/g. He has no history of angioedema or chronic cough.
Which of the following is the most appropriate initial antihypertensive therapy for this patient?

- A. Start an ACE inhibitor.
- B. Begin a thiazide diuretic.
- C. Initiate a calcium channel blocker.
- D. Prescribe an angiotensin receptor blocker (ARB) in combination with a thiazide diuretic.

The correct answer is D. Prescribe an angiotensin receptor blocker (ARB) in combination with a thiazide diuretic. This patient has hypertension with comorbid conditions of diabetes and chronic kidney disease with proteinuria. In Black patients, ACE inhibitors and ARBs are less effective as monotherapy compared to other ethnic groups, but they are still important in the presence of kidney disease, especially with proteinuria. The combination of an ARB with a thiazide diuretic is recommended to both control blood pressure and provide renal protection. The diuretic will help with volume control and potentiate the antihypertensive effect of the ARB, while the ARB will provide renal protection by reducing intraglomerular pressure and proteinuria. There is significant evidence suggesting that Black Americans have a higher likelihood of developing hypertension and are more vulnerable to its associated complications. Additionally, they may have different responses to various antihypertensive medications.

The REGARDS study highlights significant differences in stroke risk associated with elevated blood pressure between Black and White Americans aged 45-64. When systolic blood pressure was below 120 mm Hg, both groups had similar stroke risk. However, for every 10 mm Hg increase in systolic blood pressure, Black participants faced a threefold higher risk of stroke. Specifically, for those aged 45-64 with blood pressure levels between 140-159/90-99 mm Hg, Black participants had a hazard ratio of 2.35 for stroke compared to their White counterparts. This heightened vulnerability in Black individuals may be attributed to various environmental factors, such as structural racism, diet, physical activity levels, stress, or access to healthcare services. Disparities in comorbid conditions like diabetes or obesity, as well as genetic ancestry and epigenetics, may also contribute to this increased risk. It is crucial to note that these racial disparities do not stem from innate biological differences associated with race itself. Instead, further research is needed to identify the underlying causes of these variations, which are likely multifactorial and influenced by social determinants of health.

For individuals with high blood pressure, a comprehensive management plan involving education and lifestyle modifications is essential. Early introduction of combination therapy has been recommended, although there is a lack of clinical trial data to support a lower blood pressure target specifically for Black patients. Evidence suggests that angiotensin-converting enzyme (ACE) inhibitors and angiotensin receptor blockers (ARBs) may be less effective in Black patients compared to White patients. Therefore, initial antihypertensive therapy should typically include a diuretic or a diuretic in combination with a calcium channel blocker. While renin-angiotensin-aldosterone system (RAAS) inhibitors, such as ACE inhibitors and ARBs, can help reduce blood pressure in Black patients, they may be more valuable as adjunctive agents to diuretics and calcium channel blockers, particularly for patients with hypertension and specific conditions like heart failure and kidney disease (especially with proteinuria). It is important to note that Black patients are at a higher risk of developing angioedema and cough associated with ACE inhibitors. In such cases, ARBs would be the preferred choice over ACE inhibitors.

Deere BP et al. Hypertension and race/ethnicity. Curr Opin Cardiol. 2020;35:342. [PMID: 32398604]

1.5 Antihypertensive Therapy in DM Patient with CKD

Case 5

A 58-year-old woman with a 10-year history of type 2 diabetes presents for a routine follow-up. Her current medications include metformin, simvastatin, and lisinopril. Her blood pressure today is 138/86 mmHg. Her most recent laboratory tests show an HbA1c of 7.2%, serum creatinine of 1.4 mg/dL, and a urine albumin-to-creatinine ratio of 250 mg/g. She has no history of cardiovascular events but is concerned about her risk for future complications.
Which of the following is the most appropriate management to reduce her cardiovascular and renal risks?

- A. Increase the dose of lisinopril to achieve a blood pressure target below 120/70 mm Hg.
- B. Add a calcium channel blocker to better control blood pressure.
- C. Initiate treatment with canagliflozin for its cardiovascular and renal benefits.
- D. Start finerenone to improve cardiovascular outcomes and retard the progression of kidney disease.

The correct answer is C. Initiate treatment with canagliflozin for its cardiovascular and renal benefits. This patient with type 2 diabetes and hypertension has a moderately increased urine albumin-to-creatinine ratio, indicating the presence of diabetic nephropathy. The CREDENCE trial has shown that canagliflozin, an SGLT-2 inhibitor, not only improves glycemic control but also provides cardiovascular benefits and improves renal outcomes in patients with type 2 diabetes and kidney disease. Additionally, SGLT-2 inhibitors have been shown to modestly lower blood pressure, which could help this patient achieve a more optimal blood pressure target. Option A is incorrect because, according to the ACCORD study, targeting a systolic blood pressure below 120 mm Hg did not significantly reduce the rate of a composite outcome of major cardiovascular events and was associated with an increased risk of serious adverse events compared to a target of less than 140 mm Hg. Option B is incorrect because, while adding a calcium channel blocker could help in better controlling blood pressure, it does not directly address the patient's renal risk, which is significant given her diabetic nephropathy. Option D is incorrect because, although finerenone has shown benefits in patients with diabetes and chronic kidney disease, the patient's blood pressure is not far from the target, and the primary goal in this scenario should be to address both glycemic control and cardiovascular/renal risk. Canagliflozin would be more appropriate given the evidence from the CREDENCE trial. Patients with both hypertension and diabetes are at an increased risk for cardiovascular complications. The ACCORD study, which focused on patients with diabetes, demonstrated that the majority of benefits from lowering blood pressure were observed with a systolic target below 140 mm

Hg. While aiming for a lower systolic target of less than 120/70 mm Hg further reduced the risk of stroke, it also led to a higher risk of serious adverse effects.

Based on the positive impact of angiotensin-converting enzyme (ACE) inhibitors on diabetic nephropathy, current guidelines from the United States and Canada recommend a blood pressure goal of less than 130/80 mm Hg for patients with diabetes. ACE inhibitors should be included as part of the initial treatment plan. If ACE inhibitors are not well-tolerated, angiotensin receptor blockers (ARBs) or renin inhibitors can be considered as alternatives.

The ONTARGET study investigated the combination of ACE inhibitors and ARBs in patients with atherosclerosis or type 2 diabetes and end-organ damage. While this approach seemed to reduce proteinuria, it slightly increased the risk of progression to dialysis and mortality, and is therefore not recommended.

Many patients with diabetes require a combination of three to five medications to achieve their target blood pressure, typically including a diuretic and either a calcium channel blocker or beta-blocker.

In addition to traditional antihypertensive medications, certain newer agents can improve cardiovascular outcomes in patients with diabetes, despite their modest impact on blood pressure reduction. Sodium-glucose co-transporter 2 (SGLT-2) inhibitors, such as canagliflozin, are commonly used in clinical practice. In the CREDENCE trial, which included patients with diabetic nephropathy, canagliflozin improved glycemic control, slightly reduced blood pressure by 3 to 4 mm Hg, improved renal outcomes, and decreased cardiovascular risk.

Finerenone, a non-steroidal mineralocorticoid receptor antagonist that inhibits the effects of aldosterone, has a lower risk of hyperkalemia compared to spironolactone. In a study of patients with diabetes and chronic kidney disease (CKD) stages 2 to 4, finerenone reduced blood pressure by 3 mm Hg and demonstrated significant benefits in preventing cardiovascular events and potentially slowing the progression of kidney disease.

In addition to strict blood pressure management, patients with diabetes should also receive intensive treatment for other risk factors, such as dyslipidemia and hyperglycemia, to reduce their overall cardiovascular risk.

Tian L,et al. Canagliflozin for Prevention of Cardiovascular and Renal Outcomes in type2 Diabetes: A Systematic Review and Meta-analysis of Randomized Controlled Trials. Front Pharmacol. 2021 Jul 19;12:691878. PMID: 34349651

1.6 Hypertension Management in a Patient with Advanced CKD

Case 6

A 67-year-old woman with chronic kidney disease (CKD) stage 4 secondary to hypertensive nephrosclerosis presents for a routine follow-up. Her current medications include lisinopril 20 mg daily and amlodipine 10 mg daily. Her blood pressure today is 142/88 mmHg. Her laboratory tests show a serum creatinine of 3.2 mg/dL, estimated GFR of 25 mL/min, and a urine albumin-to-creatinine ratio of 400 mg/g. Her serum potassium is 4.9 mEq/L. She has no history of acute kidney injury or cardiovascular events.
Which of the following is the most appropriate next step in the management of her hypertension?

- A. Increase the dose of lisinopril.
- B. Add a loop diuretic.
- C. Transition to an angiotensin receptor blocker (ARB).
- D. Initiate treatment with patiromer to allow for an increase in the dose of lisinopril.

The correct answer is B. Add a loop diuretic. This patient with CKD stage 4 and hypertension not at goal despite being on an ACE inhibitor and a calcium channel blocker likely has volume expansion contributing to her elevated blood pressure. In patients with advanced CKD (eGFR < 30 mL/min/1.73 m^2), thiazide diuretics often lose their efficacy, and loop diuretics become necessary to control volume status and hypertension. Adding a loop diuretic would help control her blood pressure by addressing the volume component, which is often a significant factor in the hypertension associated with advanced CKD. Option A is incorrect because increasing the dose of lisinopril in a patient with advanced CKD and a serum potassium of 4.9 mEq/L could increase the risk of hyperkalemia and further decrease GFR. ACE inhibitors can be continued in CKD, but care must be taken with dosing and monitoring. Option C is incorrect because there is no evidence that transitioning to an ARB would provide a significant benefit over an ACE inhibitor in this scenario. Both classes of drugs have similar effects on the renin-angiotensin-aldosterone system and can increase the risk of hyperkalemia and worsening renal function. Option D is incorrect because while patiromer can be used to treat hyperkalemia, the patient's serum potassium is currently within the normal range. Patiromer would be considered if hyperkalemia were present and limiting the use of renin-angiotensin system blockers, which is not the case here. The prevalence of hypertension is high in patients with chronic kidney disease (CKD), affecting 40% of those with a glomerular filtration rate (GFR) of 60–90 mL/min/1.73 m^2 and 75% of those with a GFR less than 30 mL/min/1.73 m^2. Treating hypertension is crucial, as it significantly slows the progression of CKD. The SPRINT trial demonstrated that the cardiovascular risk reduction associated with lower blood pressure targets was also observed in the subgroup with a GFR less than 60 mL/min/1.73 m^2.

However, the benefit of reducing blood pressure targets on slowing the progression of CKD appears to be limited to individuals with significant proteinuria. In the SPRINT trial, the lower blood pressure goal led to a higher risk of acute kidney injury (AKI), which was usually reversible and not associated with elevated biomarkers for ischemic injury.

For patients with CKD, guidelines generally recommend a blood pressure goal of less than 130/80 mm Hg, especially if there is more than 1 g of proteinuria in 24 hours. Medications that disrupt the renin-angiotensin system, such as angiotensin-converting enzyme (ACE) inhibitors or angiotensin receptor blockers (ARBs), are the preferred initial therapy, particularly for individuals with albuminuria exceeding 300 mg/g creatinine, as they can help slow the progression of kidney disease.

As the estimated GFR (eGFR) drops below 30 mL/min/1.73 m^2, it is often necessary to switch from thiazide diuretics to loop diuretics to manage volume overload, although thiazides continue to be effective in treating hypertension in advanced CKD. ACE inhibitors remain effective and safe in kidney disease with high protein levels and serum creatinine up to 5 mg/dL (380 mcmol/L). However, the use of renin-angiotensin-aldosterone system (RAAS) blockers in patients with advanced CKD should be closely monitored by a nephrologist.

It is essential to measure kidney function and electrolytes one week after initiating treatment and then closely monitor them in patients with kidney disease. An increase in creatinine of 20–30% is considered normal and expected; more extreme changes may indicate renal artery stenosis or volume contraction.

While lower blood pressure levels are associated with acute decreases in GFR, this does not appear to lead to a higher risk of developing end-stage kidney disease (ESKD) in the long term. Continuing ACE inhibitor or ARB therapy when the serum potassium level is above 5.5 mEq/L may not be necessary, as other antihypertensive medications can still provide renoprotective effects as long as target blood pressures are achieved. Diuretics can be useful in managing mild hyperkalemia, and new cation exchange polymers like patiromer can trap potassium in the intestines, offering improved effectiveness and tolerance compared to sodium polystyrene sulfonate.

Hebert SA,et al. Hypertension Management in Patients with Chronic Kidney Disease. Methodist Debakey Cardiovasc J. 2022 Sep 6;18(4):41-49. PMID: 36132579

Case Note

Loop diuretics, such as furosemide or torsemide, are recommended for patients with advanced CKD (eGFR under 30 mL/min/1.73m^2) due to their enhanced natriuretic and diuretic effects compared to thiazide diuretics. According to the KDIGO 2021 Clinical Practice Guideline for the Management of Blood Pressure in CKD, a combination of antihypertensive agents, including a renin-angiotensin-aldosterone system (RAAS) inhibitor, a calcium channel blocker, and a diuretic, is often required to achieve optimal blood pressure control in patients with CKD.

1.7 Hypertension Management in a Patient with COPD and ACE

Case 7

A 72-year-old man with a history of chronic obstructive pulmonary disease (COPD) and hypertension presents to the clinic for a routine visit. His current medications include a thiazide diuretic and a beta-blocker. Despite adherence to his medication regimen, his blood pressure remains elevated at 155/92 mmHg. His physical examination is unremarkable except for bilateral expiratory wheezes. His serum creatinine is 1.1 mg/dL, and his serum potassium is 4.2 mEq/L. He has no history of diabetes, kidney disease, or cardiovascular events. His physician is considering adding an ACE inhibitor to his treatment regimen.
Which of the following is the most appropriate next step in managing this patient's hypertension?

- A. Initiate an ACE inhibitor and monitor serum potassium and creatinine in 1–2 weeks.
- B. Add a calcium channel blocker instead of an ACE inhibitor due to the patient's history of COPD.
- C. Increase the dose of the current medications before adding new therapy.
- D. Perform renal artery duplex ultrasonography before initiating an ACE inhibitor.

The correct answer is A. Initiate an ACE inhibitor and monitor serum potassium and creatinine in 1 to 2 weeks. This patient has hypertension that is not adequately controlled with a thiazide diuretic and a beta-blocker. Adding an ACE inhibitor is a reasonable next step given its benefits in reducing cardiovascular events and its efficacy in lowering blood pressure. It is important to monitor serum potassium and creatinine after initiating an ACE inhibitor, especially in older adults, to detect any adverse effects such as hyperkalemia or a significant increase in creatinine, which could indicate renal artery stenosis or other renal issues. Option B is incorrect because while calcium channel blockers are effective antihypertensive agents and could be considered in this patient, there is no contraindication to using an ACE inhibitor in a patient with COPD. ACE inhibitors are particularly beneficial in patients with multiple cardiovascular risk factors and can be safely used in patients with respiratory diseases, provided they are monitored for cough, which is a known side effect. Option C is incorrect because the patient's blood pressure is significantly above the target range, and merely increasing the dose of the current medications may not achieve the desired blood pressure control. Adding another class of antihypertensive medication is often necessary when blood pressure is not controlled with monotherapy or dual therapy. Option D is incorrect because there is no current indication for renal artery duplex ultrasonography in this patient. This test is typically reserved for patients with clinical clues suggesting renal artery stenosis, such as a sudden increase in serum creatinine after starting an ACE inhibitor, severe hypertension (grade 3 or higher), or hypertension that is refractory to treatment with multiple medications. Angiotensin-converting enzyme (ACE) inhibitors are the preferred choice for individuals with type 1 diabetes who have proteinuria or kidney dysfunction, as they can slow the progression to end-stage kidney disease (ESKD). Many experts have extended this recommendation to include individuals with type 1 and type 2 diabetes mellitus who have microalbuminuria, even if they do not meet the typical criteria for antihypertensive therapy. ACE inhibitors have also been shown to slow the progression of kidney disease in individuals without diabetes. The Heart Outcomes Prevention Evaluation (HOPE) trial demonstrated that the ACE inhibitor ramipril reduced cardiovascular deaths, non-fatal myocardial infarctions, and non-fatal strokes. It also lowered the incidence of new-onset heart failure, kidney problems, and new-onset diabetes in high-risk patients. Although this study did not specifically focus on hypertensive individuals, the positive outcomes were associated with a modest reduction in blood pressure, suggesting that ACE inhibitors could be beneficial for similar patient populations.

ACE inhibitors are commonly prescribed for patients with heart failure and reduced ejection fraction, often in combination with a diuretic and a beta-blocker. They are also recommended for asymptomatic patients with reduced ejection fraction.

When initiating therapy, it is crucial to measure baseline serum potassium and creatinine levels before starting medications that affect the renin-angiotensin-aldosterone system (RAAS). These levels should be rechecked 1-2 weeks after starting the therapy to monitor for hyperkalemia or a significant increase in creatinine. Slight changes in these medications rarely cause major shifts in these values. Patients with bilateral renal artery stenosis may experience severe hypotension. If serum creatinine increases by more than 25% from baseline, it may indicate volume contraction or renovascular disease, and discontinuing the ACE inhibitor can often reverse this effect.

Hyperkalemia can occur in individuals with kidney disease, type IV renal tubular acidosis (often found in those with diabetes), and older adults. A persistent dry cough is a common side effect, affecting at least 10% of patients, and may necessitate discontinuation of the medication. Skin rashes can occur with any ACE inhibitor. Angioedema is a rare but potentially serious side effect of all medications in this class due to their kininase inhibition. During the second and third trimesters of pregnancy, exposure of the fetus to ACE inhibitors has been linked to various defects caused by hypotension and reduced renal blood flow.

Mancini GBet al. Reduction of morbidity and mortality by statins, angiotensin-converting enzyme inhibitors, and angiotensin receptor blockers in patients with chronic obstructive pulmonary disease. J Am Coll Cardiol. 2006 Jun 20;47(12):2554-60. PMID: 16781387.

Table 1.1: Summary of Renin Inhibitors and Calcium Channel Blocking Agents

Drug Class	**Renin Inhibitors**
Mechanism of Action	Inhibit renin, preventing cleavage of angiotensinogen, thus effectively lowering blood pressure, reducing albuminuria, and limiting LVH.
Clinical Use	Not established as a first-line drug; large-scale prospective trial data are lacking.
Combination Therapy	Combination with ACE inhibitors or ARBs in type 2 diabetes offers no advantage and might increase the risk of adverse cardiac or renal consequences.
Drug Class	**Calcium Channel Blocking Agents**
Mechanism of Action	Cause peripheral vasodilation with less reflex tachycardia and fluid retention than other vasodilators.
Efficacy	Effective as single-drug therapy in approximately 60% of patients across all demographic groups and grades of hypertension.
Clinical Use	Equivalent to ACE inhibitors and thiazide diuretics in prevention of CHD, major cardiovascular events, cardiovascular death, and total mortality. Protective effect against stroke is well established.
Side Effects	Common side effects include headache, peripheral edema, bradycardia, and constipation. Dihydropyridine agents are more likely to produce symptoms of vasodilation. Negative inotropic effects; caution in patients with cardiac dysfunction.

1.8 Optimizing Antihypertensive Therapy in an African American Man

Case 8

A 63-year-old African American man with a history of type 2 diabetes mellitus, hypertension, and chronic kidney disease stage 3 presents to the clinic for blood pressure management. His current antihypertensive regimen includes hydrochlorothiazide and amlodipine. Despite adherence to his medication regimen, his blood pressure remains elevated at 152/94 mmHg. His physical examination is unremarkable, and his laboratory tests show a serum creatinine of 1.9 mg/dL, estimated GFR of 40 mL/min/1.73 m^2, and a urine albumin-to-creatinine ratio of 220 mg/g. His serum potassium is 4.5 mEq/L. He has no history of cardiovascular events.

Which of the following is the most appropriate next step in managing this patient's hypertension?

- A. Initiate therapy with an ACE inhibitor.
- B. Initiate therapy with an ARB.
- C. Add a beta-blocker to the current regimen.
- D. Increase the dose of amlodipine.

The correct answer is B. Initiate therapy with an ARB. This patient has hypertension that is not adequately controlled with a diuretic and a calcium channel blocker. Given his African American ethnicity and the presence of type 2 diabetes with nephropathy, an ARB would be a suitable choice. ARBs have been shown to improve cardiovascular outcomes and are effective in slowing the progression of diabetic nephropathy. They are also less likely to cause cough and angioedema compared to ACE inhibitors, which is an important consideration in this patient who may have a higher risk for these side effects. Additionally, ARBs have been shown to be effective in reducing the incidence of stroke, particularly in patients with left ventricular hypertrophy, and may have a more favorable metabolic profile with a lower incidence of new-onset diabetes. Option A is less appropriate because ACE inhibitors, while beneficial in similar clinical scenarios, may not be as effective in African American patients compared to other antihypertensive classes, as suggested by the ALLHAT trial. Additionally, ACE inhibitors have a higher incidence of cough and angioedema, which could be particularly problematic in this patient population. Option C is incorrect because beta-blockers are not typically first-line agents for the treatment of hypertension in African American patients, especially in the absence of heart failure or post-myocardial infarction. They may also adversely affect the metabolic profile in a patient with diabetes. Option D is incorrect because while increasing the dose of amlodipine could potentially lower blood pressure further, it does not address the proteinuria associated with diabetic nephropathy. In this patient with CKD and diabetes, an agent that addresses the albuminuria and has renal protective effects is preferred. ARBs are known to reduce proteinuria and have been the first-line agents in the management of diabetic nephropathy for the past 20 years. They are effective in slowing the progression of diabetic nephropathy, which is a significant risk factor for mortality, mostly from cardiovascular complications, in patients with diabetes.

ARBs are superior to other drugs like beta blockers, calcium channel blockers, and diuretics in reducing disease progression once a patient develops diabetic kidney disease. This makes them the drugs of choice for this condition.

In summary, ARBs play a crucial role in managing diabetic nephropathy by providing renoprotective effects, cardiovascular protection, and aiding in the prevention of disease progression, making them a valuable treatment option for patients with this condition.

Williams SK,et al. Hypertension Treatment in Blacks: Discussion of the U.S. Clinical Practice Guidelines. Prog Cardiovasc Dis. 2016 Nov-Dec;59(3):282-288.PMID: 27693861

Sulaica EM et al. A Review of Hypertension Management in Black Male Patients. Mayo Clin Proc. 2020 Sep;95(9):1955-1963. PMID: 32276785.

Muthuppalaniappan VMet al. Ethnic/Race Diversity and Diabetic Kidney Disease. J Clin Med. 2015 Jul 31;4(8) PMID: 26287248

1.9 Managing Systolic Hypertension in a Patient with Asthma

Case 9

A 58-year-old woman with a history of asthma and systolic hypertension presents to the clinic for a follow-up visit. She reports compliance with her current medication regimen, which includes hydrochlorothiazide and a beta-blocker. Despite this, her blood pressure remains elevated at 168/86 mmHg. She denies any chest pain, shortness of breath, or wheezing. Her physical examination is notable for a heart rate of 58 beats per minute and no respiratory distress. Her laboratory tests reveal a serum potassium of 4.3 mEq/L, and her serum creatinine is within normal limits. An electrocardiogram shows no evidence of ischemia or AV block.
Which of the following is the most appropriate next step in managing this patient's hypertension?

- A. Add amlodipine to the current regimen.
- B. Increase the dose of the beta-blocker.
- C. Initiate therapy with verapamil.
- D. Switch the beta-blocker to an ACE inhibitor.

The correct answer is A. Add amlodipine to the current regimen. This patient has isolated systolic hypertension, which is not adequately controlled with a diuretic and a beta-blocker. Adding a calcium channel blocker, such as amlodipine, is a reasonable next step. Amlodipine is a dihydropyridine calcium channel blocker that is effective in lowering systolic blood pressure and is less likely to cause bradycardia or AV block, making it a safe option in this patient with a history of asthma and a relatively low heart rate. Additionally, amlodipine has been shown to be safe in patients with heart failure, which is an important consideration in the management of hypertension. Option B is incorrect because increasing the dose of the beta-blocker may exacerbate the patient's bradycardia and is not the preferred agent for isolated systolic hypertension, especially in a patient with asthma where beta-blockers can potentially exacerbate respiratory symptoms. Option C is incorrect because verapamil, a non-dihydropyridine calcium channel blocker, has negative effects on heart rate and AV conduction. Given the patient's already low heart rate, adding verapamil could increase the risk of bradycardia and AV block. Option D is incorrect because switching the beta-blocker to an ACE inhibitor does not address the need for additional blood pressure control in the setting of isolated systolic hypertension. While an ACE inhibitor could be a component of hypertension management, it would be more appropriate to add a drug class that specifically targets systolic blood pressure, such as a calcium channel blocker. Calcium channel blockers are as effective as ACE inhibitors and thiazide diuretics in preventing CHD, major cardiovascular events, cardiovascular death, and total mortality. Calcium channel blockers (CCBs) have demonstrated a well-established protective effect against stroke, as evidenced by two major trials: the Antihypertensive and Lipid-Lowering Treatment to Prevent Heart Attack Trial (ALLHAT) and the Systolic Hypertension in Europe (Syst-Eur) trial. In these studies, CCBs appeared to be more effective than diuretic-based therapy in reducing the risk of stroke.

The protective effect of CCBs against stroke may be attributed to their mechanism of action. CCBs work by inhibiting the influx of calcium ions into cardiac and smooth muscle cells, leading to relaxation and vasodilation of blood vessels. This vasodilatory effect can reduce blood pressure, which is a major risk factor for stroke. Additionally, CCBs have been shown to possess other beneficial effects, such as reducing inflammation and oxidative stress, which may also contribute to their protective effect against stroke.

Side effects: Common side effects of calcium channel blockers include headache, peripheral edema, bradycardia, and constipation, particularly with the use of verapamil in older adults. Dihydropyridine agents like nifedipine, nicardipine, isradipine, felodipine, nisoldipine, and amlodipine are known to cause symptoms of vasodilation, such as headache, flushing, palpitations, and peripheral edema. The development of peripheral edema can be reduced by combining a CCB with an angiotensin-converting enzyme (ACE) inhibitor or an angiotensin receptor blocker (ARB).

Calcium channel blockers can have negative effects on the heart's pumping ability, so they should be used with caution in patients with pre-existing heart conditions. Among the CCBs, amlodipine is considered the safest option for patients with severe heart failure (HF).

It is important to note that while CCBs offer a protective effect against stroke, their use should be carefully considered in the context of an individual patient's overall cardiovascular risk profile, comorbidities, and potential side effects. As with any medication, the benefits and risks should be carefully weighed by the healthcare provider when prescribing CCBs for the management of hypertension or other cardiovascular conditions.

Christiansen SC, et al. Treatment of Hypertension in Patients with Asthma. N Engl J Med. 2019 Sep 12;381(11):1046-1057. doi: 10.1056/NEJMra1800345. PMID: 31509675.

Zolotareva Oet al. Comorbidity of asthma and hypertension may be mediated by shared genetic dysregulation and drug side effects. Sci Rep. 2019 Nov 8;9(1):16302. PMID: 31705029

1.10 Hypertension Management in a Patient with DM and Nephropathy

Case 10

A 65-year-old woman with a history of hypertension and type 2 diabetes mellitus presents to the clinic for a routine follow-up. She has been taking metformin and a moderate dose of a thiazide diuretic. Her blood pressure is currently 145/90 mmHg, and her hemoglobin A1c is 7.2%. She complains of recent onset of gouty arthritis, which she finds distressing. Her serum creatinine is 1.8 mg/dL, estimated GFR is 35 mL/min/1.73 m2, and her serum potassium is 4.6 mEq/L. Her urine albumin-to-creatinine ratio is within normal limits. She denies any recent use of nonsteroidal anti-inflammatory drugs or alcohol.
Which of the following is the most appropriate next step in managing this patient's hypertension?

- A. Increase the dose of the thiazide diuretic.
- B. Add a loop diuretic.
- C. Switch from the thiazide diuretic to a loop diuretic.
- D. Add a potassium-sparing diuretic.

The correct answer is C. Switch from the thiazide diuretic to a loop diuretic. This patient has chronic kidney disease (CKD) with an estimated GFR of 35 mL/min/1.73 m2, which is below the threshold at which thiazide diuretics typically lose their efficacy for blood pressure control. Loop diuretics are more effective than thiazides in patients with significant renal impairment (serum creatinine greater than 2.5 mg/dL or estimated GFR less than 30 mL/min 1.73 m2). Additionally, thiazide diuretics can increase serum uric acid levels and may precipitate gout, which this patient is experiencing. Switching to a loop diuretic may help manage both her blood pressure and her gout symptoms. Option A is incorrect because increasing the dose of the thiazide diuretic is unlikely to be effective in a patient with this level of renal impairment and may exacerbate her gout. Option B is incorrect because adding a loop diuretic to the existing thiazide diuretic would increase the risk of electrolyte imbalances and dehydration without addressing the underlying issue of thiazide-induced hyperuricemia. Option D is incorrect because while a potassium-sparing diuretic could help prevent hypokalemia, it does not address the primary issue of the thiazide diuretic being less effective in CKD and contributing to hyperuricemia. Moreover, the patient's serum potassium is already at the upper limit of normal, and adding a potassium-sparing diuretic could increase the risk of hyperkalemia. Loop diuretics, such as furosemide, have a rapid onset of action, typically within 30 to 60 minutes of oral administration. However, they also have a relatively short duration of action. For example, furosemide has a half-life of approximately 1–1.5 hours, although this can be prolonged in advanced renal dysfunction.

This rapid onset and short duration of action mean that loop diuretics can cause electrolyte and volume depletion more quickly than thiazide diuretics, which act by reducing sodium reabsorption in the distal renal tubules. The increased excretion of water and electrolytes can lead to various electrolyte imbalances, including hyponatremia (low sodium), hypokalemia (low potassium), hypomagnesemia (low magnesium), and hypochloremia (low chloride).

These electrolyte imbalances can have negative effects on the body, such as muscle weakness, fatigue, and arrhythmias. Additionally, loop diuretics can cause volume depletion, leading to dehydration and hypotension (low blood pressure).

Despite these potential adverse effects, loop diuretics are recommended for patients with kidney dysfunction, specifically those with a serum creatinine level above 2.5 mg/dL or an estimated glomerular filtration rate (eGFR) below 30 mL/min/1.73 m^2. In these patients, loop diuretics are more effective than thiazide diuretics.

Therefore, while loop diuretics are associated with a higher risk of electrolyte and volume depletion due to their rapid onset and short duration of action, they remain the preferred choice for patients with significant renal impairment. However, it is crucial to closely monitor electrolyte levels and fluid status in patients receiving loop diuretics to prevent and manage potential imbalances and depletion.

Sternlicht H,et al. Management of Hypertension in Diabetic Nephropathy: How Low Should We Go?. 2016;41(1-3):139-43. PMID: 26766168.

Colbert GB, et al. Management of Hypertension in Diabetic Kidney Disease. J Clin Med. 2023 Oct 31;12(21):6868. PMID: 37959333

Table 1.2: Summary of Diuretics

Aspect	**Description**
Mechanism of Action	Thiazide diuretics lower blood pressure initially by decreasing plasma volume, but during long-term therapy, their major hemodynamic effect is reduction of peripheral vascular resistance. Loop diuretics may lead to electrolyte and volume depletion more readily than thiazides and have short durations of action.
Clinical Use	Thiazides are the antihypertensives that have been most extensively studied and most consistently effective in clinical trials. They are effective as single-drug therapy in approximately 60% of patients in all demographic groups and all grades of hypertension. Loop diuretics should be reserved for use in patients with kidney dysfunction.
Side Effects	Common side effects include headache, peripheral edema, bradycardia, and constipation. Adverse metabolic changes, erectile dysfunction, skin rashes, and photosensitivity are less frequent. Hypokalemia, hyponatremia, and increased serum uric acid may occur.
Long-Term Effects	Long-term thiazide administration mitigates the loss of bone mineral content in older women at risk for osteoporosis. Thiazides are also useful for lowering isolated or predominantly systolic hypertension.

Table 1.3: Summary of Aldosterone Receptor Blockers

Aspect	**Description**
Clinical Use	Spironolactone and eplerenone are used in the treatment of hypertension, especially resistant hypertension, and are helpful additions to most other antihypertensive medications.
Efficacy	Effective at lowering blood pressure in Black persons and all other hypertensive patients regardless of renin level. They also ameliorate target-organ damage, including ventricular and vascular hypertrophy and renal and myocardial fibrosis.
Alternative to Surgery	Offer an alternative to adrenalectomy in primary hyperaldosteronism.
Side Effects	Spironolactone can cause breast pain and gynecomastia in men due to activity at the progesterone receptor. Hyperkalemia is a concern, especially in patients with CKD and those with pretreatment plasma potassium exceeding 4.5 mmol/L.

Table 1.4: Summary of Beta-Blocking Agents

Aspect	Description
Mechanism of Action	Decrease heart rate and cardiac output, decrease renin release. More efficacious in populations with elevated plasma renin activity.
Clinical Use	Useful in patients with angina, previous myocardial infarction, persistent sinus tachycardia, stable HF, migraine headaches, and somatic manifestations of anxiety.
Pharmacologic Properties	Differ in cardioselectivity, ability to block beta-2-receptors, lipid solubility, CNS side effects, and metabolism.
Specific Agents	Metoprolol reduces mortality in chronic stable HF with reduced EF. Carvedilol and nebivolol beneficial in HF, may reduce peripheral vascular resistance.
First-Line Use	Traditional beta-blockers should not be used as first-line agents in the treatment of hypertension without specific compelling indications.
Side Effects	Bronchospasm, sinus node dysfunction, AV conduction depression, CNS symptoms, fatigue, lethargy, erectile dysfunction. Adverse effects on lipids and glucose metabolism.
Cautions	Used cautiously in type 1 diabetes, peripheral vascular disease, and should not be used to treat hypertension arising from cocaine use or pheochromocytoma without prior alpha-blockade.
Withdrawal	Abrupt withdrawal can precipitate acute coronary events and severe increases in blood pressure.

1.11 Treatment Approach for Resistant Hypertension

Case 11

A 56-year-old man with a history of resistant hypertension, type 2 diabetes mellitus, and chronic kidney disease stage 3 is referred to you for management of his blood pressure. Despite taking maximal tolerated doses of amlodipine, a thiazide diuretic, and an ACE inhibitor, his blood pressure remains persistently elevated at 158/98 mmHg. His current medications include amlodipine 10 mg daily, hydrochlorothiazide 25 mg daily, and lisinopril 40 mg daily. His serum potassium is 4.4 mEq/L, and his estimated GFR is 45 mL/min/1.73 m2. He has no history of cardiovascular disease. On physical examination, he has no signs of volume overload, and his heart sounds are normal without murmurs, rubs, or gallops.
Which of the following is the most appropriate next step in the management of this patient's hypertension?

- A. Add spironolactone.
- B. Increase the dose of hydrochlorothiazide.
- C. Add eplerenone.
- D. Add amiloride.

The correct answer is A. Add spironolactone. This patient has resistant hypertension, which is defined as blood pressure that remains above goal despite the concurrent use of three antihypertensive agents of different classes, ideally including a diuretic. Adding an aldosterone receptor blocker such as spironolactone can be effective in patients with resistant hypertension, and it has been shown to improve outcomes in such patients. Spironolactone is particularly useful in patients with heart failure and post-myocardial infarction, but it is also effective in resistant hypertension without overt cardiac disease. The patient's serum potassium is below 4.5 mEq/L, which is a safe level to initiate therapy with spironolactone, and his GFR, while reduced, is not at a level that would contraindicate the use of spironolactone. Option B is incorrect because increasing the dose of hydrochlorothiazide is unlikely to provide additional blood pressure control in a patient who is already on a moderate dose and has resistant hypertension.Option C is incorrect because while eplerenone is a more selective aldosterone receptor blocker and less likely to cause gynecomastia, it is also less potent than spironolactone. Given the severity of this patient's hypertension, the more potent spironolactone is the preferred choice. Option D is incorrect because amiloride is a potassium-sparing diuretic that blocks the epithelial sodium channel but is not an aldosterone receptor blocker. While it can be used to treat hypertension, it is not the first choice in a patient with resistant hypertension who is already on a thiazide diuretic. Spironolactone and eplerenone, both aldosterone receptor blockers, have emerged as significant treatments for hypertension, particularly in cases of resistant hypertension, serving as valuable additions to other antihypertensive medications. These aldosterone receptor blockers are notably effective in reducing blood pressure in individuals of Black descent and others with hypertension. Aldosterone plays a pivotal role in damaging target organs, contributing to the hypertrophy of ventricular and vascular tissues, as well as fibrosis in the kidneys and heart. By antagonizing aldosterone receptors, these medications improve the outcomes of hypertension, partly independent of their blood pressure-lowering effects. Amiloride works by inhibiting aldosterone-induced activation of the epithelial sodium channel, aiding in preventing diuretic-induced hypokalemia and lowering blood pressure in cases of hyperaldosteronism and resistant hypertension.

Aldosterone receptor blockers, in conjunction with amiloride, offer a non-surgical alternative for primary hyperaldosteronism. It is important to note that spironolactone may induce breast pain and gynecomastia in men due to its interaction with the progesterone receptor, a side effect not typically associated with the more selective eplerenone.

Hyperkalemia is a concern associated with agents that inhibit aldosterone effects, particularly in patients with chronic kidney disease (CKD). Elevated plasma potassium levels exceeding 4.5 mmol/L before treatment initiation increase the risk of hyperkalemia.

Guo H, Xiao Q. Clinical efficacy of spironolactone for resistant hypertension: a meta analysis from randomized controlled clinical trials. Int J Clin Exp Med. 2015 PMID: 26221266

Acelajado MC, et al. Treatment of Resistant and Refractory Hypertension. Circ Res. 2019 Mar 29;124(7):1061-1070.PMID: 30920924

Table 1.5: Summary of Beta-Blocking Agents

Aspect	Description
Mechanism of Action	Decrease heart rate and cardiac output, decrease renin release. More efficacious in populations with elevated plasma renin activity.
Clinical Use	Useful in patients with angina, previous myocardial infarction, persistent sinus tachycardia, stable HF, migraine headaches, and somatic manifestations of anxiety.
Pharmacologic Properties	Differ in cardioselectivity, ability to block beta-2-receptors, lipid solubility, CNS side effects, and metabolism.
Specific Agents	Metoprolol reduces mortality in chronic stable HF with reduced EF. Carvedilol and nebivolol beneficial in HF, may reduce peripheral vascular resistance.
First-Line Use	Traditional beta-blockers should not be used as first-line agents in the treatment of hypertension without specific compelling indications.
Side Effects	Bronchospasm, sinus node dysfunction, AV conduction depression, CNS symptoms, fatigue, lethargy, erectile dysfunction. Adverse effects on lipids and glucose metabolism.
Cautions	Used cautiously in type 1 diabetes, peripheral vascular disease, and should not be used to treat hypertension arising from cocaine use or pheochromocytoma without prior alpha-blockade.
Withdrawal	Abrupt withdrawal can precipitate acute coronary events and severe increases in blood pressure.

1.12 Optimizing Hypertension and Heart Failure Management

Case 12

A 52-year-old man with a history of hypertension and chronic stable heart failure with reduced ejection fraction (HFrEF) presents to the clinic for a routine follow-up. He is currently taking lisinopril 20 mg daily, furosemide 40 mg daily, and eplerenone 25 mg daily. His blood pressure is 150/92 mmHg, and his heart rate is 78 beats per minute. His ejection fraction on the most recent echocardiogram was 35%. He reports no symptoms of angina, dyspnea, or claudication. His physical examination is unremarkable except for an S3 heart sound. His serum potassium is 4.8 mEq/L, and his serum creatinine is 1.2 mg/dL.
Which of the following is the most appropriate next step in the management of this patient's hypertension and heart failure?

- A. Add metoprolol succinate.
- B. Add atenolol.
- C. Add propranolol.
- D. Increase the dose of eplerenone.

The correct answer is A. Add metoprolol succinate. This patient has chronic stable heart failure with reduced ejection fraction (HFrEF) and hypertension that is not adequately controlled. Metoprolol succinate is a beta-1 selective blocker that has been shown to reduce mortality and morbidity in patients with HFrEF and is recommended in clinical guidelines for the management of such patients. It will also provide additional blood pressure control. The extended-release formulation is preferred for the management of HFrEF due to its proven benefit in large clinical trials. Option B is incorrect because atenolol, while a beta-1 selective blocker, has not been shown to reduce mortality in heart failure patients as metoprolol succinate has. Option C is incorrect because propranolol is a non-selective beta-blocker and is not the preferred agent in patients with heart failure due to its potential to exacerbate bronchospasm and its lack of proven mortality benefit in this population. Option D is incorrect because increasing the dose of eplerenone may increase the risk of hyperkalemia, especially since the patient's serum potassium is already at the upper limit of normal. Additionally, eplerenone does not have the same proven mortality benefit in HFrEF as metoprolol succinate. Metoprolol has demonstrated efficacy in reducing mortality and improving outcomes in individuals with chronic stable heart failure and reduced ejection fraction. Carvedilol and nebivolol also play a crucial role in maintaining cardiac output and providing benefits to these patients by reducing peripheral vascular resistance through distinct mechanisms.

Traditional beta-blockers, despite their limited effectiveness in preventing heart attacks and being less potent than other medications in preventing strokes and left ventricular hypertrophy (LVH), should not be the primary choice for hypertension treatment unless specific compelling reasons exist, such as active coronary artery disease (CAD).

Metoprolol, a beta-1 selective blocker, has shown mortality reduction and clinical improvement in patients with chronic stable heart failure and reduced ejection fraction (HFrEF), particularly in those with stable mild to moderate heart failure stemming from left ventricular systolic dysfunction, whether due to ischemic or dilated cardiomyopathy.

The Metoprolol in Dilated Cardiomyopathy (MDC) trial investigated the impact of metoprolol tartrate on individuals with idiopathic heart failure. While no significant difference in all-cause mortality was observed between the treatment and placebo groups, the metoprolol group exhibited notable enhancements in quality of life, ejection fraction, and exercise capacity.

In the Metoprolol CR/XL Randomized Intervention Trial in Heart Failure (MERIT-HF trial), metoprolol was linked to a 34% reduction in relative risk of all-cause mortality among patients with chronic heart failure from ischemic or dilated cardiomyopathy, significantly decreasing sudden death and death due to progressive heart failure.

Metoprolol functions by attenuating noradrenergic hormonal influences, yielding long-term benefits. It is essential to initiate beta-blockers when patients are stable without rest symptoms, as they are not intended for acute rescue. Proper dosing is crucial for optimal impact in heart failure management; doses below the target may not yield the same benefits.

Common side effects of beta blockers encompass bronchospasm, sinus node dysfunction, AV conduction depression, CNS symptoms, fatigue, lethargy, erectile dysfunction, as well as adverse effects on lipid and glucose metabolism. In the cardiovascular system, beta blockers can induce sinus node dysfunction and AV conduction depression, potentially resulting in bradycardia and hypotension. These effects may manifest as fatigue, dizziness, and in severe cases, heart failure.

Beta-blockers significantly influence the long-term prognosis of HFrEF patients and are typically the initial treatment choice for individuals with left ventricular dysfunction. Dosing should be titrated to the highest tolerated level for optimal prognostic benefits. Despite being underutilized in HFrEF patients with complex comorbidities that are not true contraindications to their use, it is crucial to consider comorbidities when prescribing -blockers and tailor treatment based on individual patient needs while understanding drug-disease interactions.

Masarone D, et al. The Use of -Blockers in Heart Failure with Reduced Ejection Fraction. J Cardiovasc Dev Dis. 2021 Aug 24;8(9):101. PMID: 34564119

Wikstrand J. MERIT-HF–description of the trial. Basic Res Cardiol. 2000;95 Suppl 1:I90-7. PMID: 11192361.

Major medical condition	**First-line Drugs**	**Added 2nd Drug (if needed to reach BP target)**	**Added 3rd Drug (if needed to reach BP target)**
Diabetes (white and other non-African ancestry)	ARB or ACEI	CCB or thiazide diuretic	Alternative 2nd drug (CCB or thiazide diuretic)
Diabetes (African ancestry)	CCB or thiazide diuretic	ARB or ACEI	Alternative 1st drug (CCB or thiazide diuretic)
Chronic kidney disease	ARB or ACEI	CCB or thiazide diuretic	Alternative 2nd drug (CCB or thiazide diuretic)
Coronary artery disease	Beta-blocker plus ARB or ACEI	CCB or thiazide diuretic	Alternative 2nd drug (CCB or thiazide diuretic)
Stroke	ACEI or ARB	CCB or thiazide diuretic	Alternative 2nd drug (CCB or thiazide diuretic)
Symptomatic heart failure	Beta-blocker plus ARB or ACEI plus diuretic plus spironolactone regardless of BP; CCB can be added if needed for BP control		

Table 1.6: Guidelines on Treatment of HTN - Patients With Major Medical Conditions

1.13 Streamlining Medication for Hypertension and BPH

> **Case 13**
>
> A 68-year-old man with a history of benign prostatic hyperplasia (BPH) and hypertension is evaluated for a recent increase in urinary frequency and difficulty with urination. His current medications include lisinopril 20 mg daily, amlodipine 5 mg daily, and tamsulosin 0.4 mg daily. His blood pressure is 142/86 mmHg. Physical examination reveals an enlarged, non-tender prostate. His serum creatinine is 1.1 mg/dL, and his prostate-specific antigen (PSA) level is within normal limits. He has no history of heart failure or stroke. The patient expresses a desire to minimize the number of medications he takes.
> Which of the following is the most appropriate next step in the management of this patient's hypertension and BPH?
>
> - A. Discontinue tamsulosin and start doxazosin.
> - B. Add prazosin to the current regimen.
> - C. Increase the dose of amlodipine.
> - D. Start finasteride for BPH and maintain the current antihypertensive regimen.

The correct answer is A. Discontinue tamsulosin and start doxazosin. This patient has both BPH and hypertension, conditions for which alpha-blockers can be beneficial. Doxazosin is an alpha-1 antagonist that can treat both hypertension and BPH. By switching from tamsulosin, which is selective for alpha-1A receptors primarily found in the prostate, to doxazosin, which blocks alpha-1 receptors in both the prostate and vasculature, the patient can potentially reduce the number of medications he takes while managing both conditions. Option B is incorrect because adding prazosin to the current regimen would not reduce the number of medications the patient takes and could increase the risk of first-dose hypotension and other side effects associated with alpha-blockers. Option C is incorrect because increasing the dose of amlodipine would address the patient's hypertension but would not improve his BPH symptoms. Additionally, higher doses of amlodipine may increase the risk of peripheral edema. Option D is incorrect because while finasteride is a treatment for BPH, it would add another medication to the patient's regimen without providing any additional blood pressure control. The patient's goal is to minimize the number of medications he takes. Prazosin, terazosin, and doxazosin function by inhibiting alpha-receptors, resulting in smooth muscle relaxation and decreased blood pressure by reducing peripheral vascular resistance. While these agents can be effective as monotherapy for certain individuals, prolonged use may lead to tachyphylaxis. Unlike specific beta-blockers and diuretics, alpha-blockers do not adversely affect serum lipid levels. They are known to elevate HDL cholesterol levels and reduce total cholesterol; however, the long-term benefits of these effects remain uncertain.

Side effects are common with alpha-blockers. Notably, a significant drop in blood pressure can occur after the initial dose, underscoring the importance of initiating treatment with a small dose at bedtime. Potential side effects post-administration include palpitations, headaches, and nervousness, which may persist during extended therapy. Doxazosin, due to its slower onset of action, may result in milder or less frequent side effects compared to other alpha-blockers.

In the ALLHAT study, individuals commencing treatment with doxazosin experienced a marked increase in heart failure hospitalizations and a higher incidence of stroke compared to those starting on diuretics. Consequently, this aspect of the research was halted. Patients exposed to alpha-blockers may face challenges during cataract surgery due to floppy iris syndrome, even after discontinuing the medication. Therefore, it is crucial to inform the ophthalmologist about the patient's medication history prior to the procedure.

Mathur RP, Nayak S, Sivaramakrishnan R, Jain V. Role of Alpha Blockers in Hypertension with Benign Prostatic Hyperplasia. J Assoc Physicians India. 2014 Sep;62(9 Suppl):40-4. PMID: 26245042

Li H,et al. Role of 1-blockers in the current management of hypertension. J Clin Hypertens (Greenwich). 2022 Sep;24(9):1180-1186. PMID: 36196467

1.14 Critical Care for Hypertensive Crisis with End-Organ Damage

Case 14

A 63-year-old woman with a history of hypertension presents to the emergency department with a severe headache, blurred vision, and confusion. Her blood pressure is 220/120 mmHg. Physical examination reveals papilledema and bilateral retinal hemorrhages. Laboratory tests show a serum creatinine of 2.2 mg/dL (up from a baseline of 1.0 mg/dL), a platelet count of 90,000/L, and evidence of hemolysis on the peripheral smear. Urinalysis shows proteinuria and hematuria. ECG shows left ventricular hypertrophy with strain pattern. There is no history of drug use, and urine toxicology is negative.
Which of the following is the most appropriate next step in the management of this patient?

- A. Administer oral amlodipine and schedule close outpatient follow-up.
- B. Begin intravenous nitroprusside infusion and admit to the intensive care unit.
- C. Prescribe oral labetalol and reassess blood pressure in 24 hours.
- D. Start intravenous furosemide for presumed pulmonary edema.

The correct answer is B. Begin intravenous nitroprusside infusion and admit to the intensive care unit. This patient is presenting with a hypertensive emergency, as evidenced by the significantly elevated blood pressure and acute end-organ damage, including hypertensive encephalopathy (headache, blurred vision, confusion), acute kidney injury (increase in serum creatinine), thrombocytopenia, hemolysis (suggestive of microangiopathic hemolytic anemia), and retinopathy (papilledema, retinal hemorrhages). Immediate blood pressure reduction is required to limit further end-organ damage. Intravenous nitroprusside is a potent vasodilator that can rapidly decrease blood pressure and is often used in hypertensive emergencies. Admission to the intensive care unit is necessary for close monitoring and titration of antihypertensive therapy. Option A is incorrect because oral amlodipine would not provide the rapid onset of blood pressure reduction needed in a hypertensive emergency and does not allow for minute-to-minute control of blood pressure. Option C is incorrect because oral labetalol would not provide the immediate blood pressure control required in this setting and does not allow for the rapid titration needed to safely reduce blood pressure in a hypertensive emergency. Option D is incorrect because, although intravenous furosemide is used in the management of pulmonary edema, there is no indication that this patient has pulmonary edema. Moreover, furosemide would not address the immediate need for controlled blood pressure reduction in the context of a hypertensive emergency. Acute hypertensive microangiopathy encompasses the association of elevated blood pressure with retinopathy (characterized by retinal hemorrhages, cotton wool spots, or papilledema), acute kidney injury, and thrombotic microangiopathy, commonly known as malignant hypertension. Approximately 10% of individuals may exhibit symptoms of hypertensive encephalopathy (such as seizures, lethargy, cortical blindness, or coma) without always displaying classic hypertensive retinopathy. The susceptibility of the posterior brain region to damage from high blood pressure stems from the absence of sympathetic nerves in this area, resulting in a limited capacity to regulate blood flow.

The microangiopathic alterations observed in conditions like hemolytic uremic syndrome (HUS) and thrombotic thrombocytopenic purpura (TTP) can present a diagnostic challenge due to the presence of thrombocytopenia, schistocytes, and elevated LDH levels. Nevertheless, the advanced retinal changes suggest that hypertension is likely the primary underlying cause, whereas the hematologic abnormalities associated with TTP or HUS tend to be more severe. TTP is notably characterized by markedly reduced levels of ADAMTS13.

Management of Hypertensive Emergencies Categorized by Type of End-Organ Damage involves a primary objective of promptly reducing blood pressure by up to 25% and gradually achieving a target level of 160/100 mm Hg within 2–6 hours. To mitigate the risk of organ ischemia resulting from significant reductions in blood pressure, it is recommended to utilize medications with a dependable, dose-dependent, transient, and gradual antihypertensive effect. In addressing this issue, it is advisable to refrain from using sublingual or oral fast-acting nifedipine formulations.

Ipek Eet al . Hypertensive crisis: an update on clinical approach and management. Curr Opin Cardiol. 2017 Jul;32(4):397-406. PMID: 28306673.

1.15 Management in CKD-Related Hypertensive Encephalopathy

Case 15

A 38-year-old woman with a history of chronic kidney disease presents to the emergency department with a two-day history of severe headaches, nausea, and visual disturbances. Her blood pressure is 220/115 mmHg. On examination, she is alert but appears anxious, and her visual acuity is reduced bilaterally. Fundoscopy reveals bilateral optic disc swelling. MRI of the brain shows hyperintense lesions in the occipital and parietal lobes on T2-weighted images, consistent with vasogenic edema. There are no signs of infarction or hemorrhage. The patient's renal function is stable compared to previous results, and there is no significant proteinuria. Which of the following is the most appropriate next step in the management of this patient's blood pressure?

- A. Administer intravenous labetalol to gradually reduce blood pressure and monitor for neurological changes.
- B. Begin intravenous nitroprusside infusion immediately to rapidly lower blood pressure.
- C. Give oral methyldopa to lower blood pressure over the next 24 hours.
- D. Start intravenous nicardipine infusion and titrate to maintain a systolic blood pressure below 160 mm Hg.

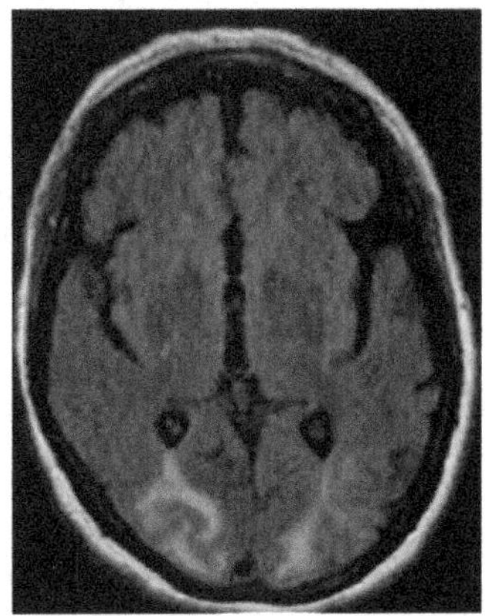

Figure 1.1: A 38-year-old woman

The correct answer is D. Start intravenous nicardipine infusion and titrate to maintain a systolic blood pressure below 160 mm Hg. This patient is presenting with symptoms and radiological findings consistent with hypertensive encephalopathy and posterior reversible encephalopathy syndrome (PRES). The goal in the management of hypertensive encephalopathy and PRES is to lower blood pressure effectively without precipitating ischemia or other complications. Intravenous nicardipine is a calcium channel blocker that can be titrated to effect and is preferred in this scenario for its ability to lower blood pressure effectively and safely. The target blood pressure in the acute setting should be a controlled reduction, aiming for a 25% reduction in the first hour, with a goal to bring the systolic blood pressure to less than 160 mm Hg. Option A is incorrect because, although intravenous labetalol is an appropriate medication for blood pressure control in hypertensive emergencies, nicardipine is preferred in PRES due to its more predictable cerebral vasodilatory effects. Option B is incorrect because intravenous nitroprusside, although a potent antihypertensive agent, is not preferred in the setting of PRES due to the risk of increasing cerebral edema and the potential for cyanide toxicity, especially in patients with renal insufficiency. Option C is incorrect because oral methyldopa would not provide the immediate blood pressure control required in the setting of hypertensive encephalopathy and PRES and does not allow for the rapid titration needed to safely reduce blood pressure. The target blood pressure in the acute setting for hypertensive encephalopathy and posterior reversible encephalopathy syndrome (PRES) is to gradually reduce blood pressure by no more than 20% to 25% in the first few hours. Hypertensive Encephalopathy is a syndrome characterized by altered mental status, headache, vision changes, or seizures that accompany elevated blood pressure. It results from a failure of cerebral autoregulation due to a sudden elevation in blood pressure, leading to endothelial injury and vasogenic edema. Radiographically, it most commonly presents with evidence of posterior-predominant T2-hyperintense lesions without significant hemorrhage. The condition shares many features with PRES, including the potential reversibility of clinical symptoms and radiographic findings with prompt blood pressure management. Posterior Reversible Encephalopathy Syndrome (PRES), on the other hand, is a neurological condition that can present with visual disturbances, seizures, encephalopathy, and a wide range of causes including hypertension, renal failure, eclampsia, and exposure to cytotoxic medications. PRES is characterized by headache, altered mental status, visual disturbances, and seizures. MRI shows edema, usually involving the posterior subcortical regions. The mechanism underlying PRES involves endothelial dysfunction, but unlike hypertensive encephalopathy, PRES can occur in patients who are normotensive or hypotensive at the initial evaluation, especially when due to medications or systemic conditions other than hypertension or eclampsia. The key differences between the two conditions include:

- Underlying Causes and Risk Factors: PRES has a broader range of causes and can occur in normotensive individuals, whereas hypertensive encephalopathy is directly related to acute elevations in blood pressure.
- Radiographic Findings: Both conditions can show similar radiographic features, but PRES is more specifically associated with vasogenic edema predominantly affecting the posterior regions of the brain.
- Clinical Presentation: While both conditions can present with similar symptoms such as headache, altered mental status, and seizures, PRES is more distinctly associated with visual disturbances and a wider variety of underlying causes.

Sudulagunta SRet al . Posterior reversible encephalopathy syndrome(PRES). Oxf Med Case Reports. 2017 Apr 3;2017(4):omx011. PMID: 28473920

1.16 Hypertension Management in Acute Intracerebral Hemorrhage

Case 16

A 52-year-old man with a history of poorly controlled hypertension presents to the emergency department with a sudden onset of right-sided weakness and difficulty speaking. His blood pressure is 200/110 mmHg. A non-contrast head CT scan shows a 30 mm left basal ganglia hemorrhage with surrounding edema but no evidence of ventricular extension. His past medical history is significant for a previous myocardial infarction and he is currently taking aspirin and atorvastatin. His heart rate is 88 beats per minute and regular. There are no signs of acute distress, and the rest of the physical examination is unremarkable.
Which of the following is the most appropriate next step in the management of this patient's blood pressure?

- A. Administer intravenous labetalol to achieve a target systolic blood pressure of 140 mm Hg.
- B. Give sublingual nifedipine to rapidly lower the systolic blood pressure to 120 mm Hg.
- C. Start oral antihypertensive therapy with amlodipine for gradual blood pressure reduction.
- D. Initiate intravenous nicardipine infusion with a target systolic blood pressure reduction of 20% from baseline within the first hour.

The correct answer is A. Administer intravenous labetalol to achieve a target systolic blood pressure of 140 mm Hg. In the setting of an acute intracerebral hemorrhage (ICH), current guidelines recommend lowering the systolic blood pressure to 140 mm Hg to help minimize hematoma expansion. Intravenous labetalol is a good choice in this scenario because it can be titrated to effect, does not significantly increase cerebral blood flow or intracranial pressure, and is appropriate for use in patients with a history of myocardial infarction. The patient's heart rate is not elevated, which makes labetalol a reasonable option. Option B is incorrect because sublingual nifedipine can cause a precipitous drop in blood pressure, which can be dangerous and is not recommended in the guidelines for the management of ICH. Option C is incorrect because oral antihypertensive therapy with amlodipine would not provide the immediate blood pressure control required in the setting of an acute ICH and does not allow for the rapid titration needed to safely reduce blood pressure. Option D is incorrect because although intravenous nicardipine is an appropriate medication for blood pressure control in ICH, the goal is not to reduce the systolic blood pressure by 20% from baseline within the first hour, but rather to target a systolic blood pressure of 140 mm Hg. In cases of acute intracerebral hemorrhage (ICH), a critical concern is the possibility of hematoma expansion, which can significantly impact patient outcomes. To address this risk, established medical guidelines provide direction on managing blood pressure during such emergencies. The primary objective is to cautiously lower systolic blood pressure to a specified target, often recommended to be below 140 mm Hg.

This target is informed by research indicating that maintaining a systolic blood pressure above 180 mm Hg may heighten the likelihood of complications like rebleeding and hematoma expansion in ICH cases. However, it is crucial to strike a balance between the imperative for swift blood pressure reduction and the potential risks of inducing ischemia or other adverse effects through overly aggressive interventions.

To navigate this delicate balance, healthcare providers frequently employ intravenous medications that enable precise control over blood pressure levels. These medications can be adjusted based on the patient's response, facilitating a gradual decrease in blood pressure towards the desired target. The specific goal of keeping systolic blood pressure below 140 mm Hg is selected to minimize the risk of further bleeding while also averting potential harm from hypoperfusion, which could result in ischemic damage to vulnerable brain tissue.

The management of blood pressure in cases of ICH demands a nuanced approach and diligent monitoring. It necessitates not only achieving a numerical target but also taking into account the patient's comprehensive clinical profile, encompassing factors such as neurological status and concurrent medical conditions.

Gioia LC et al. Blood pressure management in acute intracerebral hemorrhage: current evidence and ongoing controversies. Curr Opin Crit Care. 2015 Apr;21(2):99-106. PMID: 25689125

Arima H. Three rules for blood pressure management in acute intracerebral hemorrhage: fast, intense and stable. Hypertens Res. 2023 Jan;46(1):264-265. PMID: 36385350

Case 16B

Three days after the initial treatment with intravenous labetalol to target a systolic blood pressure of 140 mm Hg, the 52-year-old man with a history of poorly controlled hypertension and acute intracerebral hemorrhage (ICH) shows signs of clinical improvement. His right-sided weakness has slightly improved, and his speech is clearer, though still slightly slurred. His blood pressure has been maintained around 145/90 mmHg with continuous labetalol infusion, and he has been free of any new neurological deficits. However, a follow-up head CT scan reveals a slight increase in the size of the hematoma to 32 mm, with persistent surrounding edema. There is still no ventricular extension. The patient's heart rate remains stable at 85 beats per minute, and he continues to take aspirin and atorvastatin as part of his cardiac care. Given the patient's slight increase in hematoma size and his history of poorly controlled hypertension, the medical team is considering the following options for his ongoing management:

- A. Continue intravenous labetalol to maintain a target systolic blood pressure of 140 mm Hg.
- B. Pause aspirin therapy to reduce the risk of further hematoma expansion.
- C. Initiate a secondary prevention strategy with additional antihypertensive agents.
- D. Provide patient education on lifestyle modifications to control blood pressure.

bas.jpg 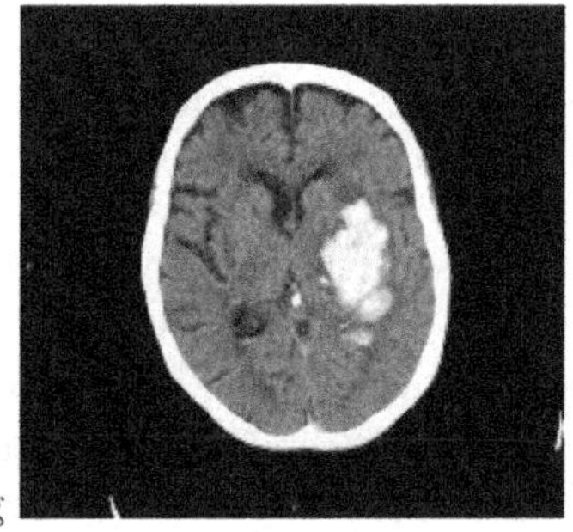

Figure 1.2: CT of A 52-year-old

The correct answer is A. Continue intravenous labetalol to maintain a target systolic blood pressure of 140 mm Hg. A. Continue intravenous labetalol: This option is appropriate as it aligns with current guidelines that recommend maintaining systolic blood pressure below 140 mm Hg to minimize hematoma expansion . The patient's blood pressure has been stable with labetalol infusion, and there is no indication of adverse effects that would necessitate a change in therapy. B. Pause aspirin therapy: Considering the patient's history of myocardial infarction, the decision to pause aspirin therapy must weigh the benefits of reducing the risk of hematoma expansion against the potential increased risk of cardiac events. The slight increase in hematoma size may justify a temporary pause in aspirin therapy, but this should be closely evaluated by the medical team. C. Initiate secondary prevention strategy: Given the patient's history of poorly controlled hypertension, introducing additional antihypertensive agents may be beneficial for long-term management and secondary prevention of ICH . This strategy should be tailored to the patient's individual needs and risk factors. D. Provide patient education: Lifestyle modifications are a critical component of hypertension management and can significantly impact blood pressure control . Educating the patient on dietary changes, exercise, smoking cessation, and alcohol intake can help prevent future hypertensive crises and cerebrovascular events. In conclusion, the most appropriate next step in the management of this patient's blood pressure would be to continue with option A, the intravenous labetalol infusion, to maintain the target systolic blood pressure of 140 mm Hg. This approach is supported by evidence suggesting that preonset antihypertensive therapy is associated with better outcomes in ICH patients . Additionally, the medical team should consider the other options as part of a comprehensive care plan tailored to the patient's evolving clinical status and long-term health goals.

1.17 Acute Ischemic Stroke Management: Pre-Thrombolysis

Case 17

A 72-year-old woman presents to the emergency department with sudden onset of left-sided weakness and slurred speech that started 1 hour ago. Her vitals show a blood pressure of 190/100 mmHg. A CT scan of her head shows no evidence of hemorrhage. The patient is currently not on any hypertensive medications and her previous blood pressure recordings have been within normal limits. Given the patient's clinical presentation and current blood pressure, which of the following is the most appropriate management strategy?

- A. Start the patient on oral antihypertensive medication and monitor blood pressure.
- B. Initiate thrombolytic therapy without any blood pressure intervention since her blood pressure will fall spontaneously.
- C. Lower the patient's blood pressure below 185/110 mmHg before administering thrombolytic therapy.
- D. Rapidly lower the patient's blood pressure to normal range using intravenous antihypertensive medications before considering thrombolytic therapy.

C. Lower the patient's blood pressure below 185/110 mmHg before administering thrombolytic therapy. The patient's symptoms suggest an acute ischemic stroke. In such cases, blood pressure often elevates acutely and will usually fall spontaneously. Antihypertensive medications are typically used only if the systolic blood pressure exceeds 180-200 mmHg. However, if thrombolytics are to be given, like in this patient who is within the therapeutic window for thrombolysis, it is crucial to maintain blood pressure at less than 185/110 mmHg during treatment and for 24 hours following treatment to minimize the risk of hemorrhagic conversion. Therefore, the most appropriate next step in this case would be to lower the patient's blood pressure below 185/110 mmHg before administering thrombolytic therapy. Blood pressure should be reduced cautiously by 10–15% over 24 hours. Acute ischemic stroke (AIS) is a medical emergency characterized by a significant reduction in cerebral blood flow (CBF), leading to neuronal death within minutes and potentially causing long-term disability or death. The area surrounding the core of the stroke, known as the penumbra, remains underperfused but viable for a limited time, making its preservation a critical goal in stroke treatment.

The Impact of Blood Pressure on Stroke Risk and Outcomes Blood pressure (BP) is a key factor in vascular function and organ perfusion, and its dysregulation can lead to vascular dysfunction, particularly in cerebral circulation. Chronic hypertension (HT) is a significant contributor to AIS, and managing BP is crucial for improving outcomes in stroke patients.

Hypertension is one of the strongest risk factors for stroke, both in the general population and specifically in individuals with type 1 diabetes. Blood pressure variables such as systolic blood pressure (SBP), diastolic blood pressure (DBP), pulse pressure (PP), and mean arterial pressure (MAP) are all independently associated with an increased risk of stroke.

The American Heart Association/American Stroke Association recommends maintaining BP below certain thresholds during the administration of intravenous thrombolysis (IVT) and mechanical thrombectomy (MT). However, the optimal BP target during MT is less clear, and the relationship between presenting BP and stroke outcome is complex, often described as a U-shaped curve where both high and low BP can lead to worse outcomes.

Cerebral autoregulation and recanalization status are key factors in this relationship, with different outcomes observed in patients who achieve recanalization compared to those who do not. High BP is common in AIS patients, and while BP typically decreases spontaneously over the first week, managing it is still critical. Studies have shown that substantial drops in intra-procedural BP are associated with worse neurological outcomes.

The Role of Combined Therapies Combining MT with IVT has been shown to improve prognosis for AIS patients without increasing the risk of hemorrhagic transformation (HT) compared to MT alone. This combination therapy significantly improves functional independence (FI), excellent outcomes, and reduces mortality risk.

Beyond hypertension, other systemic factors contribute to stroke risk, including high cholesterol, heart disorders, diabetes, obesity, sickle cell disease, poor diet, lack of physical activity, excessive alcohol consumption, and tobacco use. Genetic predispositions, age, gender, and ethnicity also play roles in stroke susceptibility.

Managing blood pressure is a cornerstone of AIS treatment and prevention. While hypertension remains a major risk factor, the complexity of BP management during acute stroke treatment underscores the need for individualized care. The combination of MT and IVT therapies offers promising outcomes, but further research is needed to optimize BP targets for different stages of stroke management.

Gasecki D et al. Blood Pressure Management in Acute Ischemic Stroke. Curr Hypertens Rep. 2020 Dec 10;23(1):3. PMID: 33305339

Guo QH et al. Blood Pressure Goals in Acute Stroke. Am J Hypertens. 2022 Jun 16;35(6):483-499. PMID: 35323883

Boulanger JM et al. Canadian Stroke Best Practice Recommendations for Acute Stroke Management: Prehospital, Emergency Department, and Acute Inpatient Stroke Care, 6th Edition, Update 2018. Int J Stroke. 2018 Dec;13(9):949-984. PMID: 30021503

Case Note

Key Points to Remember:

1. Acute Hypertensive Microangiopathy: The goal is to reduce blood pressure to 160/100 mm Hg within 2-6 hours, with an initial reduction of no more than 25% within minutes to 1-2 hours. Medications with predictable, dose-dependent, transient, and progressive effects should be used, and sublingual or oral fast-acting nifedipine should be avoided. It's important to monitor for organ ischemia resulting from excessive blood pressure reductions .
2. Acute Ischemic Stroke: The blood pressure goal is less than 185/110 mm Hg if thrombolytics are to be given, with a 10-15% reduction over 24 hours. If systolic blood pressure exceeds 180-200 mm Hg, a cautious reduction is recommended. Blood pressure usually falls spontaneously, so excessive reduction should be avoided.
3. Intracerebral Hemorrhage: The goal is to reduce blood pressure to 140 mm Hg within the first 6 hours, with a gradual reduction. Nonsedating agents that do not increase cerebral blood flow or intracranial pressure should be used. The aim is to minimize bleeding while maintaining cerebral perfusion

Table 1.7: Therapeutic Strategies for Hypertensive Emergencies with Specific End-Organ Damage

Condition	Blood Pressure Goal	Initial BP Reduction	Medication Considerations	Special Considerations
Acute hypertensive microangiopathy	160/100 mm Hg within 2-6 hours	No more than 25% within minutes to 1-2 hours	Predictable, dose-dependent, transient, and progressive agents. Avoid sublingual or oral fast-acting nifedipine	Monitor for organ ischemia from excessive BP reductions
Acute ischemic stroke	Less than 185/110 mm Hg if thrombolytics are to be given	10-15% over 24 hours	Cautious reduction if systolic BP exceeds 180-200 mm Hg	BP usually falls spontaneously; avoid excessive reduction
Intracerebral hemorrhage	140 mm Hg within first 6 hours	Gradual reduction	Nonsedating agents that do not increase cerebral blood flow or intracranial pressure	Minimize bleeding, balance with maintaining cerebral perfusion
Acute aortic dissection	Below 120 mm Hg and heart rate less than 60 bpm within 30 minutes	Rapid reduction	Combination of vasodilation and beta-blockade	Prevent further bleeding while maintaining cerebral perfusion

1.18 Management of Scleroderma Renal Crisis

Case 18

A 56-year-old woman with a 10-year history of systemic sclerosis presents to the emergency department with acute onset of shortness of breath, severe hypertension, and decreased urine output. Her blood pressure is 190/120 mmHg. Physical examination reveals diffuse skin thickening, and bilateral crackles are heard at the lung bases. Laboratory tests show a serum creatinine of 2.5 mg/dL, increased from a baseline of 1.0 mg/dL a month ago, and a urinalysis with proteinuria and microscopic hematuria. There is no evidence of hemolytic anemia, and her platelet count is normal. An echocardiogram shows normal left ventricular function with no signs of pulmonary hypertension.
Which of the following is the most appropriate next step in the management of this patient's hypertensive crisis?

- A. Administer intravenous nitroglycerin to rapidly lower blood pressure.
- B. Begin oral captopril therapy and titrate to effect based on blood pressure response.
- C. Start intravenous enalaprilat and adjust the dose to achieve gradual blood pressure control.
- D. Give intravenous furosemide to manage volume overload and hypertension.

The correct answer is C. Start intravenous enalaprilat and adjust the dose to achieve gradual blood pressure control. This patient is presenting with a scleroderma renal crisis, a life-threatening complication of systemic sclerosis characterized by acute onset of severe hypertension and rapidly progressive renal failure. Angiotensin-converting enzyme (ACE) inhibitors, such as captopril or intravenous enalaprilat, are the treatment of choice for scleroderma renal crisis due to their efficacy in reducing blood pressure and improving renal function. Intravenous enalaprilat is particularly useful in the acute setting for its rapid onset and short duration of action, which allows for careful titration of blood pressure in a closely monitored setting. Option A is incorrect because intravenous nitroglycerin is primarily used for the management of ischemic chest pain and has a more significant effect on preload reduction than afterload; it is not the first-line treatment for scleroderma renal crisis. Option B is incorrect because, although oral captopril is an appropriate treatment for scleroderma renal crisis, in the acute setting with severe hypertension and evidence of end-organ damage, intravenous administration of an ACE inhibitor allows for more precise blood pressure control. Option D is incorrect because, while intravenous furosemide can be used to manage volume overload, it does not address the underlying pathophysiology of scleroderma renal crisis and may not adequately control severe hypertension. Additionally, aggressive diuresis can potentially worsen renal function if the patient is not volume overloaded. The recommended drug options and combinations for various types of hypertensive emergencies, as well as drugs that should be avoided in each scenario. The goal is to provide guidance on the most effective and safe pharmacological interventions based on the specific clinical situation.

1. Acute hypertensive microangiopathy: Labetalol or Nicardipine are recommended due to their efficacy in rapidly controlling blood pressure without causing significant adverse effects.
2. Hypertensive encephalopathy and posterior reversible encephalopathy syndrome (PRES): Labetalol and Nicardipine are preferred for their ability to lower blood pressure effectively. Drugs like Nitroprusside, Methyldopa, Clonidine, and Nitroglycerin are to be avoided due to their potential to exacerbate the condition or cause additional complications.
3. Myocardial ischemia and infarction: Combinations such as Nicardipine with Esmolol, Nitroglycerin with Labetalol, or Nitroglycerin with Esmolol are recommended for their complementary actions in reducing blood pressure and controlling heart rate. Drugs like Hydralazine, Diazoxide, Minoxidil, and Nitroprusside should be avoided because they may cause rapid changes in blood pressure or have other adverse cardiac effects.
4. Acute kidney injury: Fenoldopam, Nicardipine, and Clevidipine are suitable choices due to their renal protective effects and ability to manage blood pressure without worsening kidney function.
5. Aortic dissection: Combinations of Esmolol with Nicardipine or Clevidipine, as well as Labetalol or Esmolol with Nitroprusside, are recommended to achieve rapid and controlled blood pressure reduction while avoiding excessive dilation that could worsen the dissection. Drugs like Hydralazine, Diazoxide, and Minoxidil are to be avoided due to their unpredictable effects on blood pressure.
6. Acute pulmonary edema with left ventricular (LV) systolic dysfunction: Nicardipine combined with Nitroglycerin and a loop diuretic, or Clevidipine with the same combination, are recommended to manage both blood pressure and pulmonary congestion. Drugs like Hydralazine, Diazoxide, and Beta-blockers should be avoided due to their potential to worsen pulmonary edema or cardiac function.
7. Acute pulmonary edema with diastolic dysfunction: Esmolol combined with low-dose Nitroglycerin and a loop diuretic, or Labetalol with the same combination, are recommended to manage blood pressure while avoiding exacerbation of diastolic dysfunction.
8. Ischemic stroke with systolic blood pressure above 180–200 mm Hg: Nicardipine, Clevidipine, and Labetalol are preferred for their ability to lower blood pressure in a controlled manner. Drugs like Nitroprusside, Methyldopa, Clonidine, and Nitroglycerin should be avoided due to their potential to cause rapid fluctuations in blood pressure or other adverse effects.
9. Intracerebral hemorrhage with systolic blood pressure above 140–160 mm Hg: Nicardipine, Clevidipine, and Labetalol are recommended for their effectiveness in reducing blood pressure without causing a rapid decrease that could compromise cerebral perfusion.
10. Hyperadrenergic states, including cocaine use: Nicardipine or Clevidipine combined with a benzodiazepine, or Phentolamine, are recommended for their ability to manage the sympathetic overactivity without causing unopposed alpha-adrenergic effects. Labetalol and Beta-blockers should be avoided due to the risk of worsening hypertension.
11. Preeclampsia, eclampsia: Labetalol and Nicardipine are recommended for their safety profile in pregnancy. Diuretics and ACE inhibitors are to be avoided due to their potential adverse effects on the fetus.
12. Scleroderma renal crisis: Captopril or intravenous Enalaprilat are recommended for their efficacy in managing the hypertensive crisis associated with systemic sclerosis.

1.19 Management of Cocaine-Induced Hypertension and Hyperadrenergic State

Case 19

A 33-year-old man is brought to the emergency department with chest pain, palpitations, and a headache. He has a history of recreational drug use and admits to using cocaine earlier in the day. His blood pressure is 180/110 mmHg, heart rate is 120 beats per minute, and he is diaphoretic and restless. An electrocardiogram shows sinus tachycardia without ischemic changes. Initial blood tests including cardiac biomarkers are pending. The patient is agitated and reports feeling extremely anxious. Which of the following is the most appropriate next step in the management of this patient's hypertension?

- A. Administer intravenous labetalol to control blood pressure and heart rate.
- B. Begin intravenous nitroglycerin to relieve chest pain and lower blood pressure.
- C. Start intravenous nicardipine and give a benzodiazepine for agitation and sympathetic suppression.
- D. Give oral metoprolol to target the tachycardia and hypertension.

The correct answer is C. Start intravenous nicardipine and give a benzodiazepine for agitation and sympathetic suppression. This patient is presenting with a hyperadrenergic state secondary to cocaine use. Cocaine induces sympathetic overactivity by inhibiting the reuptake of norepinephrine, leading to both alpha and beta-adrenergic effects. The management of hypertension in this setting should focus on medications that do not cause unopposed alpha-adrenergic effects, which can worsen hypertension. Nicardipine, a calcium channel blocker, is effective for blood pressure control without increasing the risk of coronary vasospasm. Benzodiazepines are used to reduce central sympathetic outflow, which can help control both blood pressure and heart rate, as well as alleviate the patient's agitation. Option A is incorrect because labetalol, although it has both alpha and beta-blocking effects, should be avoided as it may not adequately block the alpha effects of cocaine and can potentially lead to unopposed alpha-adrenergic effects and worsening hypertension. Option B is incorrect because nitroglycerin is primarily used for the management of ischemic chest pain and does not adequately address the sympathetic overactivity associated with cocaine use. Option D is incorrect because beta-blockers like metoprolol should be avoided in acute cocaine intoxication due to the risk of unopposed alpha-adrenergic effects, which can lead to a paradoxical increase in blood pressure. In the scenario of acute cocaine intoxication, the administration of beta-blockers can trigger a phenomenon termed unopposed alpha-stimulation. This phenomenon arises when the equilibrium between alpha and beta receptors in the body is disrupted, resulting in elevated blood pressure and/or exacerbated coronary artery vasoconstriction. Activation of alpha-1 receptors in the adrenergic system induces smooth muscle contraction and vasoconstriction, while stimulation of beta-1 receptors enhances heart rate, conduction, and contractility. On the other hand, beta-2 receptor activation promotes smooth muscle relaxation. Typically, a harmonious interplay between alpha-1 and beta-2 stimulation regulates vascular tone. However, the use of a non-selective beta-blocker tilts this balance towards alpha-1 stimulation, favoring vasoconstriction.

Cocaine impacts both alpha and beta receptors by heightening sympathetic activity through norepinephrine reuptake inhibition, resulting in combined alpha and beta-adrenergic effects. When a beta-blocker is introduced in this context, the absence of counteracting effects on alpha receptors can lead to compromised myocardial blood flow and coronary vasoconstriction. In individuals experiencing myocardial ischemia, this could exacerbate the condition by further reducing coronary blood flow.

Furthermore, concurrent use of beta-blockers with cocaine can intensify blood vessel constriction, diminishing oxygen availability and causing a surge in blood pressure. This outcome contradicts the intended effects of beta-blockers, which aim to dilate blood vessels, slow heart rate, and reduce blood pressure. Consequently, although beta-blockers are fundamental in managing traditional acute coronary syndromes, they are generally contraindicated in cases of acute cocaine intoxication due to concerns regarding coronary vasoconstriction and the potential for an acute rise in blood pressure stemming from unopposed alpha-receptor stimulation.

Hollander JE. Cocaine intoxication and hypertension. Ann Emerg Med. 2008 Mar;51(3 Suppl):S18-20. PMID: 18191302

2

PERICARDIUM/MYOCARDIUM

2.1 A Case of Chest Pain and ECG Changes

Case 20

A 47-year-old male with no significant past medical history presents to the emergency department with a 2-day history of sharp, retrosternal chest pain that worsens when lying flat and improves with sitting up and leaning forward. He denies any recent illness or trauma. On examination, his blood pressure is 130/80 mmHg, heart rate is 95 beats per minute, and he is afebrile. A faint pericardial friction rub is auscultated. An ECG is performed and shows diffuse ST-elevation with a concave-upwards contour and PR-segment depression, without reciprocal ST-segment depression. There is no evidence of pericardial effusion on the echocardiogram. Which of the following is the most appropriate next step in the management of this patient?

- A. Immediate pericardiocentesis due to suspicion of cardiac tamponade.
- B. High-dose aspirin therapy and initiation of colchicine.
- C. Empirical antibiotic therapy for suspected bacterial pericarditis.
- D. Urgent cardiac catheterization to rule out acute myocardial infarction.

The correct answer is B. High-dose aspirin therapy and initiation of colchicine. The patient presents with classic signs and symptoms of acute pericarditis, including chest pain that improves with leaning forward, a pericardial friction rub, and ECG changes consistent with acute pericarditis (diffuse ST-elevation and PR-segment depression) . The absence of pericardial effusion on echocardiogram and the lack of hemodynamic instability make cardiac tamponade unlikely . Therefore, pericardiocentesis (option A) is not indicated. Empirical antibiotics (option C) are not warranted without evidence of bacterial infection, which is rare in developed countries . Urgent cardiac catheterization (option D) is not the first-line investigation for acute pericarditis, especially in the absence of dynamic ECG changes or cardiac biomarkers suggestive of acute myocardial infarction. The combination of high-dose aspirin or nonsteroidal anti-inflammatory drugs (NSAIDs) with colchicine is recommended for the treatment of acute pericarditis to reduce inflammation and prevent recurrence. In acute pericarditis, experts recommend limiting physical activity until symptoms resolve. Athletes should refrain from exercise until symptoms resolve, and all laboratory tests return to normal, typically around 3 months. The 2015 European Society of Cardiology (ESC) guidelines suggest the following treatment:

- Aspirin: 750–1000 mg every 8 hours for 1–2 weeks,

followed by a taper by decreasing the dose by 250–500 mg every 1–2 weeks.

- Ibuprofen: 600 mg every 8 hours for 1–2 weeks, followed by a taper by decreasing the dose by 200–400 mg every 1–2 weeks.

Gastroprotection should be considered when using high-dose anti-inflammatory medications.

The addition of colchicine during the acute episode can help prevent future recurrences. Colchicine should be added to the NSAID at a dose of:

- 0.5–0.6 mg once daily for patients less than 70 kg
- 0.5–0.6 mg twice daily for patients more than 70 kg

Colchicine should be continued for at least 3 months. In the final week, the dose can be tapered by decreasing every other day for patients under 70 kg or once a day for those over 70 kg.

For post-myocardial infarction (MI) pericarditis (Dressler syndrome), aspirin and colchicine are recommended instead of NSAIDs to avoid negative impact on myocardial healing. The recommended treatment is:

- Aspirin: 750–1000 mg three times daily for 1–2 weeks
- Colchicine: 3 months

Even with initial treatment, about 30% of patients experience recurrence. In refractory cases and recurrent pericarditis, colchicine should be used for a minimum of 6 months, and therapy may need to be extended. C-reactive protein (CRP) is utilized to evaluate treatment effectiveness, and tapering begins once it returns to normal levels.

In recurrent pericarditis, indomethacin (25–50 mg every 8 hours) can also be considered in place of ibuprofen.

In severe cases, refractory situations, or immune-mediated causes, systemic corticosteroids may be considered. However, this treatment may increase the risk of recurrence and potentially prolong the illness.

The main causes of acute pericarditis include viral infections (e.g., coxsackieviruses, influenza, Epstein-Barr virus, varicella, hepatitis, mumps, and HIV), autoimmune syndromes, uremia, neoplasms, radiation, drug toxicity, hemopericardium, and post-cardiac surgery or myocardial inflammation. Pericarditis and myocarditis often occur together in 20–30% of cases. Diagnosis mainly involves ruling out acute myocardial infarction and identifying the underlying cause.

Adler Y et al. 2015 ESC Guidelines for the diagnosis and management of pericardial diseases: The Task Force for the Diagnosis and Management of Pericardial Diseases of the European Society of Cardiology (ESC) Eur Heart J. 2015 Nov 7;36(42):2921-2964. PMID: 26320112

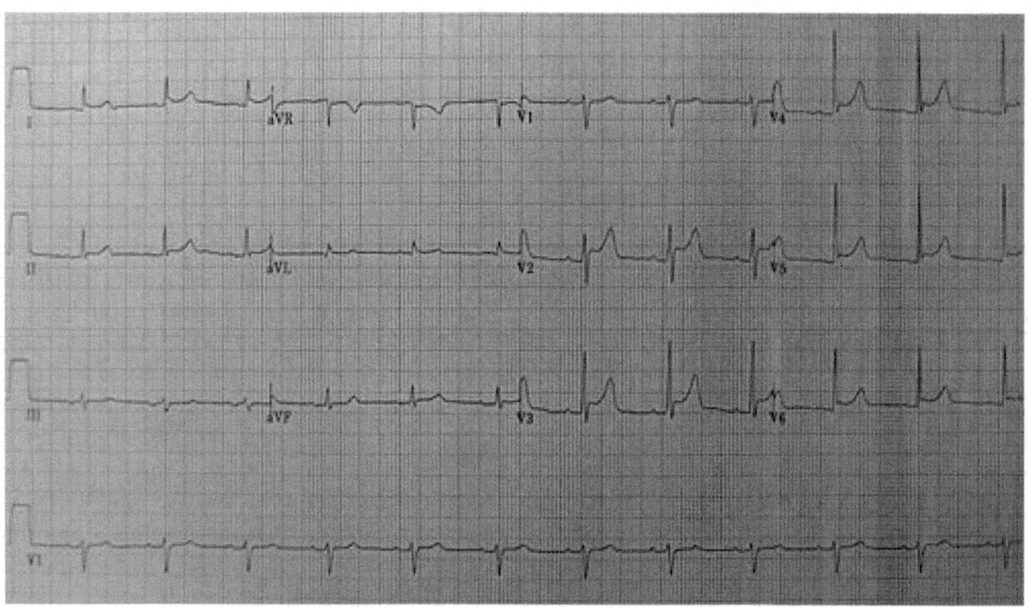

Figure 2.1: A 47-year-old male ECG

Type of Pericarditis	Symptoms and Signs
Inflammatory Pericarditis	Chest pain (pleuritic and postural), substernal pain radiating to neck, shoulders, back, or epigastrium, dyspnea, fever, pericardial friction rub
Tuberculous Pericarditis	Subacute presentation, nonspecific symptoms (fever, night sweats, fatigue) for days to months
Bacterial Pericarditis	Similar to other types of inflammatory pericarditis, patients appear toxic and critically ill
Uremic Pericarditis	Can present with or without symptoms, fever is absent
Neoplastic Pericarditis	Often painless, symptoms relate to hemodynamic compromise or the primary disease, large pericardial effusion
Post-MI or Postcardiotomy Pericarditis (Dressler Syndrome)	Recurrence of pain with pleural-pericardial features, rub often audible, large effusions uncommon, spontaneous resolution usually occurs in a few days
Radiation Pericarditis	Clinical onset usually within the first year but may be delayed for many years

Table 2.1: Symptoms and Signs of Different Types of Pericarditis

2.2 A Post-MI Pleuritic Chest Pain, Fever Case Study

Case 21

A 62-year-old male with a history of a recent myocardial infarction (MI) 3 weeks ago presents to the clinic with a new onset of pleuritic chest pain and low-grade fever. The chest pain is sharp, worsens with inspiration, and is relieved by sitting up and leaning forward. On examination, his blood pressure is 125/75 mmHg, heart rate is 88 beats per minute, and temperature is 37.8C (100F). A pericardial friction rub is heard on auscultation. An ECG shows diffuse ST elevations and PR depressions. Laboratory tests reveal a slight elevation in white blood cell count and erythrocyte sedimentation rate. An echocardiogram shows no evidence of pericardial effusion. Which of the following is the most appropriate next step in the management of this patient?

- A. Initiate high-dose ibuprofen and colchicine for suspected post-MI pericarditis.
- B. Perform urgent coronary angiography to rule out recurrent myocardial infarction.
- C. Start broad-spectrum antibiotics for suspected bacterial pericarditis.
- D. Schedule pericardiocentesis to evaluate for possible purulent pericarditis.

The correct answer is A. High-dose aspirin therapy and initiation of colchicine. The correct answer is A. Initiate high-dose ibuprofen and colchicine for suspected post-MI pericarditis. The patient's presentation is consistent with post-MI pericarditis, also known as Dressler syndrome, which is an inflammatory response to myocardial necrosis that typically occurs weeks to months after an MI. The clinical features include pleuritic chest pain, fever, pericardial friction rub, and ECG changes of pericarditis. The absence of a new pericardial effusion on echocardiogram and the timing of symptoms following an MI support this diagnosis. The treatment of choice is anti-inflammatory therapy with NSAIDs, such as ibuprofen, and colchicine to reduce inflammation and prevent recurrence. Option B is incorrect because the patient's clinical presentation and ECG findings are not suggestive of an acute recurrent MI, and the timing of the symptoms is more consistent with Dressler syndrome. Option C is incorrect because there is no strong evidence of bacterial infection, which is a rare cause of pericarditis in developed countries, especially in the post-MI setting without evidence of an effusion or sepsis. Option D is incorrect because pericardiocentesis is not indicated in the absence of a significant pericardial effusion or cardiac tamponade. Dressler's syndrome, also known as post-myocardial infarction (post-MI) syndrome or post-pericardiotomy syndrome, typically develops days to weeks, or even several months, following a myocardial infarction or open heart surgery. It can reoccur, and it is likely an immunological response to myocardial injury. Patients with Dressler's syndrome exhibit characteristic symptoms such as chest discomfort, fever, fatigue, and an elevated white blood cell count. Occasionally, additional symptoms of an autoimmune illness, like joint pain and fever, may manifest.

Post-MI syndrome is a rare complication of myocardial infarction. Although estimates vary, even before the advent of coronary revascularization, studies suggested an incidence rate of 3 to 5%. With the widespread availability of prompt revascularization as the mainstay of acute MI treatment, the occurrence of post-MI syndrome has decreased even further and is now estimated to occur in only about 1% of patients following MI.

The combination of pleuritic chest pain, pericardial effusion, and specific ECG changes in a patient after a myocardial infarction is characteristic of post-MI syndrome. However, it is crucial for clinicians to note that this triad has low sensitivity and is found in only a small number of patients. In a study of patients with post-MI syndrome, it was discovered that classic ECG changes were present in only about 25% of cases, while pericardial effusion was found to be absent in nearly 20%.

Although usually not life-threatening, severe complications like cardiac tamponade have been reported in Dressler's syndrome. Both pain and fatigue can significantly affect the quality of life for patients experiencing persistent or recurrent symptoms, which is why treatment with colchicine and nonsteroidal anti-inflammatory drugs (NSAIDs) is often warranted.

Cardiac tamponade is uncommon in Dressler's syndrome following a myocardial infarction but is more likely to occur after open heart surgery. For quicker diagnosis of post-MI syndrome, clinicians need to be vigilant when assessing patients who show new chest pain, fatigue, or signs of inflammation after a myocardial infarction. Additional laboratory tests to assess inflammation, such as the erythrocyte sedimentation rate or C-reactive protein, can be crucial in confirming the diagnosis. It is also advisable to assess for pericardial effusion and to exclude any signs of hemodynamically significant effusion or other structural issues.

Aten K et al. Dressler Syndrome: Not Just a Relic of the Past. Cureus. 2022 Oct 25;14(10):e30670. PMID: 36426326

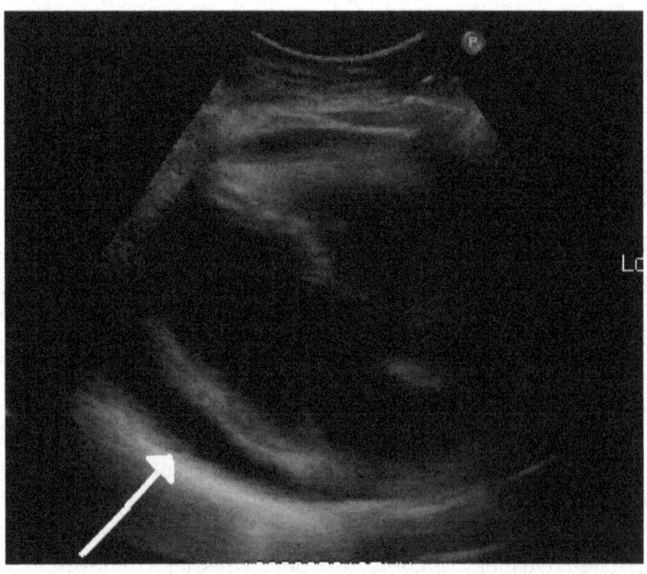

Figure 2.2: Pericarditis

Type of Pericarditis	Laboratory Findings and Diagnostic Studies
Viral Pericarditis	Leukocytosis often present, slightly elevated cardiac enzymes, echocardiogram often normal or reveals only a trivial amount of extra fluid
Tuberculous Pericarditis	Acid-fast bacilli found elsewhere, small or moderate pericardial effusions, low yield of mycobacterial organisms by pericardiocentesis
Bacterial Pericarditis	Diagnostic pericardiocentesis can be confirmatory
Uremic Pericarditis	Incidence of pericarditis correlates with the level of BUN and creatinine, "shaggy" pericardium, hemorrhagic and exudative effusion
Neoplastic Pericarditis	Cytologic examination of the effusion or pericardial biopsy, large pericardial effusions
Post-MI or Postcardiotomy Pericarditis	High ESR, large pericardial effusions and accompanying pleural effusions are frequent

Table 2.2: Laboratory Findings and Diagnostic Studies for Different Types of Pericarditis

2.3 Case of Atypical Chest Pain In Advanced CKD Patient

Case 22

A 57-year-old female with a history of chronic kidney disease stage 5 presents to the emergency department with sharp, substernal chest pain that radiates to the back and is relieved by sitting forward. She has not initiated dialysis yet. Her blood pressure is 145/90 mmHg, heart rate is 102 beats per minute, and she is afebrile. On examination, a pericardial friction rub is audible. Laboratory results show a blood urea nitrogen (BUN) of 112 mg/dL and creatinine of 9.8 mg/dL. An echocardiogram reveals a small pericardial effusion without signs of tamponade. An ECG shows diffuse, nonspecific ST-segment and T-wave changes.
Which of the following is the most appropriate next step in the management of this patient?

- A. Initiate hemodialysis immediately to address uremic pericarditis.
- B. Administer intravenous broad-spectrum antibiotics to cover for potential bacterial pericarditis.
- C. Perform pericardiocentesis to relieve the pericardial effusion.
- D. Prescribe high-dose nonsteroidal anti-inflammatory drugs (NSAIDs) for pain management.

The correct answer is A. Initiate hemodialysis immediately to address uremic pericarditis. This patient with advanced chronic kidney disease presents with symptoms suggestive of uremic pericarditis, which is associated with a high level of BUN and creatinine. The "shaggy" appearance of the pericardium and hemorrhagic effusion are characteristic of uremic pericarditis. The most effective treatment for uremic pericarditis is to reduce the uremic state, which is best accomplished by initiating hemodialysis. This can alleviate the symptoms and prevent the progression of the pericarditis. Option B is incorrect because there is no evidence of bacterial infection, and the patient's presentation is more consistent with uremic pericarditis due to her advanced kidney disease. Option C is incorrect because pericardiocentesis is not indicated in the absence of cardiac tamponade or a large effusion causing hemodynamic compromise. Option D is incorrect because NSAIDs are generally avoided in patients with advanced chronic kidney disease due to the risk of further renal injury and because they do not address the underlying uremic condition. Uremic pericarditis is a condition that develops due to inflammation of the pericardium caused by toxins and immune complexes in individuals with kidney disease. Pericarditis and acute coronary syndrome can have similar initial clinical presentations, with overlapping electrocardiogram (ECG) findings, making the diagnosis challenging.

In the evaluation of suspected uremic pericarditis, regular blood tests should include inflammatory markers, white blood cell (WBC) count with differential, creatine kinase, troponins, and assessments of renal and liver function. Elevated levels of C-reactive protein and erythrocyte sedimentation rate are frequently observed in uremic pericarditis. Leukocytosis occurs in 40% to 60% of individuals with uremic and dialysis-associated pericarditis. It is important to note that cardiac enzymes can be elevated in patients with end-stage renal disease (ESRD), suggesting myocardial damage even in those with normal kidney function. However, there is no significant difference in blood urea nitrogen levels between patients with or without uremic or dialysis pericarditis.

The pericardial fluid in uremic and dialysis-associated pericarditis is typically exudative and contains mononuclear cells on fluid analysis. Pericardial biopsy can reveal various findings, such as necrotizing or non-necrotizing fibrinous pericarditis, chronic fibrous thickening in constrictive pericarditis, or a normal state.

If acute pericarditis is suspected, echocardiography is the preferred diagnostic procedure. It aids in evaluating pericarditis and can also detect myocarditis with changes in ventricular function or constriction. Additional imaging techniques, such as cardiac magnetic resonance imaging (MRI) and computed tomography (CT), can be used to diagnose complex or uncertain cases of pericarditis. However, gadolinium-based contrast agents are not recommended for patients with advanced renal disease (estimated glomerular filtration rate under 30 mL/min per 1.73 m^2) due to the potential risk of nephrogenic systemic fibrosis.

The management of uremic pericarditis requires collaboration among internists, cardiologists, and nephrologists. The incidence of uremic pericarditis has decreased since the implementation of renal replacement therapy, and dialysis remains the primary treatment option for these patients.

Sadjadi SA et al. Uremic pericarditis: a report of 30 cases and review of the literature. Am J Case Rep. 2015 Mar 22;16:169-73. PMID: 25796283

Rehman KAet al. Uremic pericarditis, pericardial effusion, and constrictive pericarditis in end-stage renal disease: Insights and pathophysiology. Clin Cardiol. 2017 Oct;40(10):839-846. PMID: 28873222

Symptom/Sign or Characteristic	Description
Pain	May be associated with pain if part of an acute inflammatory process; often painless in neoplastic or uremic effusion
Dyspnea and Cough	Common, especially with tamponade
Cardiac Tamponade	Life-threatening; evidenced by tachycardia, hypotension, pulsus paradoxus, raised JVP, muffled heart sounds, decreased ECG voltage or electrical alternans
Prognosis	Depends on the cause; large idiopathic chronic effusions have a 30 to 35% risk of progression to tamponade
Pericardial Friction Rub	May be present even with large effusions
Tachycardia	Fast heart rate
Tachypnea	Rapid breathing
Narrow Pulse Pressure	Small difference between systolic and diastolic blood pressure
Pulsus Paradoxus	Decline of ¿10 mm Hg in systolic pressure during inspiration
CVP (Central Venous Pressure)	Elevated central venous pressure
Ventricular Filling	Inhibited throughout diastole in tamponade
Edema or Ascites	Rare in tamponade; suggests a more chronic process

Table 2.3: Symptoms, Signs, and Characteristics of Pericardial Effusion and Cardiac Tamponade

2.4 Management Approach to Recurrent Pericarditis

Case 23

A 46-year-old male with a history of idiopathic acute pericarditis presents to the clinic with sharp, pleuritic chest pain that improves when sitting up and leaning forward. He has had two previous episodes of pericarditis in the past year. His current medications include colchicine and high-dose ibuprofen. On physical examination, a pericardial friction rub is audible. An ECG shows diffuse ST-segment elevations. A transthoracic echocardiogram reveals a small pericardial effusion without evidence of tamponade. Laboratory tests show elevated inflammatory markers. The patient mentions that he has been experiencing gastrointestinal side effects from the colchicine.
Given the patient's history and current presentation, what is the most appropriate next step in the management of this patient's recurrent pericarditis?

- A) Increase the dose of colchicine and continue high-dose ibuprofen.
- B) Initiate therapy with an interleukin-1 receptor antagonist such as anakinra.
- C) Perform surgical pericardial stripping immediately.
- D) Switch to a different NSAID and discontinue colchicine.

orrect Answer: B) Initiate therapy with an interleukin-1 receptor antagonist such as anakinra. The patient presents with recurrent pericarditis, as evidenced by multiple episodes of pericarditis, characteristic chest pain, a pericardial friction rub, ECG changes, and a pericardial effusion. The recurrence of symptoms despite the use of colchicine and NSAIDs, along with the development of gastrointestinal side effects from colchicine, suggests the need for an alternative treatment approach. Anakinra, an interleukin-1 receptor antagonist, has been shown to be beneficial in managing recurrent pericarditis, particularly in cases where traditional therapies such as colchicine and NSAIDs are not effective or not tolerated. Anakinra works by blocking the inflammatory effects of interleukin-1, a cytokine involved in the pathogenesis of pericarditis.

Surgical pericardial stripping is considered a last resort for recurrent pericarditis cases that are refractory to medical therapy and is typically not indicated unless there is evidence of constrictive pericarditis, which this patient does not have. Therefore, option C is not appropriate at this stage.

Switching to a different NSAID may not provide additional benefit and does not address the need for more potent immunosuppression due to the recurrent nature of the disease. Increasing the dose of colchicine is not advisable due to the patient's gastrointestinal side effects.

In conclusion, the most appropriate next step in management for this patient with recurrent pericarditis and intolerance to colchicine is to initiate therapy with anakinra (option B), which targets the underlying pathophysiology of the disease and has been shown to be effective in such cases.

Recurrent pericarditis (RP) appears to result from an abnormal immune reaction. Inadequate initial treatment, whether in terms of drug selection, dosage, treatment duration, or tapering, has been demonstrated to increase the likelihood of recurrences. During a recurrent episode, symptoms, physical examination findings, and electrocardiographic changes are typically milder than the initial episode, making imaging a valuable tool for confirming the diagnosis of RP. Cardiac magnetic resonance imaging (MRI) is increasingly preferred due to its ability to identify active pericardial inflammation. Utilizing inflammatory biomarkers can help evaluate the likelihood of recurrences and guide treatment adjustments.

The initial treatment for RP involves non-steroidal anti-inflammatory drugs (NSAIDs) and colchicine. NSAIDs help manage pain, while colchicine can reduce the risk of future recurrences. Glucocorticoids are frequently utilized as second-line medications, yet they are associated with a high frequency of recurrent episodes.

Interleukin-1 inhibitors, such as anakinra and rilonacept, have been shown to significantly decrease the likelihood of recurrences in patients with RP during treatment. These medications target the underlying inflammatory process and may offer a more effective approach in managing recurrent pericarditis.

It is essential to recognize and appropriately treat recurrent pericarditis, as uncontrolled inflammation can lead to chronic or constrictive pericarditis, which can have significant consequences on cardiac function and overall health. A multidisciplinary approach, involving rheumatologists, cardiologists, and other relevant specialists, may be necessary to optimize the management of these challenging cases. The potential side effects of Anakinra, as reported by various sources, include:

1. Injection Site Reactions: The most common side effects are related to the site of injection, including redness, itching, rash, pain, bleeding, blistering, burning, coldness, discoloration of the skin, feeling of pressure, hives, infection, inflammation, lumps, numbness, pain, rash, redness, scarring, soreness, stinging, swelling, tenderness, tingling, ulceration, or warmth.
2. Serious Infections: Anakinra may lower the body's ability to fight infections, leading to serious infections such as skin/bone/joint infections and pneumonia. Symptoms of infection include sore throat that doesn't go away, fever/chills, cough with mucus, and spreading redness/swelling/tenderness of the skin.
3. Allergic Reactions: Serious allergic reactions, including anaphylaxis or angioedema, which can be life-threatening and require immediate medical attention. Symptoms include rash, itching/swelling (especially of the face/tongue/throat), severe dizziness, and trouble breathing.
4. Blood Cell Count Changes: Anakinra may lower the number of some types of blood cells in the body, increasing the risk of infections.
5. Elevated Cardiac Enzymes: In patients with end-stage renal disease (ESRD), cardiac enzymes can be elevated, suggesting myocardial damage.
6. Adverse Pregnancy Outcomes: While the available data from anakinra-exposed pregnancies have not identified a clear association with miscarriage or adverse maternal or fetal outcomes, the risk cannot be definitively established or excluded.

Vecchiè A et al. Recurrent pericarditis: an update on diagnosis and management. Panminerva Med. 2021 Sep;63(3):261-269.PMID 33618510.

Correia ETO et al. Anakinra in Recurrent Pericarditis: Current Evidence on Clinical Use, Effectiveness, and Safety. J Cardiovasc Pharmacol. 2020 Jul;76(1):42-49 PMID: 32265370.

Case Note

The top five advantages of anakinra: effectiveness in stubborn cases, fast action, reduced chance of recurrence, easy steroid withdrawal, and improved side effect profile compared to standard treatment. Considering the evidence provided, physicians should consider trying anakinra if conventional treatments with NSAIDs, colchicine, and steroids are ineffective or if the patient experiences recurrent pericarditis.

2.5 Post-Radiation Lung Cancer Patient with Dyspnea

Case 24

A 68-year-old male with a history of non-small cell lung cancer treated with mediastinal radiation therapy 8 months ago presents with dyspnea on exertion and orthopnea. He denies chest pain. On physical examination, his blood pressure is 110/70 mmHg, heart rate is 110 beats per minute, and jugular venous pressure is elevated. A pericardial knock is heard, and there is a paradoxical pulse. An echocardiogram shows a large pericardial effusion with evidence of right atrial and ventricular diastolic collapse consistent with cardiac tamponade. Which of the following is the most appropriate next step in the management of this patient?

- A. Immediate pericardiocentesis to relieve cardiac tamponade.
- B. Initiation of nonsteroidal anti-inflammatory drugs (NSAIDs) for presumed radiation pericarditis.
- C. Pericardial window procedure to provide continuous drainage of the effusion.
- D. Systemic chemotherapy for suspected recurrence of lung cancer.

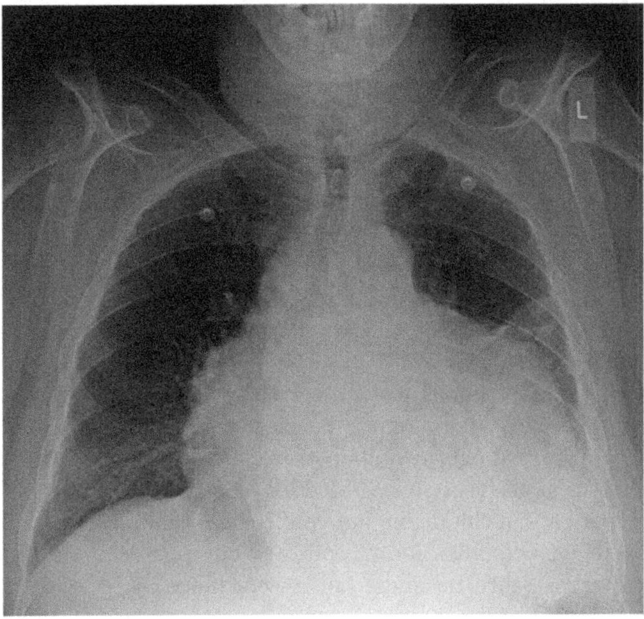

Figure 2.3: A 68-year-old

The correct answer is A. Immediate pericardiocentesis to relieve cardiac tamponade. The patient presents with signs and symptoms of cardiac tamponade, which is a life-threatening condition requiring urgent intervention. The echocardiographic findings of right atrial and ventricular collapse during diastole are diagnostic of tamponade physiology. Immediate pericardiocentesis is indicated to relieve the pressure on the heart and restore normal hemodynamics. Option B is incorrect because, although the patient has a history of mediastinal radiation, the presence of cardiac tamponade is an acute emergency and NSAIDs will not provide the immediate relief needed. Option C, a pericardial window, is a surgical intervention that may be considered for recurrent effusions or as a longer-term solution but is not the first-line treatment in an emergency setting of cardiac tamponade. Option D is incorrect because, while the patient has a history of lung cancer, the immediate life-threatening issue is cardiac tamponade. While systemic chemotherapy may be a consideration for cancer treatment, it does not address the acute cardiac emergency. Pericardial effusions can be linked to pain in acute inflammatory situations or may be painless, especially with neoplastic or uremic effusion. Shortness of breath and cough are frequent symptoms, particularly in cases of cardiac tamponade. Cardiac tamponade is a serious condition that can be identified by the following symptoms: rapid heartbeat, low blood pressure, paradoxical pulse (a decline in systolic blood pressure of more than 10 mmHg during inspiration), elevated jugular venous pressure, muted heart sounds, and changes in electrocardiogram (ECG) readings. Additional symptoms may arise from the underlying condition causing the tamponade.

The outcome of cardiac tamponade depends on the underlying etiology. Extended idiopathic chronic pericardial effusions (lasting over 3 months) carry a 30–35% risk of progressing to cardiac tamponade.

A pericardial friction rub may be present despite the presence of large pericardial effusions. Cardiac tamponade typically presents with tachycardia, tachypnea, a narrow pulse pressure, and a relatively preserved systolic blood pressure.

Pulsus paradoxus, a hallmark sign of cardiac tamponade, is characterized by a decrease of more than 10 mmHg in systolic blood pressure during inspiration. When the pericardial effusion is significant, the right ventricle (RV) enlarges during inspiration, causing septal motion towards the left ventricular (LV) chamber. This reduces LV filling, leading to an accentuated drop in stroke volume and systemic blood pressure with inspiration, known as the paradoxical pulse.

Central venous pressure (CVP) is elevated in cardiac tamponade, and since the intrapericardial and intracardiac pressures are elevated at the beginning of diastole, there is no visible y descent in the hemodynamic tracings of the right atrium, right ventricle, or left ventricle. These tracings show that pericardial pressure hinders early ventricular filling. In contrast to constrictive pericarditis, the RV and LV fill mostly during early diastole (rapid y descent), with ventricles unable to fill completely until mid to late diastole. In tamponade, ventricular filling is hindered throughout diastole. The presence of edema or ascites is uncommon in cardiac tamponade; these signs typically indicate a more chronic condition.

Adler Yet al. Cardiac tamponade. Nat Rev Dis Primers. 2023 Jul 20;9(1):36. PMID: 37474539.

2.6 Post-Radiation Lymphoma Patient with Progressive Dyspnea

Case 24B

A 70-year-old male with a history of radiation therapy for Hodgkin's lymphoma 15 years ago presents with progressive dyspnea on exertion, peripheral edema, and abdominal distension over the past 6 months. Physical examination reveals elevated jugular venous pressure with a prominent y-descent, Kussmaul's sign, and pericardial knock. There is no pulsus paradoxus. A chest radiograph shows normal heart size without pericardial calcification. An echocardiogram demonstrates normal systolic function, septal bounce, and respiration-related septal shift with an inspiratory reduction in mitral inflow Doppler pattern of greater than 25%. Cardiac MRI shows no pericardial thickening but confirms septal bounce and ventricular interdependence. Right heart catheterization reveals equalization of end-diastolic pressures in all four chambers, a dip-and-plateau pattern on ventricular pressure tracings, and discordance of RV and LV systolic pressures with inspiration.
Which of the following is the most appropriate next step in the management of this patient?

- A. Initiate treatment with diuretics and sodium restriction for symptomatic relief.
- B. Perform endomyocardial biopsy to differentiate from restrictive cardiomyopathy.
- C. Schedule pericardiectomy given the evidence of constrictive pericarditis.
- D. Start high-dose corticosteroids for presumed inflammatory pericardial disease.

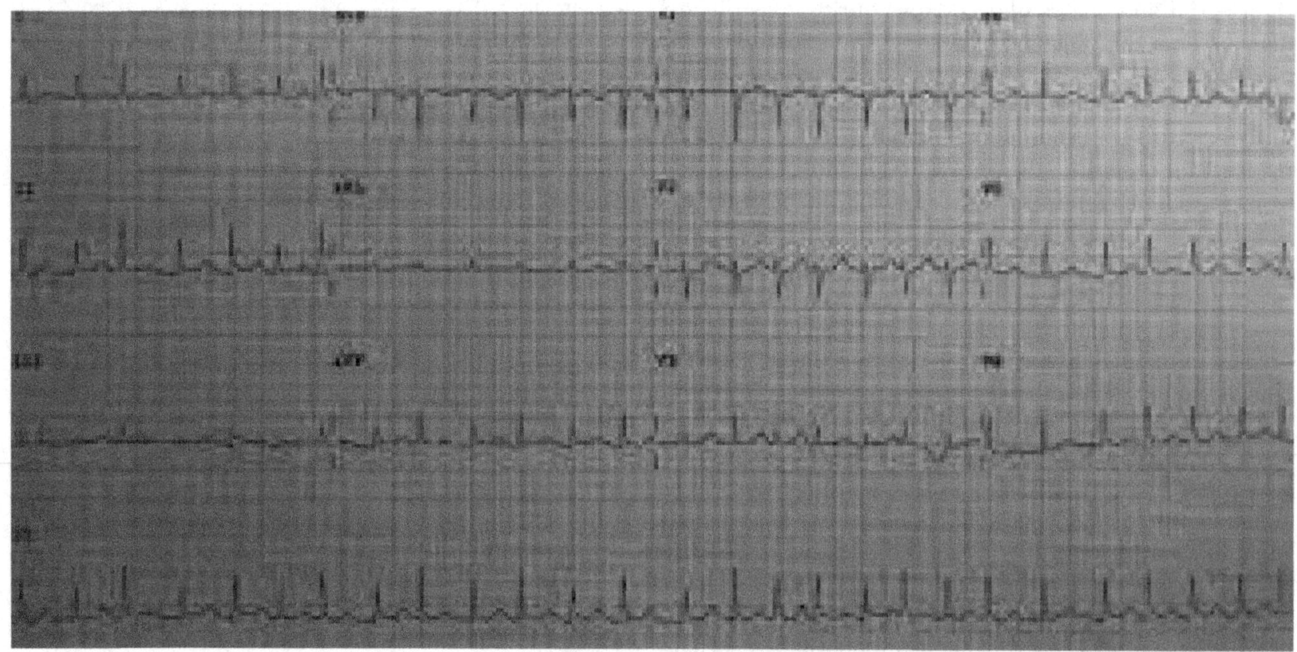

Figure 2.4: Electrical Alternans ECG

The correct answer is A. Immediate pericardiocentesis to relieve cardiac tamponade. The patient's clinical presentation and findings from echocardiography, cardiac MRI, and right heart catheterization are consistent with constrictive pericarditis. The history of radiation therapy, the presence of a septal bounce, ventricular interdependence, equalization of end-diastolic pressures, and discordance of RV and LV systolic pressures with inspiration are all supportive of this diagnosis. Pericardiectomy is the definitive treatment for constrictive pericarditis and can lead to symptomatic improvement and normalization of hemodynamics. Option A is incorrect because while diuretics and sodium restriction may provide symptomatic relief, they do not address the underlying pathophysiology of constrictive pericarditis and are not definitive treatments. Option B is incorrect because the clinical and hemodynamic findings are consistent with constrictive pericarditis rather than restrictive cardiomyopathy, making an endomyocardial biopsy unnecessary in this context. Option D is incorrect because there is no evidence of active inflammation that would respond to corticosteroids, and the patient's history and findings are not suggestive of an inflammatory pericardial disease but rather post-radiation constrictive pericarditis. A chest X-ray can indicate chronic pericardial effusion by showing an enlarged cardiac silhouette with a globular shape, but it might appear normal in acute cases. On an electrocardiogram (ECG), there are usually nonspecific T-wave changes and decreased QRS voltage. Electrical alternans, which is considered pathognomonic for pericardial effusion, is only occasionally present and is thought to be due to the heart swinging within the large effusion. Echocardiography is the primary diagnostic tool for demonstrating pericardial effusion and is highly sensitive. If cardiac tamponade is present, the high intrapericardial pressure can compress low-pressure cardiac structures like the right atrium (RA) and right ventricle (RV). Cardiac computed tomography (CT) and magnetic resonance imaging (MRI) can show pericardial fluid, pericardial thickening, and any related lesions in the chest. Diagnostic pericardiocentesis or pericardial biopsy may be necessary for microbiologic and cytologic studies. A pericardial biopsy can be performed through a small subxiphoid incision or using a video-assisted thoracoscopic surgical procedure. Unfortunately, the quality of the pericardial fluid itself rarely leads to a definitive diagnosis, and any type of fluid (serous, serosanguinous, bloody, etc.) can be seen in most pericardial diseases. Pericardial fluid analysis is most helpful in ruling out a bacterial cause and can sometimes provide insights into malignancies. Effusions caused by hypothyroidism or lymphatic obstruction may contain cholesterol or be chylous in nature, respectively.

In the evaluation of suspected cardiac tamponade, observing the jugular venous pressure (JVP) and testing for the presence of a paradoxical pulse are important. A common cause of a paradoxical pulse is severe pulmonary disease, particularly asthma, due to significant changes in intrapleural pressures during breathing. Serial echocardiograms are recommended if no immediate intervention is planned.

In the management of cardiac tamponade, vasodilators and diuretics should be avoided. If tamponade is present, immediate pericardiocentesis or cardiac surgery is necessary. Due to the curvilinear and upsloping pressure-volume relationship in the pericardial fluid, removing a small amount of fluid can lead to a significant drop in intrapericardial pressure and immediate hemodynamic improvement. However, complete drainage with a catheter is recommended. Additional drainage may be necessary, particularly in cases of malignant effusions.

Pericardial windows created through video-assisted thoracoscopy have shown great success in preventing recurrences, even when the initial cause of the effusion remains. They have proven to be more effective than other methods such as needle pericardiocentesis, subxiphoid surgical windows, or percutaneous balloon pericardiotomy. Effusions related to recurrent inflammatory pericarditis can be managed as described in the section on acute inflammatory pericarditis. The presence of pericardial fluid in individuals with pulmonary hypertension indicates a poor prognosis.

Study	Description
CXR	May suggest chronic effusion by an enlarged cardiac silhouette; normal in acute situations
ECG	Nonspecific T wave changes, reduced QRS voltage, electrical alternans occasionally
Echocardiography	Primary method for demonstrating pericardial effusion; sensitive
Cardiac CT and MRI	Show pericardial fluid, thickening, and contiguous lesions
Pericardiocentesis/Biopsy	For microbiologic and cytologic studies; fluid analysis most useful in excluding bacterial causes and occasionally helpful in malignancies
Fluid Analysis	May contain cholesterol in hypothyroidism or be chylous in lymphatic obstruction

Table 2.4: Diagnostic Studies for Pericardial Effusion

2.7 Post-Radiation Breast Cancer Patient With Progressive Dyspnea

Case 25

A 60-year-old female with a history of radiation therapy for breast cancer presents with progressive dyspnea on exertion and peripheral edema. Physical examination reveals elevated jugular venous pressure with a prominent y-descent, Kussmaul's sign, and bilateral pitting edema. The chest radiograph shows normal heart size without pericardial calcification. An echocardiogram demonstrates normal systolic function, septal bounce, and respiratory variation in mitral inflow velocities greater than 25%. Cardiac MRI shows no pericardial thickening but confirms septal bounce and ventricular interdependence. The patient undergoes cardiac catheterization, which reveals equalization of end-diastolic pressures in all four chambers, a dip-and-plateau pattern in ventricular pressure tracings, and discordance between RV and LV systolic pressures with inspiration. Based on the clinical scenario and diagnostic findings, what is the most likely diagnosis for this patient?

- A) Constrictive pericarditis
- B) Restrictive cardiomyopathy
- C) Pericardial effusion with impending tamponade
- D) Left ventricular aneurysm

Correct Answer: A) Constrictive pericarditis The patient's clinical presentation and diagnostic findings are consistent with constrictive pericarditis. The history of radiation therapy increases the risk of developing constrictive pericarditis. The physical examination findings of elevated jugular venous pressure with a prominent y-descent, Kussmaul's sign, and peripheral edema are suggestive of impaired right-sided heart function due to a non-compliant pericardium. The echocardiographic findings of a septal bounce and significant respiratory variation in mitral inflow velocities are characteristic of constrictive pericarditis, indicating ventricular interdependence due to a rigid pericardium. Although the cardiac MRI did not show pericardial thickening, which can be absent in 20 to 25% of constrictive pericarditis cases, it confirmed the septal bounce and ventricular interdependence. The definitive diagnostic feature in this scenario is the cardiac catheterization, which shows equalization of end-diastolic pressures across all cardiac chambers, a dip-and-plateau pattern in ventricular pressure tracings (the "square-root" sign), and discordance between RV and LV systolic pressures with inspiration. These hemodynamic findings are pathognomonic for constrictive pericarditis and are not seen in restrictive cardiomyopathy, where there is concordance of RV and LV systolic pressures with inspiration. Option B, restrictive cardiomyopathy, is less likely given the discordance of RV and LV systolic pressures with inspiration and the presence of a

Kussmaul sign, which are not typical features of restrictive cardiomyopathy. Option C, pericardial effusion with impending tamponade, is not supported by the hemodynamic findings of equalization of end-diastolic pressures and the absence of echocardiographic evidence of a significant effusion. Option D, left ventricular aneurysm, is not consistent with the patient's hemodynamic profile or imaging findings, and the absence of pericardial calcification at the LV apex on the chest radiograph makes this diagnosis unlikely. In conclusion, the most likely diagnosis for this patient, given the history, physical examination, and combination of noninvasive and invasive diagnostic findings, is constrictive pericarditis (option A). The major symptoms of constrictive pericarditis are fatigue and lack of energy. Chronic swelling, liver congestion, and fluid buildup are typically observed. Ascites frequently appears disproportionate to the amount of swelling in the limbs. During the physical examination, these signs are revealed along with a characteristically elevated jugular venous pressure (JVP) and a rapid y descent. This can be identified at the bedside by closely observing the jugular pulse and noticing a noticeable increase in the pulse wave at the end of ventricular systole (caused by the accentuation of the v wave during the rapid y descent). The Kussmaul sign, which is the failure of the JVP to decrease with inspiration, is also a common finding. The apex may retract during systole, and a pericardial sound may be heard in early diastole. Pulsus paradoxus is uncommon. Atrial fibrillation is a prevalent condition.

Echocardiography rarely shows a thickened pericardium in constrictive pericarditis. However, it is quite common to observe a rapid early filling and a septal "bounce". Right ventricular (RV) and left ventricular (LV) interaction can be demonstrated by an inspiratory maneuver, which typically shows a decrease in the mitral inflow Doppler pattern by more than 25%, similar to cardiac tamponade. The initial mitral inflow into the left ventricle is usually very rapid, which is also evident in the Doppler inflow (E wave) pattern. Additional echocardiographic characteristics, such as the ratio of the medial and lateral mitral annular motion (e' velocity), respiration-related septal shift, and hepatic vein expiratory diastolic reversal ratio, indicate constrictive physiology.

Cardiac computed tomography (CT) and magnetic resonance imaging (MRI) tests are only occasionally beneficial in the diagnosis of constrictive pericarditis. To establish the diagnosis, there must be pericardial thickening of more than 4 mm, although this is not demonstrable in 20–25% of patients with constrictive pericarditis. Some MRI techniques can show the septal bounce and provide additional evidence of ventricular interaction.

Anasari-Gilani K et al. Multimodality approach to the diagnosis and management of constrictive pericarditis. Echocardiography. 2020;30:632. [PMID: 32240548]

Case Note

The diagnostic process for constrictive pericarditis involves a careful integration of clinical findings, echocardiographic features, and, in some cases, advanced imaging modalities like CT and MRI. Early recognition and appropriate management are crucial, as constrictive pericarditis can have significant hemodynamic consequences if left untreated.

2.8 Management of Refractory Constrictive Pericarditis

Case 26

A 68-year-old male with a history of chronic renal insufficiency and a remote history of tuberculosis presents with fatigue, abdominal swelling, and lower extremity edema. He denies chest pain or recent infections. Physical examination reveals elevated jugular venous pressure, Kussmaul's sign, and ascites. Laboratory tests show a serum sodium level of 130 mEq/L, creatinine of 2.5 mg/dL, and normal liver enzymes. An echocardiogram demonstrates normal left ventricular systolic function, thickened pericardium, and septal bounce. Cardiac catheterization confirms the diagnosis of constrictive pericarditis with equalization of end-diastolic pressures and a dip-and-plateau pattern in ventricular pressure tracings. Despite aggressive diuretic therapy with intravenous furosemide, the patient's symptoms and edema persist.
What is the most appropriate next step in the management of this patient's constrictive pericarditis?

- A) Increase the dose of intravenous furosemide.
- B) Initiate anti-tuberculosis therapy.
- C) Refer for surgical pericardiectomy.
- D) Start an aldosterone antagonist.

Correct Answer: C) Refer for surgical pericardiectomy. This patient with constrictive pericarditis has evidence of right heart failure, as indicated by elevated jugular venous pressure, Kussmaul's sign, ascites, and peripheral edema. The history of tuberculosis suggests a possible etiology for his constrictive pericarditis. However, there is no mention of active tuberculosis or ongoing inflammation, and the patient's symptoms are primarily hemodynamic rather than inflammatory. Therefore, anti-tuberculosis therapy (option B) would not be indicated unless there was evidence of active disease. The patient has not responded to aggressive diuretic therapy, as evidenced by persistent symptoms and edema despite the use of intravenous furosemide. Increasing the dose of intravenous furosemide (option A) is unlikely to be beneficial at this point, given the refractory nature of his fluid overload. While adding an aldosterone antagonist (option D) could be considered in the management of right heart failure, especially in the presence of ascites and liver congestion, this patient's renal insufficiency and hyponatremia increase the risk of hyperkalemia and worsening renal function with the use of such agents. Given the patient's refractory symptoms and the confirmation of constrictive pericarditis by cardiac catheterization, the most appropriate next step is to refer for surgical pericardiectomy (option C). This procedure is indicated when medical therapy fails to control symptoms. Although the patient has several poor prognostic factors, including renal insufficiency and a history of tuberculosis, the persistence of symptoms despite optimal medical therapy suggests that surgical intervention is necessary to improve his quality of life. Cardiac catheterization is commonly utilized to confirm or establish a diagnosis in complex cases where echocardiographic findings are inconclusive or diverse. Generally, pulmonary pressure is lower in cases of constriction compared to restrictive cardiomyopathy. When managing constrictive pericarditis, it is crucial to incorporate simultaneous measurement of both left ventricular (LV) and right ventricular (RV) pressure tracings during cardiac catheterization to demonstrate the interaction between RV and LV with inspiration and expiration. This dynamic can be visualized using cardiac MRI. Hemodynamically, patients with constriction typically exhibit equalization of end-diastolic pressures across cardiac chambers, experience rapid early filling followed by a sudden rise in diastolic pressure (resembling a "square-root" sign), have RV end-diastolic pressure exceeding one-third of systolic pressure, demonstrate discordant RV and LV systolic pressure measurements during inspiration (RV increases while LV decreases), and often present with a Kussmaul sign (right atrial pressure fails to decrease with inspiration). In contrast, restrictive cardiomyopathy shows alignment of RV and LV systolic pressures with inspiration.

Pericardiectomy carries significant morbidity and mortality risks, especially in patients with substantial comorbidities; however, it can offer remarkable relief from symptoms.The decision to proceed with surgery should involve a multidisciplinary team comprising cardiologists, cardiothoracic surgeons, and potentially infectious disease specialists, considering the patient's tuberculosis history. In conclusion, the most appropriate next step for this patient with refractory symptoms of constrictive pericarditis is to refer for surgical pericardiectomy (option C), as it offers the best chance for symptomatic improvement when medical therapy has failed.

Goldstein JA et al. Hemodynamics of constrictive pericarditis and restrictive cardiomyopathy. Catheter Cardiovasc Interv. 2020;95:1240. [PMID: 31904891]

2.9 Post-COVID-19 Chest Pain: Decoding a Diagnostic Dilemma

Case 27

A 42-year-old male with no significant past medical history presents to the emergency department with chest pain and shortness of breath. He tested positive for COVID-19 two weeks ago and has been experiencing a low-grade fever and fatigue since then. His temperature is 37.8C, blood pressure is 130/85 mmHg, heart rate is 110 beats per minute, and respiratory rate is 20 breaths per minute. Physical examination reveals a pericardial friction rub. Laboratory tests show elevated troponin I levels, and an ECG demonstrates diffuse ST elevations. Echocardiography reveals global hypokinesis with a left ventricular ejection fraction of 45%. There is no evidence of pericardial effusion. The patient is hemodynamically stable.
Which of the following is the most appropriate next step in the management of this patient?

- A) Initiate high-dose aspirin and colchicine for presumed pericarditis.
- B) Begin intravenous immunoglobulin (IVIG) and corticosteroids for suspected myopericarditis.
- C) Perform an endomyocardial biopsy to confirm the diagnosis of myocarditis.
- D) Start empiric broad-spectrum antibiotics and admit to the hospital for suspected bacterial endocarditis.

Correct Answer: B) Begin intravenous immunoglobulin (IVIG) and corticosteroids for suspected myopericarditis. The patient presents with signs and symptoms suggestive of myopericarditis, which is an inflammatory condition of the myocardium and pericardium. The recent history of COVID-19, the presence of a pericardial friction rub, elevated cardiac enzymes, and diffuse ST elevations on ECG are consistent with this diagnosis. The echocardiographic findings of global hypokinesis and reduced ejection fraction further support the presence of myocardial involvement. In the context of COVID-19, myopericarditis is thought to be mediated by direct viral injury to cardiomyocytes and an excessive immune response, leading to inflammation and cardiac injury. The management of myopericarditis in COVID-19 patients includes supportive care and may involve the use of immunomodulatory therapies such as IVIG and corticosteroids (B). These treatments aim to reduce the immune response and inflammation associated with the condition. High-dose aspirin and colchicine (A) are typically used in the treatment of acute pericarditis. While they may be beneficial in cases of pericarditis without significant myocardial involvement, the presence of myocarditis with cardiac dysfunction in this patient suggests that a more aggressive anti-inflammatory approach is warranted. An endomyocardial biopsy (C) is the gold standard for the diagnosis of myocarditis. However, it is an invasive procedure and is not typically performed as an initial step in the management, especially when the clinical presentation is strongly suggestive of myopericarditis and the patient is hemodynamically stable. Empiric broad-spectrum antibiotics (D) would be indicated if there was a high suspicion of bacterial endocarditis. However, the clinical scenario does not provide evidence of bacterial infection, and the recent history of COVID-19 makes myopericarditis a more likely diagnosis. In summary, the most appropriate next step in the management of this patient with suspected myopericarditis secondary to COVID-19 is to begin treatment with IVIG and corticosteroids to modulate the immune response and reduce inflammation. This approach addresses the underlying pathophysiology of the condition and can improve outcomes in patients with COVID-19–associated cardiac involvement. Primary myocarditis typically arises from either an acute viral infection or a subsequent immune response, while secondary myocarditis is a result of inflammation triggered by nonviral pathogens, medications, chemicals, physical agents, hypersensitivity reactions, or inflammatory conditions such as systemic lupus erythematosus (SLE).

During the COVID-19 pandemic, myopericarditis caused by the coronavirus has emerged as a significant concern. Managing this condition parallels the approach to myocarditis. There is speculation that the spike protein of SARS-CoV-2 may bind to the ACE-2 membrane receptor on cardiomyocytes, leading to direct cellular injury and T-lymphocyte-mediated cytotoxicity, potentially exacerbated by a cytokine storm, T-cell activation, and subsequent cytokine release.

The diagnosis of myocarditis relies on biopsies and involves the observation of a specific quantity of lymphocytes and monocytes, along with CD3-positive T lymphocytes. The nature of injury can be sudden, insidious, or prolonged. Both cellular and humoral inflammatory processes contribute to the progression of chronic injury, with certain subgroups potentially benefiting from immunosuppression. In some cases, genetic predisposition may influence the development of myocarditis. Autoimmune myocarditis, such as giant cell myocarditis, can manifest without an identifiable viral infection. The diverse clinical presentations and the incomplete understanding of immunopathology make it challenging to fully comprehend the underlying mechanisms. Myocarditis can manifest following SARS-CoV-2 infection or occasionally post-vaccination. In both scenarios, younger male individuals appear to face a higher risk of this rare occurrence. Regarding vaccination-related myocarditis, the CDC reports incidence rates ranging from 5 to 97 cases per million individuals aged 18 to 45 years, with indications that rates may be higher following the Moderna vaccine compared to the Pfizer-BioNTech vaccine.

Sayegh MN et al. Presentations, Diagnosis, and Treatment of Post-COVID Viral Myocarditis in the Inpatient Setting: A Narrative Review. Cureus. 2023 May 22;15(5):e39338 PMID: 37378093

2.10 Progressive Cardiac Symptoms Following a Flu-like Illness

Case 28

A 28-year-old female presents to the emergency department with a 1-week history of progressive shortness of breath, fatigue, and a recent onset of palpitations. She reports a flu-like illness 2 weeks prior. On examination, she is tachycardic with a heart rate of 120 beats per minute, blood pressure is 100/70 mmHg, and she has a low-grade fever of 37.8C (100F). Cardiac auscultation reveals a soft S1 and S3 gallop without murmurs. Lung fields are clear. Laboratory tests show an elevated white blood cell count, increased erythrocyte sedimentation rate (ESR), and C-reactive protein (CRP). Troponin T levels are elevated, and B-type natriuretic peptide (BNP) is significantly increased. An echocardiogram shows global hypokinesis with a left ventricular ejection fraction of 35%. Cardiac MRI with gadolinium enhancement reveals spotty areas of myocardial injury consistent with myocarditis. The patient is hemodynamically stable but continues to have symptomatic palpitations and chest discomfort despite optimal medical therapy including beta-blockers and ACE inhibitors. Which of the following is the most appropriate next step in the management of this patient?

- A. Initiate high-dose corticosteroids for presumed autoimmune myocarditis.
- B. Perform coronary angiography to exclude ischemic heart disease.
- C. Obtain an endomyocardial biopsy to confirm the diagnosis of myocarditis.
- D. Start empirical antiviral therapy targeting the most likely viral etiology.

The correct answer is C. Obtain an endomyocardial biopsy to confirm the diagnosis of myocarditis. According to the AHA/ACC/ESC class I recommendations, an endomyocardial biopsy is indicated in patients with heart failure symptoms, a normal-sized or dilated left ventricle (LV), and hemodynamic compromise that occurs less than 2 weeks after the onset of symptoms, or in patients with a dilated LV 2 weeks to 3 months after the onset of symptoms who have new ventricular arrhythmias, AV nodal block, or who do not respond to usual care after 1–2 weeks. In this case, the patient has heart failure symptoms with a reduced ejection fraction and persistent arrhythmias despite medical therapy, making her a candidate for an endomyocardial biopsy to confirm the diagnosis and potentially guide specific treatment. Option A is incorrect because high-dose corticosteroids for presumed autoimmune myocarditis should not be initiated without histologic confirmation of the diagnosis due to potential side effects and the possibility of worsening certain viral myocarditis. Option B is incorrect because the patient's presentation is more consistent with myocarditis rather than ischemic heart disease, and the cardiac MRI findings support this diagnosis. Coronary angiography is not indicated unless there is a high suspicion of concomitant coronary artery disease, which is less likely given the patient's age, gender, and clinical presentation. Option D is incorrect because empirical antiviral therapy is not typically recommended without specific evidence of a viral etiology. Moreover, the efficacy of antiviral therapy in myocarditis is uncertain and not part of standard care. Confirmation of myocarditis often relies on histologic evidence. Guidelines suggest considering a biopsy in specific heart failure and ventricular scenarios, although these recommendations may lack robust support and should be contemplated following imaging modalities like MRI, particularly when a potentially treatable cause is suspected. In cases where inflammation is detected without viral genomes via PCR, immunosuppression might offer benefits.

Given the sporadic nature of cardiac involvement, the diagnosis may be overlooked in up to half of cases, even with a biopsy. Laboratory findings lack consistency, but typically reveal elevated white blood cell (WBC) counts, along with increased erythrocyte sedimentation rate (ESR) and C-reactive protein (CRP) levels. Troponin I or T levels are elevated in around one-third of patients, while creatine kinase-MB (CK-MB) elevation is observed in only 10%. Additional biomarkers like B-type natriuretic peptide (BNP) and N-terminal pro-BNP are commonly elevated. Echocardiography serves as a convenient tool for evaluating cardiac function and excluding other conditions. An MRI with gadolinium enhancement highlights scattered areas of myocardial damage.

Ammirati E et al. Diagnosis and Treatment of Acute Myocarditis: A Review. JAMA. 2023 Apr 4;329(13):1098-1113. PMID: 37014337

2.11 Sudden Cardiac Distress In An Athlete

Case 29

A 32-year-old male professional athlete presents to the emergency department with acute onset of severe dyspnea, chest pain, and palpitations after a high-intensity training session. He has no significant past medical history but reports a mild upper respiratory tract infection 2 weeks ago. On examination, he is diaphoretic, with a blood pressure of 85/50 mmHg, heart rate of 130 beats per minute, and oxygen saturation of 88% on room air. Physical examination reveals jugular venous distension, muffled heart sounds, and no significant murmurs. There is no peripheral edema. An ECG shows sinus tachycardia with diffuse ST elevations. Troponin I levels are markedly elevated. Echocardiography demonstrates a left ventricular ejection fraction (LVEF) of 30%, with no ventricular dilatation but with global hypokinesis and normal valvular function. The patient rapidly deteriorates into cardiogenic shock.
Which of the following is the most appropriate next step in the management of this patient?

- A. Initiate high-dose intravenous corticosteroids and intravenous immunoglobulin (IVIG).
- B. Begin treatment with nonsteroidal anti-inflammatory drugs (NSAIDs) and colchicine for myopericarditis.
- C. Start empirical antiviral therapy with pleconaril for suspected enteroviral myocarditis.
- D. Provide aggressive short-term support with an intra-aortic balloon pump (IABP) or left ventricular assist device (LVAD), and consider extracorporeal membrane oxygenation (ECMO) if severe pulmonary infiltrates are present.

The correct answer is D. Provide aggressive short-term support with an intra-aortic balloon pump (IABP) or left ventricular assist device (LVAD), and consider extracorporeal membrane oxygenation (ECMO) if severe pulmonary infiltrates are present. The patient is presenting with signs of fulminant myocarditis, which is characterized by acute onset of severe cardiac dysfunction leading to cardiogenic shock, often without significant ventricular dilatation. In such cases, aggressive hemodynamic support is critical to maintain end-organ perfusion and allow time for the myocardium to recover. Mechanical circulatory support devices like IABP or LVAD can provide this support, and ECMO may be necessary if there is associated severe respiratory failure. Option A is incorrect because, while corticosteroids and IVIG are used in some cases of myocarditis, controlled trials have not consistently shown benefit, and they are not the first-line treatment in the setting of cardiogenic shock due to fulminant myocarditis. Option B is incorrect because NSAIDs and colchicine are used for myopericarditis-related chest pain and pericarditis, respectively, but they are not appropriate in the acute management of fulminant myocarditis with hemodynamic compromise. Option C is incorrect because empirical antiviral therapy is not indicated without a confirmed viral etiology, and there is no evidence to support the routine use of pleconaril or other antivirals in the setting of fulminant myocarditis. Individuals with severe myocarditis may exhibit symptoms of sudden heart failure. Acute myocarditis is considered a potential cause of sudden death in 5 to 20% of cases in athletes under 35 years old. The ventricles are typically not enlarged but thickened (potentially due to myxedema). The diagnosis of myocarditis involves assessing symptoms, elevated biomarkers such as troponins, ST segment changes on electrocardiogram, and abnormalities in echocardiographic wall motion or thickness. A definitive diagnosis typically requires cardiac MRI or biopsy. Treatment strategies vary depending on the urgency, severity, symptom presentation, and underlying cause of the condition. Approximately 75% of hospitalized myocarditis patients follow a straightforward course with a relatively low mortality rate. Conversely, acute myocarditis complicated by acute heart failure or ventricular arrhythmias carries a 12% risk of in-hospital mortality or necessitating a heart transplant. Between 2% to 9% of patients may experience hemodynamic instability, requiring inotropic agents or mechanical circulatory support like extracorporeal life support to aid recovery, with a 28% mortality or heart transplant rate at 60 days. Treatment primarily addresses the clinical scenario, utilizing ACE inhibitors and beta blockers if left ventricular ejection fraction (LVEF) is below 40%. Nonsteroidal anti-inflammatory drugs (NSAIDs) are recommended for myopericarditis-related chest pain, while colchicine may be considered for predominant pericarditis. Supportive care is typically employed for COVID-19-related myocardial inflammation. Among various therapies studied in a 2020 review, corticosteroids were associated with improved outcomes compared to other treatments like remdesivir, glucocorticoids, IL-6 inhibitors (e.g., tocilizumab), intravenous immunoglobulin (IVIG), and colchicine. In cases where a specific infecting agent is identified, antimicrobial therapy is essential. Exercise restriction during recovery is advised, with caution recommended regarding the use of digoxin due to limited efficacy. Studies on immunosuppressive therapies like corticosteroids and IVIG have not shown significant benefits universally; however, some experts suggest IVIG administration at a dose of 2 g/kg over 24 hours in confirmed cases. Preliminary trials suggest a potential supportive role for interferon and empirical testing of antiviral medications like pleconaril for enteroviruses. Determining the optimal duration of treatment cessation upon patient improvement remains an area requiring further research. Severe cases of myocarditis may necessitate intensive short-term support such as an intra-aortic balloon pump (IABP) or left ventricular assist device (LVAD). In instances where fulminant myocarditis coexists with severe lung infiltrates, temporary extracorporeal membrane oxygenation (ECMO) support may be crucial and has demonstrated significant efficacy.

Tschöpe C et al Nat Rev Cardiol. 2021 Mar;18(3):169-193. PMID: 33046850

Table 2.5: Noninfectious Myocarditis Summary

Risk Factor	Description
Medications/Drugs	Phenothiazines, lithium, chloroquine, etc. cause ECG changes, arrhythmias, or HF. Cocaine may cause coronary artery spasm, MI, arrhythmias, and myocarditis.
Radiation	Can cause acute inflammatory reaction and chronic fibrosis of heart muscle, usually with pericarditis.
Systemic Disorders	Giant cell myocarditis, eosinophilic myocarditis, celiac disease, etc. are associated with myocarditis.
Cancer Chemotherapy Agents	Anthracyclines may result in cardiotoxicity and heart failure.
HIV	Indirectly responsible for HIV cardiomyopathy, with other factors often implicated.
Precautions	Avoid NSAIDs, alcohol, and strenuous physical exercise. Monitor for early signs of cardiotoxicity.

3 CORONARY HEART DISEASE

3.1 Management of Dyslipidemia in Coronary Heart Disease (CHD)

Case 30

A 63-year-old male with a history of hypertension and smoking presents to the clinic for a follow-up after being discharged from the hospital for an acute myocardial infarction (MI) one month ago. He has been adherent to his medications, which include aspirin, a beta-blocker, and a high-intensity statin. His current LDL cholesterol level is 85 mg/dL. He has no history of diabetes or peripheral artery disease. He reports that he quit smoking immediately after his MI. His blood pressure today is 132/84 mmHg. He inquires about additional strategies to further reduce his risk of another coronary event.
Which of the following is the most appropriate next step in the management of this patient's dyslipidemia?

- A) Increase the dose of the current statin to achieve an LDL cholesterol level below 70 mg/dL.
- B) Add ezetimibe to the current statin therapy to achieve an LDL cholesterol level below 70 mg/dL.
- C) Initiate PCSK9 inhibitor therapy in addition to the current statin to achieve an LDL cholesterol level below 70 mg/dL.
- D) Continue current management as the LDL cholesterol level is already below 100 mg/dL.

Correct Answer: B) Add ezetimibe to the current statin therapy to achieve an LDL cholesterol level below 70 mg/dL. The patient has a history of acute myocardial infarction and is currently on high-intensity statin therapy with an LDL cholesterol level of 85 mg/dL. According to current guidelines, for patients with a history of cardiovascular events (secondary prevention), it is recommended to aim for an LDL cholesterol level below 70 mg/dL to further reduce the risk of recurrent coronary events. Increasing the dose of the current statin (A) could be considered, but the patient is already on high-intensity statin therapy, and there may be diminishing returns in efficacy and an increased risk of side effects with higher doses of statins. Adding ezetimibe to the current statin therapy (B) is a well-established strategy to further lower LDL cholesterol levels. The IMPROVE-IT trial demonstrated that the addition of ezetimibe to statin therapy provided additional cardiovascular benefits compared to statin therapy alone in patients who had experienced an acute coronary syndrome. Initiating PCSK9 inhibitor therapy(C) in addition to the current statin could be an option, especially for patients who do not achieve LDL cholesterol goals with maximally tolerated statin and ezetimibe therapy or for those who are statin intolerant. However, PCSK9 inhibitors are expensive and are typically not first-line agents for further LDL reduction after high-intensity statin therapy. Continuing current management (D) without further intervention may not be the best option for this patient, as the LDL cholesterol level is above the recommended target for secondary prevention, and there is evidence that further reduction can provide additional cardiovascular benefits. In summary, the most appropriate next step in the management of this patient's dyslipidemia is to add ezetimibe to the current statin therapy to achieve an LDL cholesterol level below 70 mg/dL . This approach is supported by evidence from clinical trials and is consistent with current guidelines for secondary prevention in patients with a history of coronary heart disease. Modifying risk factors for coronary heart disease (CHD), such as smoking cessation, managing dyslipidemia, and reducing blood pressure, can help prevent and slow the progression of coronary artery disease. Lowering LDL cholesterol levels can decelerate the advancement of atherosclerosis and, in some cases, lead to regression. In individuals with clinical evidence of vascular disease, fewer new lesions develop, endothelial function may be restored, and the risk of coronary events is significantly reduced, even without regression. Numerous clinical trials have demonstrated the efficacy of statin medications in reducing mortality, coronary events, and strokes. Beneficial effects have been observed in individuals with a history of heart events (secondary prevention), those at high risk for events such as patients with diabetes and peripheral artery disease, those with high cholesterol but few other risk factors, and those without vascular disease or diabetes but with elevated high-sensitivity C-reactive protein (hsCRP) levels and normal LDL levels. The cholesterol treatment guidelines recommend the benefits of moderate- and high-dose statin therapy, as mentioned in the previous section on risk factors for coronary artery disease and hyperlipidemia. The IMPROVE-IT trial showed that adding 10 mg of ezetimibe daily to simvastatin provided a modest additional benefit in reducing the risk of heart attack and ischemic stroke, but not in reducing mortality, in patients who had experienced an acute coronary syndrome and were stable. Ezetimibe may be used in conjunction with statin therapy for individuals who have not achieved their target cholesterol level for secondary prevention or cannot tolerate high-dose statin therapy. The benefits of statins were observed regardless of age, race, baseline cholesterol levels, or hypertension status. Statins provide benefits for patients with vascular disease, including those with normal cholesterol levels. Furthermore, higher-dose statin therapy is associated with greater benefits. Patients at high risk for vascular events should be prescribed a statin, irrespective of their cholesterol levels. Experts recommend that individuals who have experienced cardiovascular events should aim to reduce their LDL cholesterol levels to below 70 mg/dL. Monoclonal antibodies that inhibit PCSK9 (proprotein convertase subtilisin/kexin type 9) can lower LDL cholesterol levels. A trial showed that adding the PCSK9 inhibitor evolocumab to statin therapy reduced atherothrombotic events by 20% without affecting mortality.

The ODYSSEY Outcomes trial demonstrated that alirocumab reduced cardiovascular events in patients with acute coronary syndromes. Alirocumab and evolocumab are approved by the FDA for patients with familial hypercholesterolemia and atherosclerotic vascular disease who are already on the highest tolerable dose of statins and require additional lowering of LDL cholesterol levels. Inclisiran, a short interfering RNA that targets the liver to decrease PCSK9 synthesis, is being studied as a biennial (every two years) injection. Research has shown a reduction in LDL levels, resulting in FDA approval in early 2022.

Byrne P et al. Evaluating the Association Between Low-Density Lipoprotein Cholesterol Reduction and Relative and Absolute Effects of Statin Treatment: A Systematic Review and Meta-analysis. JAMA Intern Med. 2022 May 1;182(5):474-481. PMID: 35285850

Case Note

According to current guidelines, for patients with a history of cardiovascular events (secondary prevention), it is recommended to aim for an LDL cholesterol level below 70 mg/dL to further reduce the risk of recurrent coronary events.

3.2 Management ofHypertriglyceridemia in Coronary Heart Disease (CHD)

Case 31

A 58-year-old female with a history of type 2 diabetes mellitus, hypertension, and stable ischemic heart disease is seen in the clinic for routine follow-up. Her current medications include metformin, lisinopril, and atorvastatin. Despite good adherence to her medication regimen and lifestyle modifications, her fasting lipid panel reveals an LDL cholesterol of 68 mg/dL, HDL cholesterol of 40 mg/dL, and triglycerides of 280 mg/dL. Her last HbA1c was 7.2%, and her blood pressure today is 135/85 mmHg.
Which of the following is the most appropriate addition to this patient's treatment regimen to reduce her cardiovascular risk?

- A) Initiate icosapent ethyl to target elevated triglycerides.
- B) Add extended-release niacin to increase HDL cholesterol.
- C) Prescribe fibrate therapy to specifically lower triglycerides.
- D) Increase the dose of atorvastatin to further lower LDL cholesterol.

Correct Answer: A) Initiate icosapent ethyl to target elevated triglycerides. The patient has stable ischemic heart disease, type 2 diabetes, and persistently elevated triglycerides despite being on statin therapy and making lifestyle modifications. The REDUCE-IT trial demonstrated that icosapent ethyl, a highly purified form of eicosapentaenoic acid (EPA), significantly reduced cardiovascular events in patients with elevated triglyceride levels who were already taking statins. Given the patient's elevated triglycerides and existing cardiovascular disease, adding icosapent ethyl to their treatment regimen would be an appropriate choice to further reduce their cardiovascular risk. Icosapent ethyl, a highly concentrated form of EPA administered at a high dose, showed positive effects in the REDUCE-IT trial. There was a notable 26% reduction in the risk of cardiovascular death, myocardial infarction (MI), and stroke, as well as a 20% decrease specifically in cardiovascular death. The FDA has approved icosapent ethyl to be used in combination with statin therapy to reduce the risk of heart attack, stroke, coronary revascularization procedures, or unstable angina in patients with elevated triglyceride levels and either established cardiovascular disease or diabetes with additional risk factors. While extended-release niacin has been used in the past to increase HDL cholesterol levels, recent studies such as AIM-HIGH and HPS2-THRIVE have shown that adding niacin to statin therapy did not reduce cardiovascular events and may cause harm, making it an inappropriate choice for this patient. The HPS2-THRIVE trial found that combining extended-release niacin (2 g) with laropiprant did not provide any benefits but instead caused significant harm in over 25,000 individuals with vascular disease who were already on simvastatin. Fibrate therapy can be effective in lowering triglycerides and is sometimes used in patients with very high triglyceride levels to reduce the risk of pancreatitis. However, fibrates have not consistently shown a benefit in reducing cardiovascular events when added to statin therapy, especially in patients with only moderately elevated triglyceride levels, as is the case here. Increasing the dose of atorvastatin may further lower LDL cholesterol, but the patient's LDL is already well-controlled at 68 mg/dL. The primary lipid abnormality that needs to be addressed is the elevated triglycerides. Moreover, there is no evidence that increasing statin dosage in this context would address the elevated triglycerides or result in additional cardiovascular risk reduction. Attempts to raise HDL levels have not been found to be advantageous.

The AIM-HIGH study found no benefit in adding niacin to individuals with vascular disease and an LDL level of 70 mg/dL who were already taking statin medication.

In summary, the most appropriate addition to this patient's treatment regimen to reduce their cardiovascular risk is to initiate icosapent ethyl. This recommendation is based on the patient's profile and the evidence from the REDUCE-IT trial, which showed a significant reduction in cardiovascular events with icosapent ethyl in patients with elevated triglycerides who were on statin therapy.

Xu J et al. Treatment of Hypertriglyceridemia: A Review of Therapies in the Pipeline. J Pharm Pract. 2023 Jun;36(3):650-661.PMID: 34720008

3.3 Antiplatelet Therapy in Chronic Coronary Artery Disease

Case 32

A 67-year-old male with a history of chronic stable coronary artery disease (CAD) presents to the clinic for a routine follow-up. He underwent percutaneous coronary intervention (PCI) with stent placement in his left anterior descending artery 2 years ago. He has been on dual antiplatelet therapy with aspirin 81 mg and clopidogrel 75 mg daily since the procedure. His other medical conditions include well-controlled hypertension and hyperlipidemia. He has no history of diabetes or smoking. His current medications include lisinopril, atorvastatin, and metoprolol. He has no history of bleeding disorders or gastrointestinal bleeding. His 10-year atherosclerotic cardiovascular disease (ASCVD) risk score is calculated at 12%.
Given the patient's history and current treatment regimen, which of the following is the most appropriate management of his antiplatelet therapy?

- A) Continue dual antiplatelet therapy with aspirin and clopidogrel indefinitely.
- B) Discontinue clopidogrel and maintain aspirin 81 mg daily for secondary prevention.
- C) Increase the dose of aspirin to 325 mg daily and continue clopidogrel.
- D) Discontinue both aspirin and clopidogrel and initiate monotherapy with a novel oral anticoagulant (NOAC).

Correct Answer: B) Discontinue clopidogrel and maintain aspirin 81 mg daily for secondary prevention. In patients with chronic stable CAD who are beyond the initial period following PCI with stent placement, the benefits of dual antiplatelet therapy (DAPT) need to be weighed against the increased risk of bleeding. The current guidelines recommend DAPT for a period of 6 to 12 months following PCI, depending on the type of stent placed and the patient's bleeding risk. Beyond this period, continuation of DAPT should be individualized based on the patient's risk of ischemic events versus the risk of bleeding. In this case, the patient is 2 years post-PCI and has been on DAPT since the procedure. Given that he has no history of bleeding and is well beyond the recommended duration for DAPT, it would be appropriate to discontinue clopidogrel and maintain aspirin 81 mg daily for secondary prevention (B). This is supported by the ADAPTABLE trial, which found that 81 mg of aspirin was as effective as 325 mg for reducing cardiovascular events and had a lower risk of bleeding. Increasing the dose of aspirin to 325 mg daily (C) is not supported by the evidence from the ADAPTABLE trial, which showed no additional benefit in terms of cardiovascular event reduction and a higher risk of bleeding with the higher dose of aspirin. Continuing DAPT indefinitely (A) is not recommended in this patient due to the increased risk of bleeding without a clear ongoing benefit in reducing ischemic events, especially as he is 2 years post-PCI and has stable CAD. Initiating monotherapy with a NOAC (D) is not indicated in this scenario as NOACs are not recommended for monotherapy in secondary prevention of CAD in patients without an indication for anticoagulation, such as atrial fibrillation or venous thromboembolism. In summary, the most appropriate management of this patient's antiplatelet therapy is to discontinue clopidogrel and maintain aspirin 81 mg daily for secondary prevention. This approach minimizes the patient's bleeding risk while continuing to provide protection against thrombotic events. The benefits of aspirin for primary prevention of cardiovascular events are modest, even for patients with diabetes, and it is not recommended for most people. In 2022, the U.S. Preventive Services Task Force (USPSTF) issued recommendations on the use of aspirin for primary prevention of cardiovascular events. Individuals aged 40 to 59 years with a 10-year atherosclerotic cardiovascular disease (ASCVD) risk of 10% or more should weigh the potential benefits and harms of initiating aspirin therapy for primary prevention. The statement also recommends that individuals aged 60 years and older should not start taking aspirin for primary prevention of cardiovascular disease.

The use of antiplatelet therapy is highly effective for preventing further complications, and individuals with established cardiovascular disease should be prescribed aspirin. A study was conducted to assess the effects of different doses of aspirin in patients with chronic coronary artery disease (CAD), specifically comparing 81 mg versus 325 mg, within a large pragmatic trial known as ADAPTABLE. The unique clinical trial design showed that a daily dose of 81 mg of aspirin had a more favorable effect on the risk of cardiovascular events and bleeding compared to a daily dose of 325 mg.

Clopidogrel was beneficial in preventing vascular events for 9–12 months after acute coronary syndromes (ACS) and showed benefits in extending dual antiplatelet therapy following coronary stenting. However, in the CHARISMA study, clopidogrel in combination with aspirin did not provide additional long-term benefits. The study included individuals with stable atherothrombosis or multiple risk factors, all of whom received aspirin therapy and were followed for a median of 28 months.

Siasos G et al. Antithrombotic Treatment in Coronary Artery Disease. Curr Pharm Des. 2023;29(35):2764-2779. PMID: 37644793

Bakhru MR et al Interpreting the CHARISMA study. What is the role of dual antiplatelet therapy with clopidogrel and aspirin? Cleve Clin J Med. 2008 Apr;75(4):289-95. PMID: 18491435

3.4 Antithrombotic Therapy in CAD and PVD

Case 33

A 72-year-old male with a history of stable coronary artery disease (CAD) and peripheral artery disease (PAD) presents to the clinic for a routine cardiovascular risk assessment. He underwent coronary artery bypass grafting (CABG) 5 years ago and has a history of intermittent claudication that is managed with supervised exercise therapy. His current medications include aspirin 81 mg daily, atorvastatin 40 mg daily, and lisinopril 10 mg daily. His blood pressure is 130/80 mmHg, and his physical examination is unremarkable except for diminished but palpable pedal pulses bilaterally. His most recent laboratory tests show normal renal function, a hemoglobin level of 14 g/dL, and no previous history of bleeding disorders. His cardiovascular risk factors are well-controlled, and he has no other significant medical issues.
Considering the patient's history and current clinical status, which of the following is the most appropriate management of his antithrombotic therapy?

- A) Continue aspirin 81 mg daily without additional antithrombotic therapy.
- B) Replace aspirin with clopidogrel 75 mg daily for dual antiplatelet therapy.
- C) Add rivaroxaban 2.5 mg twice daily to the current aspirin therapy.
- D) Discontinue aspirin and initiate anticoagulation with warfarin, targeting an INR of 2-3.

Correct Answer: C) Add rivaroxaban 2.5 mg twice daily to the current aspirin therapy. The COMPASS trial demonstrated that in stable patients with CAD and PAD, the addition of low-dose rivaroxaban (2.5 mg twice daily) to aspirin reduced the risk of cardiovascular death, myocardial infarction, and stroke by 24% compared to aspirin alone [[C]]. There was an associated increase in bleeding, but the benefits in terms of reducing severe cardiovascular events and overall mortality were significant. This combination therapy is recommended for patients at high risk for severe cardiac events who have a low risk of bleeding, which fits the profile of the patient in this scenario. Continuing aspirin 81 mg daily without additional antithrombotic therapy (A) would not provide the same level of protection against cardiovascular events as the combination of aspirin with low-dose rivaroxaban in this patient with both CAD and PAD. Replacing aspirin with clopidogrel 75 mg daily for dual antiplatelet therapy (B) is not supported by the evidence for patients in the context described. While clopidogrel may be used in place of aspirin in patients with aspirin intolerance, the COMPASS trial specifically showed a benefit with the combination of low-dose rivaroxaban and aspirin. Discontinuing aspirin and initiating anticoagulation with warfarin (D) is not indicated in this scenario. Warfarin is not superior to aspirin for secondary prevention in patients with CAD and PAD without other indications for anticoagulation, such as atrial fibrillation or mechanical heart valves. Moreover, the COMPASS trial did not compare rivaroxaban with warfarin in this patient population.

In summary, the most appropriate management of this patient's antithrombotic therapy is to add rivaroxaban 2.5 mg twice daily to the current aspirin therapy. This approach is based on the evidence from the COMPASS trial and is recommended for patients like the one described, who have stable CAD and PAD and are at high risk for severe cardiac events but have a low risk of bleeding.

Eikelboom JW et al. Rivaroxaban with or without Aspirin in Stable Cardiovascular Disease. N Engl J Med. 2017 Oct 5;377(14):1319-1330. PMID: 28844192

Case Note

The COMPASS trial demonstrated that adding rivaroxaban, a direct factor Xa inhibitor, to aspirin therapy provided additional cardiovascular benefits in stable patients with coronary artery disease and peripheral arterial disease. Specifically, the addition of 2.5 mg of rivaroxaban twice daily to 100 mg of aspirin reduced the risk of cardiovascular death, myocardial infarction, and stroke by 24% compared to using 100 mg of aspirin alone. While there was a small increase in bleeding events, an 18% reduction in overall mortality was also observed. Based on these findings, the combination of rivaroxaban and aspirin has been approved by the FDA for long-term management of patients with coronary artery disease (CAD) and peripheral artery disease who are at high risk for major cardiovascular events but have a low risk of bleeding complications.

3.5 Pharmacotherapy in Cardiovascular Risk Management

Case 34

A 56-year-old male with a history of well-controlled hypertension and hypercholesterolemia presents to the clinic for an annual check-up. He has no history of diabetes, smoking, or known coronary artery disease. His current medications include hydrochlorothiazide 25 mg daily and atorvastatin 20 mg daily. His blood pressure today is 128/78 mmHg, and his physical examination is unremarkable. His fasting lipid panel shows an LDL cholesterol of 90 mg/dL, HDL cholesterol of 55 mg/dL, and triglycerides of 150 mg/dL. His 10-year ASCVD risk score is calculated at 7.5%. He mentions that he sometimes forgets to take his medications and is interested in simplifying his regimen to improve adherence.
Based on the patient's clinical profile and interest in simplifying his medication regimen, which of the following is the most appropriate next step in management?

- A) Initiate a polypill containing aspirin, ramipril, and atorvastatin.
- B) Continue current medications without changes.
- C) Add ramipril to the patient's regimen for cardiovascular risk reduction.
- D) Switch hydrochlorothiazide to a combination pill of hydrochlorothiazide and ramipril.

Correct Answer: B) Continue current medications without changes. The patient in this scenario is considered to be at intermediate risk for atherosclerotic cardiovascular disease (ASCVD) with a 10-year risk score of 7.5%. The HOPE and EUROPA trials have shown that angiotensin-converting enzyme (ACE) inhibitors like ramipril and perindopril can reduce vascular events in high-risk patients. However, there is no clear evidence that ACE inhibitors provide substantial benefits for primary prevention in patients who are at low to intermediate risk and do not have clinical evidence of atherosclerotic disease. While the SECURE study found that a polypill containing aspirin, ramipril, and atorvastatin improved medication adherence and reduced the occurrence of major adverse cardiovascular events, this approach is generally more appropriate for patients who are at high risk or have established cardiovascular disease. In this patient with intermediate risk and no history of cardiovascular events, the addition of aspirin and ramipril may not be justified due to the potential risks associated with polypharmacy and the lack of evidence for benefit in this specific risk group. Continuing the current medications without changes is the most appropriate next step because the patient's blood pressure and lipid levels are well-controlled on his current regimen, and his ASCVD risk does not warrant the addition of an ACE inhibitor or aspirin for primary prevention. Switching hydrochlorothiazide to a combination pill of hydrochlorothiazide and ramipril could be considered if the patient had a higher ASCVD risk or if there were other indications for ACE inhibitor therapy, such as diabetes with proteinuria or heart failure. However, in the absence of such indications, it is not necessary to add an ACE inhibitor solely for the purpose of cardiovascular risk reduction in this patient.

In summary, the most appropriate management for this patient is to continue his current medications without changes. This decision is based on the patient's intermediate ASCVD risk, the lack of evidence for the benefit of ACE inhibitors in primary prevention for such patients, and the well-controlled nature of his hypertension and hypercholesterolemia.

Sleight P. The HOPE Study (Heart Outcomes Prevention Evaluation). J Renin Angiotensin Aldosterone Syst. 2000 Mar;1(1):18-20.PMID: 11967789

3.6 Managing Recurrent Chest Discomfort:Evaluating the Next Steps

Case 35

A 55-year-old man with a history of hypertension and hyperlipidemia presents to the clinic complaining of recurrent chest discomfort for the past 2 months. He describes the discomfort as a pressure-like sensation in the center of his chest, which occurs during his morning walks and resolves within minutes of resting. The discomfort also arises when he is angry or after a heavy meal, lasting up to 15 minutes. He denies any symptoms at rest or at night. He has not tried any medications for these symptoms. His current medications include lisinopril and atorvastatin. On examination, his blood pressure is 138/86 mmHg, heart rate is 78 beats per minute, and the cardiovascular examination is unremarkable. An electrocardiogram (ECG) shows no significant ST-T wave changes.
Which of the following is the most appropriate next step in the management of this patient?

- A. Prescribe sublingual nitroglycerin and schedule a stress test.
- B. Start a calcium channel blocker and reassess symptoms in 4 weeks.
- C. Refer for immediate coronary angiography.
- D. Advise lifestyle modifications and reassess in 6 months.

The correct answer is A. Prescribe sublingual nitroglycerin and schedule a stress test. The patient's symptoms are consistent with stable angina pectoris, which is typically precipitated by exertion or emotional stress and relieved by rest. The use of sublingual nitroglycerin can help alleviate symptoms when they occur and also serves as a diagnostic tool, as relief with nitroglycerin supports the diagnosis of angina. Additionally, scheduling a stress test is appropriate to evaluate the presence and extent of ischemia, assess functional capacity, and guide further management, including the need for coronary angiography or revascularization. Option B is incorrect because, while calcium channel blockers can be used to treat angina, the first step should be to confirm the diagnosis and assess the severity of ischemic heart disease with a stress test before initiating therapy. Option C is incorrect because immediate coronary angiography is not typically indicated in stable patients without evidence of acute coronary syndrome (ACS) or high-risk features. Non-invasive stress testing is the preferred initial approach to risk stratification in stable angina.Option D is incorrect because, although lifestyle modifications are an important part of managing coronary artery disease, this patient's symptoms warrant further investigation with a stress test to guide management. Simply advising lifestyle modifications without further diagnostic evaluation may delay necessary treatment and increase the risk of adverse cardiac events. Angina pectoris typically results from stable coronary artery disease (CAD) or chronic coronary syndromes, often caused by atherosclerotic heart disease. Coronary vasospasm can occur at the site of a lesion or, less commonly, in vessels that appear normal. Rare causes like congenital anomalies, emboli, arteritis, or dissection can also lead to coronary artery obstruction, resulting in ischemia or infarction. Angina can also occur without coronary artery blockage due to conditions like severe myocardial hypertrophy, severe aortic stenosis or regurgitation, or in situations of increased metabolic demands such as hyperthyroidism, significant anemia, or paroxysmal tachycardias with rapid ventricular rates.

The diagnosis of angina pectoris relies heavily on the patient's history, which should cover specific details such as the triggers and relieving factors for angina, the nature of the discomfort, its location and radiation, the duration of episodes, and the effect of nitroglycerin.

Angina typically occurs during physical exertion and is relieved by rest. Patients may prefer to remain upright rather than lying down, as a reclined position can increase the workload on the heart. The level of activity needed to trigger angina can remain stable in similar situations or fluctuate daily. The angina threshold typically decreases after meals, during emotional stress, or in cold weather. It is typically lower in the morning or after strong emotions; the latter can trigger attacks without physical activity. Additionally, discomfort may arise during sexual activity, at rest, or at night due to coronary spasm.

Characteristics of the discomfort:

- Patients often describe angina as a sensation of tightness, squeezing, burning, pressing, choking, aching, bursting, "gas," indigestion, or an ill-characterized discomfort. It is commonly described by clenching a fist over the mid-chest.
- The discomfort is typically not sharply localized and does not occur in spasms.
- The discomfort may vary widely among patients but is usually consistent for each patient unless unstable angina or myocardial infarction (MI) occurs.
- Usually, the discomfort is felt behind or slightly to the left of the mid-sternum. When it starts further to the left or, occasionally, on the right, it typically moves centrally towards the center of the sternum.
- Angina can radiate to any dermatome from C8 to T4, but it most commonly radiates to the left shoulder and upper arm, often extending down the inner volar aspect of the arm to the elbow, forearm, wrist, or fourth and fifth fingers. It might also spread to the right shoulder or arm, the lower jaw, the neck, or even the back.

Duration of angina attacks:

1. The duration of angina attacks is typically brief and resolves completely without any lingering discomfort.
2. If the attack occurs due to physical activity and the patient quickly stops to rest, it typically lasts less than 3 minutes.
3. Episodes triggered by a large meal or strong emotions typically last for 15–20 minutes.
4. Attacks lasting over 30 minutes are uncommon and may indicate the development of an acute coronary syndrome (ACS) with unstable angina, MI, or a different diagnosis.
5. The impact of nitroglycerin on the diagnosis of angina pectoris is confirmed when sublingual nitroglycerin rapidly relieves an attack and when preventive nitrates allow for increased activity or prevent angina altogether.

Knuuti J et al. 2019 ESC Guidelines for the diagnosis and management of chronic coronary syndromes. Eur Heart J. 2020;41:407. PMID: 31504439

3.7 "Managing Angina in a Hypertensive Diabetic Patient

Case 36

A 65-year-old woman with a history of type 2 diabetes mellitus and hypertension presents with a 3-month history of intermittent chest discomfort. The discomfort is described as a pressure sensation in the mid-chest, occurring during her daily walks and resolving with rest. She has not experienced this discomfort at rest. Her current medications include metformin, lisinopril, and atorvastatin. Physical examination reveals a blood pressure of 145/90 mmHg, a regular pulse of 78 beats per minute, and no murmurs, gallops, or rubs on auscultation. Her resting ECG shows nonspecific ST-T wave changes, and her fasting lipid profile is within therapeutic targets.

Which of the following is the most appropriate next step in the management of this patient?

- A. Initiate a beta-blocker and reassess in 4 weeks.
- B. Perform an exercise ECG stress test.
- C. Conduct a pharmacologic stress imaging study.
- D. Refer for immediate coronary angiography.

Category	Description
Procedure	Exercise ECG testing is a noninvasive procedure used to evaluate inducible ischemia in patients with angina. It can be performed on a motorized treadmill or a bicycle ergometer. The most common protocol is the Bruce protocol, which increases treadmill speed and elevation every 3 minutes until the patient is limited by symptoms.
Precautions and Risks	The risk of exercise testing is about one infarction or death per 1000 tests. Patients with pain at rest or minimal activity are at higher risk and should not be tested. Symptomatic aortic stenosis is a relative contraindication.
Indications	Exercise testing is used to confirm the diagnosis of angina, determine the severity of activity limitation due to angina, assess prognosis in patients with known coronary disease, and evaluate responses to therapy. It should only be done for asymptomatic individuals whose occupations place them or others at special risk.
Interpretation	The usual ECG criterion for a positive test is 1-mm horizontal or downsloping ST-segment depression measured 80 msec after the J point. Patients exhibiting more severe ST-segment depression at low workloads or heart rates, limited duration of exercise, or hypotension during the test have more severe disease and a poorer prognosis. Such patients should be referred for coronary arteriography and possible revascularization.
False Positives	False positives are uncommon when a 2-mm depression is present. However, less impressive positive tests in asymptomatic patients are often "false positives". Exercise testing results that do not conform to the clinical suspicion should be confirmed by stress imaging.

Table 3.1: Summary of Exercise ECG Testing

The correct answer is C. Conduct a pharmacologic stress imaging study. Myocardial stress imaging is recommended in various situations such as when the resting ECG complicates the interpretation of an exercise ECG, to confirm exercise ECG results that contradict clinical assessment, to pinpoint the area of ischemia, differentiate between ischemic and infarcted myocardium, evaluate revascularization after surgery or angioplasty, and as a prognostic tool for patients with coronary disease. This patient has diabetes mellitus, which is a coronary artery disease (CAD) risk equivalent, and presents with symptoms suggestive of stable angina. Given her diabetes and nonspecific ST-T wave changes on the resting ECG, which may interfere with the interpretation of an exercise ECG stress test, a pharmacologic stress imaging study (such as stress echocardiography or nuclear stress test) is more appropriate. This will provide information on the presence and extent of inducible ischemia and myocardial function without the confounding effects of the ECG changes. Additionally, patients with diabetes have a higher prevalence of silent ischemia, making an imaging study more informative than an exercise ECG alone. Option A is incorrect because, while beta-blockers are a treatment for angina, the diagnosis and extent of ischemia should be confirmed with a stress imaging study before initiating therapy, especially in a patient with diabetes and nonspecific ST-T wave changes. Option B is incorrect because an exercise ECG stress test may not be as diagnostic in this patient due to her nonspecific ST-T wave changes at rest, which can obscure the interpretation of exercise-induced ECG changes. Option D is incorrect because immediate coronary angiography is an invasive procedure and is not typically the first-line investigation for a patient with suspected stable angina without evidence of high-risk features or failure of initial noninvasive testing.

Myocardial Perfusion Imaging (MPI)—Also known as nuclear stress testing or radionuclide imaging, this diagnostic test provides images where the uptake of a radioactive tracer is proportional to the blood flow at the time of injection. The test yields positive results in approximately 75 to 90% of cases with significant coronary artery disease and in 20 to 30% of those without. There are instances where other conditions such as infiltrative diseases (e.g., sarcoidosis, amyloidosis), left bundle branch block, and dilated cardiomyopathy can produce resting or persistent perfusion abnormalities. False results in MPI can occur due to diaphragmatic attenuation or, in women, breast tissue attenuation. To decrease the likelihood of these artifacts, tomographic imaging (single-photon emission computed tomography [SPECT]) is utilized.

Radionuclide Ventriculography—This procedure uses radioactive tracers to generate images of the left ventricle (LV) and measure its ejection fraction (EF) and wall motion. Resting abnormalities typically indicate infarction, whereas abnormalities that appear only during stress tests suggest stress-induced ischemia in coronary artery disease. The sensitivity of radionuclide ventriculography is similar to that of myocardial perfusion imaging, but specificity may decrease in older individuals and those with different heart diseases. Due to the accuracy of LVEF measurement, it is also used to monitor patients undergoing treatments that may have cardiotoxic effects, such as chemotherapy.

Stress Echocardiography—This technique involves performing echocardiograms during supine exercise or immediately after upright exercise. The aim is to detect exercise-induced segmental wall motion abnormalities, which serve as markers of ischemia. In well-established laboratories, the test accuracy is comparable to that achieved with scintigraphy, but a higher number of tests may yield technically inadequate results. Exercise is the preferred method of stress testing due to the additional information it provides. In certain cases, pharmacological stress using high-dose dobutamine (20–40 mcg/kg/min) can serve as an alternative to exercise.

Category	Description
Indications	Myocardial stress imaging is indicated for various reasons, including when the resting ECG makes an exercise ECG difficult to interpret, for confirmation of exercise ECG results contrary to clinical impression, to localize the region of ischemia, to distinguish ischemic from infarcted myocardium, to assess the completeness of revascularization, and as a prognostic indicator in patients with known coronary disease.
Myocardial Perfusion Scintigraphy	This test provides images in which radionuclide uptake is proportionate to blood flow at the time of injection. It is positive in about 75–90% of patients with anatomically significant coronary disease and in 20–30% of those without it. False-positive radionuclide tests may occur due to various conditions, and tomographic imaging can reduce the severity of artifacts.
Radionuclide Angiography	This procedure uses radionuclide tracers to image the LV and measures its EF and wall motion. It is used to detect resting abnormalities representing infarction and stress-induced ischemia.
Stress Echocardiography	This test demonstrates exercise-induced segmental wall motion abnormalities as an indicator of ischemia. It is comparable in accuracy to scintigraphy but may have a higher proportion of technically inadequate tests. Pharmacologic stress with high-dose dobutamine can be used as an alternative to exercise.

Table 3.2: Summary of Myocardial Stress Imaging

3.8 Chest Discomfort in a Hypertensive Smoker

Case 37

A 58-year-old male with a history of smoking and controlled hypertension presents with exertional chest discomfort. He reports that the discomfort is a squeezing sensation that occurs when climbing two flights of stairs and resolves with rest. He has no symptoms at rest. His medications include hydrochlorothiazide and amlodipine. Physical examination is unremarkable, and resting ECG shows no abnormalities. He undergoes an exercise ECG stress test, and at 5 minutes into the Bruce protocol, he develops 2.5-mm horizontal ST-segment depression in leads II, III, and aVF, which persists for 5 minutes into recovery. His blood pressure increases from 130/85 mmHg at rest to 150/90 mmHg at peak exercise, and he does not experience any chest pain during the test.
Which of the following is the most appropriate next step in the management of this patient?

- A. Initiate high-dose statin therapy and reassess in 6 weeks.
- B. Perform coronary computed tomography angiography (CCTA).
- C. Refer for coronary angiography.
- D. Prescribe a beta-blocker and schedule a follow-up in 3 months.

The correct answer is C. Refer for coronary angiography. The patient's exercise ECG stress test shows significant ST-segment depression at a low workload, which is indicative of severe ischemia and suggests a high likelihood of significant coronary artery disease (CAD). The presence of ST-segment depression greater than 2 mm, especially at a low workload and persisting into recovery, is associated with a poorer prognosis and indicates that the patient may have more severe disease. In such cases, coronary angiography is warranted to directly visualize the coronary arteries and assess for the presence and severity of CAD, which may require revascularization. Option A is incorrect because, while high-dose statin therapy is important in the management of CAD, the severity of the findings on the stress test in this patient warrants further diagnostic evaluation with coronary angiography rather than just initiating or adjusting medical therapy. Option B is incorrect because, although CCTA is a useful non-invasive imaging modality for the assessment of coronary artery disease, the severity of the stress test findings in this patient suggests that he is at high risk for significant CAD, and direct visualization with coronary angiography is more appropriate to guide potential revascularization. Option D is incorrect because prescribing a beta-blocker, while potentially beneficial for symptom management and improving prognosis, does not address the need for immediate and definitive assessment of the coronary anatomy given the high-risk findings on the stress test. CT angiography may be useful when evaluating patients with a low probability of significant coronary artery disease (CAD). Compared to conventional care, its use has been associated with a lower 5-year mortality rate in patients with stable chest pain. Similar to radionuclide single-photon emission computed tomography (SPECT) imaging, CT angiography can be utilized to assess suspected acute coronary syndrome (ACS) and chest symptoms with reduced radiation exposure. In the large randomized comparative effectiveness PROMISE trial, the outcomes of patients with stable chest pain who underwent anatomic imaging with CT angiography were comparable to those who underwent functional testing (stress electrocardiogram, stress radionuclide, or stress echocardiography).

CT-derived fractional flow reserve (CT-FFR), or CT angiography with non-invasive functional assessment of coronary stenosis, has also been applied to patients with a low-to-intermediate probability of CAD. It has been demonstrated that CT-FFR decreases the proportion of non-CAD patients who require invasive angiography. CT-FFR has received clinical approval and is utilized in clinical practice throughout the United States and Europe. The 2021 ACC/AHA Guideline for the Evaluation and Diagnosis of Chest Pain has endorsed the use of CT-FFR with a level IIa recommendation for intermediate-risk patients with chest pain and no prior history of CAD who have a 40 to 90% stenosis on CT imaging to determine the need for revascularization.

Rønnow Sand NP et al. Prediction of Coronary Revascularization in Stable Angina: Comparison of FFRCT With CMR Stress Perfusion Imaging. JACC Cardiovasc Imaging. 2020 Apr;13(4):994-1004 PMID: 31422146.

Lu MT,et al. Noninvasive FFR Derived From

Coronary CT Angiography: Management and Outcomes in the PROMISE Trial. JACC Cardiovasc Imaging. 2017 Nov;10(11):1350-1358. PMID: 28412436

3.9 Asymptomatic Patient with Family History of CAD

Case 38

A 54-year-old male with a family history of coronary artery disease (CAD) presents for a routine check-up. He is asymptomatic but concerned about his risk for heart disease. His blood pressure is 135/85 mmHg, and his total cholesterol is 210 mg/dL with an HDL of 35 mg/dL. He does not smoke, has a sedentary lifestyle, and his 10-year atherosclerotic cardiovascular disease (ASCVD) risk score is calculated to be 12%. He is currently not on any lipid-lowering therapy.
Which of the following is the most appropriate next step in the management of this patient?

- A. Initiate high-intensity statin therapy.
- B. Order an electron beam CT (EBCT) to assess for coronary calcium score.
- C. Recommend lifestyle modifications and reassess in 6 months.
- D. Prescribe a moderate-intensity statin and re-evaluate lipid profile in 3 months.

The correct answer is A. Initiate high-intensity statin therapy. According to the American Heart Association (AHA) guidelines, for patients with a 10-year atherosclerotic cardiovascular disease (ASCVD) risk score of 7.5% or higher, initiation of statin therapy is recommended to reduce the risk of cardiovascular events. This patient has an intermediate ASCVD risk of 12% and a family history of coronary artery disease (CAD), which may not be fully accounted for in the risk score, potentially underestimating his true risk. Therefore, initiating high-intensity statin therapy is appropriate to reduce his LDL cholesterol levels and overall cardiovascular risk. The other options are less appropriate in this case. While electron beam computed tomography (EBCT) can be used to refine risk assessment in intermediate-risk patients, this patient's risk score and family history already provide sufficient evidence to justify the initiation of statin therapy without the need for further risk stratification. Lifestyle modifications are an important part of managing cardiovascular risk; however, this patient's risk level and family history warrant the initiation of statin therapy in addition to lifestyle changes, not as an alternative to pharmacotherapy. Given the patient's intermediate risk and family history of CAD, high-intensity statin therapy is preferred over moderate-intensity statin therapy to achieve a greater reduction in LDL cholesterol and subsequent cardiovascular risk. The 2018 ACC/AHA Guideline on the Treatment of Blood Cholesterol to Reduce Atherosclerotic Cardiovascular Risk in Adults recommends statin therapy for four specific populations: patients with (1) clinical atherosclerotic disease, (2) LDL cholesterol 190 mg/dL, (3) diabetes aged 40 to 75 years, and (4) an estimated 10-year atherosclerotic risk of 7.5% or more aged 40 to 75 years. The guidelines do not suggest treating to a specific target LDL cholesterol level.

Individuals falling into these categories should receive treatment with a moderate- or high-intensity statin, with high-intensity statins recommended for populations at greater risk. The 2022 U.S. Preventive Services Task Force (USPSTF) Lipid Recommendations also advocate for statin therapy for primary prevention of cardiovascular disease in individuals aged 40 to 75 with one or more risk factors and a 10-year estimated CVD risk of 10% or higher. The main differences between the 2018 ACC/AHA cholesterol treatment guidelines and the 2022 USPSTF lipid recommendations are as follows:

1. Eligibility for Statin Therapy:The 2018 ACC/AHA guidelines recommend statin therapy for patients with clinical atherosclerotic cardiovascular disease (ASCVD), LDL cholesterol levels above or 190 mg/dL, diabetes patients aged 40 to 75 years, and individuals aged 40 to 75 years with an estimated 10-year ASCVD risk of 7.5% or higher.
2. The 2022 USPSTF recommendations suggest prescribing statins for primary prevention of cardiovascular disease in adults aged 40 to 75 years who have one or more cardiovascular disease risk factors and a 10-year estimated CVD risk of 10% or higher. The USPSTF also recommends that clinicians selectively offer statins to adults without prior CVD events who have a 10-year CVD risk of 7.5% to less

than 10%, indicating a smaller likelihood of benefit.

3. Specificity and Individualization: The ACC/AHA guidelines provide a more individualized approach to statin therapy, taking into account a broader range of risk factors and patient characteristics.
4. The USPSTF guidelines serve as a broader roadmap for populations, focusing on specific risk thresholds to guide statin therapy.
5. Age Considerations:The ACC/AHA guidelines do not set an upper age limit for statin therapy consideration, whereas the USPSTF suggests that current evidence is insufficient to assess the balance of benefits and harms of initiating statins in adults 76 years or older.
6. Risk Assessment Tools:The ACC/AHA guidelines utilize the Pooled Cohort Equations for risk assessment, while the USPSTF calls for more research on improving the accuracy of CVD risk prediction across populations.
7. Treatment Goals:The ACC/AHA guidelines do not recommend treating to a specific target LDL cholesterol level, while the USPSTF emphasizes that the magnitude of the benefits of statin use is proportional to a person's CVD risk level.
8. Evidence and Recommendations:Both guidelines are based on evidence assessing the benefits and harms of statin use, but they differ in their interpretation and application of this evidence to clinical practice

Delabays B et al. Comparison of the European and US guidelines for lipid-lowering therapy in primary prevention of cardiovascular disease. Eur J Prev Cardiol. 2023 Nov 30;30(17):1856-1864. PMID: 37290056.

3.10 Exertional Chest Discomfort Next Step Evaluation

Case 39

A 60-year-old male with a history of hypertension and hyperlipidemia presents with a 4-month history of exertional chest discomfort. The discomfort is described as a pressure sensation in the chest that occurs during his daily walks and resolves with rest. He denies any symptoms at rest. His blood pressure is controlled at 130/80 mmHg with lisinopril, and his LDL cholesterol is 100 mg/dL on atorvastatin. A resting ECG shows no significant abnormalities. His 10-year ASCVD risk score is calculated to be 15%. He is referred for further evaluation of his chest pain.
Which of the following is the most appropriate next step in the evaluation of this patient?

- A. Initiate high-intensity statin therapy and reassess in 6 weeks.
- B. Perform exercise ECG stress testing.
- C. Order multislice CT angiography with CT-FFR.
- D. Refer for invasive coronary angiography.

The correct answer is C. Order multislice CT angiography with CT-FFR. This patient has stable chest pain with exertional symptoms and a moderate to high likelihood of CAD based on his risk factors and clinical presentation. Multislice CT angiography with CT-FFR is a non-invasive imaging modality that can provide both anatomic and functional assessment of coronary stenosis. It is particularly useful in patients with a low to intermediate likelihood of CAD, as it can help to rule out significant coronary disease and reduce the number of unnecessary invasive angiographies. Given the patient's intermediate risk and the absence of prior CAD, this approach aligns with the 2021 ACC/AHA Guideline for the Evaluation and Diagnosis of Chest Pain, which gives a level IIa recommendation for such patients. Option A is incorrect because the patient is already on statin therapy, and the primary issue is the evaluation of his new exertional chest discomfort, which requires further diagnostic workup rather than an adjustment in his lipid management. Option B is incorrect because, while exercise ECG stress testing is a common initial test for CAD, the patient's intermediate risk and the availability of more advanced non-invasive imaging modalities that provide both anatomic and functional information make CT angiography with CT-FFR a better choice. Option D is incorrect because invasive coronary angiography is typically reserved for patients with a high likelihood of CAD, those with high-risk findings on non-invasive testing, or those with acute coronary syndromes. This patient's presentation does not yet warrant an invasive approach without prior non-invasive imaging.

Rønnow Sand NP et al. Prediction of Coronary Revascularization in Stable Angina: Comparison of FFRCT With CMR Stress Perfusion Imaging. JACC Cardiovasc Imaging. 2020 Apr;13(4):994-1004 PMID: 31422146.

Lu MT,et al. Noninvasive FFR Derived From Coronary CT Angiography: Management and Outcomes in the PROMISE Trial. JACC Cardiovasc Imaging. 2017 Nov;10(11):1350-1358. PMID: 28412436

3.11 Chronic Stable Angina with Chest Pain

Case 40

A 67-year-old female with a history of hypertension, diabetes, and chronic stable angina presents with increasing frequency of chest pain over the past 2 months. The pain is typically retrosternal, precipitated by walking two blocks or climbing one flight of stairs, and relieved by rest or nitroglycerin. She is currently on maximal medical therapy including high-dose statins, beta-blockers, ACE inhibitors, and aspirin. Despite this, her angina has become more limiting, and she is now experiencing symptoms with minimal exertion. A recent echocardiogram shows normal left ventricular function with no wall motion abnormalities. She has not undergone any prior coronary revascularization procedures.
Which of the following is the most appropriate next step in the management of this patient?

- A. Increase the dose of her current beta-blocker.
- B. Refer for coronary arteriography.
- C. Initiate ranolazine and reassess in 4 weeks.
- D. Schedule a myocardial perfusion imaging study.

The correct answer is B. Refer for coronary arteriography. This patient has life-limiting stable angina despite an adequate medical regimen, which is an indication for coronary arteriography according to the guidelines. The purpose of the arteriography in this case would be to assess the coronary anatomy to determine if percutaneous transluminal coronary angioplasty (PTCA) or bypass surgery is a consideration. Given the progression of her symptoms to the point of limiting her daily activities, despite maximal medical therapy, invasive evaluation is warranted to potentially improve her symptoms and quality of life through revascularization. Option A is incorrect because the patient is already on maximal medical therapy, including beta-blockers, and her angina is not well controlled, indicating that further increasing the dose is unlikely to provide significant additional benefit. Option C is incorrect because, although ranolazine can be used for symptom control in chronic angina, this patient's symptoms are not controlled despite maximal medical therapy. Therefore, the next step is to evaluate for revascularization options rather than adding another anti-anginal medication. Option D is incorrect because, while myocardial perfusion imaging is a useful non-invasive test for the assessment of ischemia, this patient's clinical presentation and failure to respond to medical therapy indicate that she is likely to benefit from revascularization. Therefore, direct visualization of the coronary arteries through arteriography is more appropriate to guide potential revascularization. Coronary angiography is the principal diagnostic procedure for coronary artery disease (CAD). It can be performed with minimal risk of mortality (around 0.1%) and morbidity (1–5%). However, due to its invasive nature and cost, it is recommended only for individuals with a high likelihood of CAD. Coronary angiography should be performed in the following situations, if percutaneous coronary intervention (PCI) or coronary artery bypass graft (CABG) surgery is being considered:

1. Stable angina that persists despite appropriate medical treatment.
2. Clinical presentation (unstable angina, postinfarction angina, etc) or noninvasive testing indicates high-risk disease (see Indications for Revascularization).
3. A study on aortic valve disease and angina pectoris to investigate if the angina is caused by coronary disease.

4. Asymptomatic elderly patients having valve surgery with the possibility of concomitant bypass if the anatomy allows.
5. Recurrence of symptoms after coronary revascularization to assess occlusion of bypass grafts or native vessels.
6. Cardiac failure when a surgically correctable issue is suspected, such as LV aneurysm, mitral regurgitation, or reversible ischemic dysfunction.
7. Survivors of sudden death, symptomatic, or life-threatening arrhythmias when CAD may be a correctable cause.
8. Chest pain of unknown origin or cardiomyopathy of uncertain etiology.
9. Urgently conducted cardiac catheterization with the goal of performing primary percutaneous coronary intervention (PCI) in patients with suspected acute MI.

A reduction of more than 50% of the luminal diameter is considered hemodynamically (and clinically) significant, with most lesions causing ischemia associated with narrowing exceeding 70%. For individuals with highly positive exercise electrocardiograms (ECGs) or scintigraphic studies, the presence of three-vessel or left main coronary artery disease may be found in 75–95% of cases, depending on the criteria used.Intravascular ultrasound (IVUS) can be helpful in evaluating the outcomes of percutaneous coronary intervention (PCI) or stenting. Moreover, IVUS is the preferred invasive diagnostic method for assessing ostial left main lesions and coronary dissections.

Fractional flow reserve (FFR) is a valuable tool for assessing the hemodynamic significance of coronary stenosis. During FFR measurement, a pressure wire is used to measure the pressure drop across a coronary lesion following adenosine-induced hyperemia. Revascularization guided by abnormal FFR leads to better clinical outcomes than revascularization of all angiographically stenotic lesions. FFR has become the standard method for evaluating borderline lesions when assessing the clinical and hemodynamic significance of a coronary stenosis. Furthermore, the measurement of distal and proximal pressures during the wave-free period in diastole has been proven to yield comparable clinical results to FFR, without the need for adenosine.

Left ventricular (LV) angiography is typically performed concurrently with coronary angiography. It allows for the visualization of global and regional left ventricular function, as well as the assessment of any mitral regurgitation that may be present. LV function significantly impacts the prognosis of coronary heart disease (CHD).

Darmoch F et al Intravascular Ultrasound Imaging-Guided Versus Coronary Angiography-Guided Percutaneous Coronary Intervention: A Systematic Review and Meta-Analysis. J Am Heart Assoc. 2020 Mar 3;9(5):e013678.PMID: 32075491

3.12 Case of Atypical Chest Pain

Case 41

A 45-year-old female with no significant past medical history presents with a 3-week history of intermittent chest pain. The pain is described as a sharp, stabbing sensation localized to the left side of the chest, which worsens with deep breathing and certain movements of the torso. She denies any exertional component to the pain. On physical examination, there is tenderness to palpation over the second and third left costochondral junctions. There are no other abnormalities noted on examination, and vital signs are within normal limits. An electrocardiogram (ECG) shows no abnormalities.
Which of the following is the most appropriate next step in the management of this patient?

- A. Prescribe a high-dose proton pump inhibitor and reassess in 4 weeks.
- B. Order a stress echocardiogram to evaluate for inducible ischemia.
- C. Administer a trial of nonsteroidal anti-inflammatory drugs (NSAIDs) and reassess in 2 weeks.
- D. Refer for cervical and thoracic spine MRI to evaluate for disk disease.

The correct answer is C. Administer a trial of nonsteroidal anti-inflammatory drugs (NSAIDs) and reassess in 2 weeks. The patient's clinical presentation is suggestive of costochondritis, also known as Tietze syndrome, which is characterized by pain and tenderness at the costochondral or costosternal junctions. This condition is a common cause of chest pain and can be differentiated from cardiac causes by the reproducibility of pain with palpation and the lack of association with exertion. Treatment typically involves NSAIDs for pain relief and reduction of inflammation. The patient should be reassessed to ensure improvement with this therapy. Option A is incorrect because there is no history of gastrointestinal symptoms such as heartburn or acid regurgitation to suggest reflux esophagitis, and the pain's relation to movement and palpation makes a GI cause less likely. Option B is incorrect because the patient's pain lacks an exertional component and is reproducible with palpation and movement, which is not characteristic of angina pectoris. Therefore, a stress echocardiogram is not indicated at this time. Option D is incorrect because the patient's pain is localized to the costochondral junctions and there are no symptoms suggestive of cervical or thoracic spine disease, such as radiating arm pain or paresthesias in a dermatomal pattern. Disorders of the cervical or thoracic spine affecting the dorsal roots can cause intense chest pain that mimics the location and radiation pattern of angina pectoris. The pain is triggered by certain movements of the neck or spine, lying down, and exertional activities such as straining or lifting. Pain from cervical or thoracic disk disease affects the outer aspect of the arm, thumb, and index fingers, rather than the ring and little fingers. Gastrointestinal conditions such as reflux esophagitis, peptic ulcer, chronic cholecystitis, esophageal spasm, and functional gastrointestinal disorders can cause symptoms similar to angina pectoris. The clinical picture can be confusing as ischemic pain can also be associated with upper gastrointestinal symptoms, and esophageal motility disorders may respond to nitrates and calcium channel blockers. Evaluating esophageal motility can be beneficial in these cases. Injury and inflammation in the left shoulder and thoracic outlet syndromes can lead to chest pain caused by nerve irritation or muscle compression. Symptoms typically occur with movements of the arm and shoulder and may be accompanied by abnormal sensations. Pulmonary conditions such as pneumonia, pulmonary embolism, and spontaneous pneumothorax can result in both chest pain and shortness of breath. Thoracic aortic dissection can also cause severe chest pain, typically felt in the back. The pain starts suddenly, peaks abruptly, and may be accompanied by changes in pulses. Various cardiac conditions, such as mitral valve prolapse, hypertrophic cardiomyopathy (HCM), myocarditis, pericarditis, aortic valve disease, or right ventricular hypertrophy (RVH), can lead to atypical chest pain or myocardial ischemia.

3.13 Use of Nitrate in Stable Angina

Case 42

A 68-year-old male with a history of chronic stable angina is being evaluated for optimization of his anti-anginal therapy. He is currently taking aspirin, a beta-blocker, and sublingual nitroglycerin as needed for chest pain. Despite these medications, he reports having angina that typically occurs during his daily afternoon walks. His last dose of the beta-blocker is in the morning, and he uses the sublingual nitroglycerin approximately twice a week. His blood pressure is well-controlled, and he has no history of erectile dysfunction or use of phosphodiesterase inhibitors. He is interested in a medication regimen that could prevent his angina without the need for frequent dosing.

Which of the following is the most appropriate addition to this patient's anti-anginal regimen?

- A. Prescribe isosorbide dinitrate 30 mg orally three times daily with the last dose after dinner.
- B. Prescribe isosorbide mononitrate 120 mg once daily in a sustained-release preparation in the morning.
- C. Prescribe transdermal nitroglycerin patch 0.4 mg/hour rate to be applied in the morning and removed after 12 hours.
- D. Prescribe oral sustained-release nitroglycerin preparations 6.25 mg four times daily.

Atypical Feature	Possible Cause
Prolonged duration (hours or days), darting or knifelike pains at the apex or over the precordium	Less likely to be ischemia
Sharply localized tenderness of the intercostal muscles	Anterior chest wall syndrome
Diffuse chest pain reproduced by local pressure	Inflammation of the chondrocostal junctions (Tietze syndrome)
Sudden sharp, severe chest pain related to specific movements of the neck or spine, recumbency, and straining or lifting	Cervical or thoracic spine disease involving the dorsal roots
Pain involves the outer or dorsal aspect of the arm and the thumb and index fingers rather than the ring and little fingers	Cervical or thoracic disk disease
Pain suggestive of angina pectoris	Reflux esophagitis, peptic ulcer, chronic cholecystitis, esophageal spasm, and functional GI disease
Chest pain due to nerve irritation or muscular compression, usually precipitated by movement of the arm and shoulder and associated with paresthesias	Degenerative and inflammatory lesions of the left shoulder and thoracic outlet syndromes
Chest pain as well as dyspnea	Pneumonia, pulmonary embolism (PE), and spontaneous pneumothorax
Severe chest pain commonly felt in the back, sudden in onset, reaches maximum intensity immediately, and may be associated with changes in pulses	Dissection of the thoracic aorta
Atypical chest pain or even myocardial ischemia	Other cardiac disorders, such as mitral valve prolapse, hypertrophic cardiomyopathy (HCM), myocarditis, pericarditis, aortic valve disease, or right ventricular hypertrophy (RVH)

Table 3.3: Summary of Atypical Chest Pain Features and Possible Causes

The correct answer is C. Prescribe transdermal nitroglycerin patch 0.4 mg/hour rate to be applied in the morning and removed after 12 hours. This patient has chronic stable angina and is experiencing breakthrough symptoms despite the use of a beta-blocker and sublingual nitroglycerin. The addition of a long-acting nitrate can help prevent anginal episodes. The transdermal nitroglycerin patch provides a consistent delivery of medication throughout its wear time and can be timed to cover the patient's period of greatest activity when he is most likely to experience angina. Importantly, the patch should be removed after 12 hours to prevent the development of nitrate tolerance, which is a common limitation of long-term nitrate therapy. This regimen allows for a nitrate-free interval overnight when the patient is less likely to exert himself and therefore less likely to experience angina. Option A is incorrect because dosing isosorbide dinitrate three times daily may not provide a sufficient nitrate-free interval to prevent tolerance, which is a key consideration in long-term nitrate therapy. Option B is incorrect because taking a sustained-release preparation of isosorbide mononitrate in the morning would not provide the necessary nitrate-free interval, as the medication would be active throughout the 24-hour period. Option D is incorrect because oral sustained-release nitroglycerin preparations dosed four times daily would not allow for an adequate nitrate-free interval and could lead to tolerance. Sublingual nitroglycerin is the preferred medication for the immediate treatment of angina pectoris, taking effect within 1-2 minutes. At the onset of an angina attack, a new nitroglycerin tablet is placed under the tongue. Nitroglycerin buccal spray, which comes in a metered-dose delivery system with a dosage of 0.4 mg, is offered as a more convenient alternative for those who struggle with handling pills, and it provides more consistent absorption. The primary limitation of long-term nitrate therapy is the development of tolerance, which can be mitigated by implementing a treatment regimen that incorporates a daily nitrate-free interval of at least 8 to 10 hours. Isosorbide dinitrate can be administered three times a day, with the final dose taken after dinner, or alternatively, longer-acting isosorbide mononitrate can be taken once daily. Most patients should remove transdermal nitrate formulations overnight. Headache is a frequent side effect that limits the use of nitrate therapy. Additional adverse effects include nausea, dizziness, and hypotension. Phosphodiesterase inhibitors, particularly those used for the treatment of erectile dysfunction, should not be taken within 24 hours of using nitrates due to the risk of severe hypotension.

Wei J et al Nitrates for stable angina: a systematic review and meta-analysis of randomized clinical trials. Int J Cardiol. 2011 Jan 7;146(1):4-12. PMID: 20557963.

3.14 Beta-blockers In Asthma and Angina Case

Case 43

A 58-year-old male with a history of chronic stable angina and previous myocardial infarction is seen for a routine follow-up. He is currently on aspirin, a high-intensity statin, and sublingual nitroglycerin as needed. He reports experiencing chest pain with moderate exertion, such as climbing two flights of stairs, which is relieved by rest or nitroglycerin. His last exercise stress test six months ago showed no evidence of inducible ischemia. His other medical problems include well-controlled asthma, for which he uses an inhaled corticosteroid and occasional albuterol, and a history of depression. His current medications do not include a beta-blocker. His blood pressure is 132/84 mmHg, heart rate is 78 bpm, and respiratory rate is 14 breaths per minute. On examination, his lungs are clear to auscultation, and there are no signs of heart failure.
Which of the following is the most appropriate addition to this patient's medication regimen?

- A. Initiate metoprolol succinate extended-release, titrate to maximum tolerated dose.
- B. Initiate pindolol to improve exertional angina symptoms.
- C. Initiate amlodipine to reduce the frequency of angina episodes.
- D. Initiate ivabradine to reduce heart rate and angina frequency.

The correct answer is A. Initiate metoprolol succinate extended-release, titrate to maximum tolerated dose. Beta-blockers are recommended as first-line therapy for patients with chronic stable angina, particularly in those with a history of myocardial infarction, as they have been shown to prolong life in this patient population. Metoprolol succinate extended-release is a beta-blocker without intrinsic sympathomimetic activity (ISA) and is appropriate for patients with chronic stable angina. It should be titrated to the maximum tolerated dose to achieve optimal heart rate control and angina relief. The patient's well-controlled asthma does not necessarily contraindicate the use of beta-blockers, especially cardioselective ones, which have a lower risk of bronchospasm. Option B is incorrect because beta-blockers with intrinsic sympathomimetic activity, such as pindolol, are less desirable for the treatment of angina, particularly in patients with a history of myocardial infarction, as they may exacerbate angina and have not been shown to be effective in secondary prevention trials. Option C is incorrect because, while amlodipine, a calcium channel blocker, can be used to treat chronic stable angina, beta-blockers should be considered first-line therapy in this patient with a history of myocardial infarction. Calcium channel blockers are generally considered when beta-blockers are contraindicated or not tolerated. Option D is incorrect because ivabradine is indicated for symptomatic stable angina in patients who are intolerant to or have contraindications for beta-blockers. In this patient, there is no contraindication to beta-blockers, and they have not yet been tried. Beta-blockers are the sole antianginal medications proven to extend the lifespan of people with coronary disease following a heart attack. Beta-blockers are indicated as the initial treatment for most individuals with chronic angina according to the guidelines for stable ischemic heart disease. Beta-blockers with intrinsic sympathomimetic activity, like pindolol, are not preferred due to their potential to worsen angina in certain persons and their lack of efficacy in secondary prevention trials. Regardless of variations in cardioselectivity, vasodilation, and lipid solubility, all beta-blockers appear to be equally effective in treating stable ischemic heart disease. Severe bronchospastic illness, bradyarrhythmias, and decompensated heart failure are the main contraindications.

Shu de F et al . Long-term beta blockers for stable angina: systematic review and meta-analysis. Eur J Prev Cardiol. 2012 Jun;19(3):330-41. PMID: 22779086

Case Note

Regardless of variations in cardioselectivity, vasodilation, and lipid solubility, all beta-blockers appear to be equally effective in treating stable ischemic heart disease. Severe bronchospastic illness, bradyarrhythmias, and decompensated heart failure are the main contraindications.

3.15 Managing Angina and Ranolazine

Case 44

A 63-year-old male with a history of hypertension, hyperlipidemia, and chronic stable angina is seen in the clinic for a routine follow-up. He is currently on aspirin, atorvastatin, lisinopril, and metoprolol. Despite these medications, he reports having angina with less exertion than previously, now occurring with walking one block or climbing a flight of stairs. He denies any episodes of syncope or palpitations. His current medications do not include any antianginal therapy other than metoprolol. His blood pressure is 138/82 mmHg, heart rate is 60 bpm, and ECG shows normal sinus rhythm with no QT prolongation. His current regimen of medications does not include any CYP450 3A inhibitors or inducers, and he has no history of ventricular arrhythmias or acute coronary syndromes.
Which of the following is the most appropriate addition to this patient's medication regimen to manage his angina?

- A. Initiate ranolazine 500 mg orally twice a day.
- B. Increase the dose of metoprolol.
- C. Initiate amlodipine.
- D. Initiate sotalol.

The correct answer is A. Initiate ranolazine 500 mg orally twice a day. Ranolazine is indicated for the treatment of chronic stable angina and can be used when patients continue to experience angina despite optimal doses of first-line antianginal medications such as beta-blockers. Ranolazine has been shown to prolong exercise duration and time to angina without affecting heart rate or blood pressure. This patient's heart rate is controlled, and he is not on any medications that would contraindicate the use of ranolazine, such as potent CYP450 3A inhibitors or other QT-prolonging drugs. Option B is incorrect because the patient's heart rate is already at the lower limit of normal, and increasing the dose of metoprolol may lead to bradycardia without providing additional antianginal benefit. Option C is incorrect because, while amlodipine could be considered for additional antianginal effect, ranolazine is a more appropriate choice given the patient's persistent symptoms despite beta-blocker therapy and the absence of contraindications to ranolazine. Option D is incorrect because sotalol is a class III antiarrhythmic that can prolong the QT interval and is not indicated for the treatment of stable angina. It is also contraindicated in patients taking ranolazine. Ranolazine is a medication prescribed for chronic angina. Clinical trials have shown that Ranolazine can effectively prolong exercise duration and delay the onset of angina symptoms, all while maintaining stable heart rate and blood pressure levels. This beneficial impact is consistent whether Ranolazine is used as a standalone treatment or in conjunction with traditional antianginal therapies. Importantly, Ranolazine can be safely combined with medications for erectile dysfunction. The typical recommended dosage is 500 mg taken orally twice daily. However, it is crucial to note that due to the potential risk of QT prolongation, Ranolazine should not be administered to individuals with pre-existing QT prolongation, those currently taking QT-prolonging medications like quinidine, dofetilide, or sotalol, or those using potent or moderate CYP450 3A inhibitors such as clarithromycin and rifampin.The mechanism of action of Ranolazine in treating chronic angina involves several key processes. At therapeutic levels, Ranolazine inhibits the late phase of inward sodium channels in ischemic cardiac myocytes. This inhibition leads to a reduction in intracellular sodium concentration, subsequently decreasing intracellular calcium influx via the Na-Ca channel. By reducing intracellular calcium levels, Ranolazine helps decrease ventricular wall tension, thereby lowering oxygen consumption without affecting blood pressure or heart rate. Moreover, at higher concentrations, Ranolazine also inhibits the rapid delayed rectifier potassium current, which delays action potential and prolongs the QT interval. Additionally, Ranolazine inhibits fatty acid oxidation, promoting glucose oxidation, reducing lactic acid production, and enhancing heart function.

Wilson SR et al. Efficacy of ranolazine in patients with chronic angina observations from the randomized, double-blind, placebo-controlled MERLIN-TIMI . J Am Coll Cardiol. 2009 Apr 28;53(17):1510-6. PMID: 19389561

Case Note

Despite the QT prolongation, there is a lower rate of ventricular arrhythmias with its use following ACSs, as demonstrated in the MERLIN trial.

3.16 Calcium Channel Blockers Treatment In Angina

Case 45

A 72-year-old female with a history of hypertension, type 2 diabetes mellitus, and recent non-ST elevation myocardial infarction (NSTEMI) is seen in the outpatient clinic for follow-up. She was discharged one week ago and is currently on aspirin, clopidogrel, atorvastatin, metoprolol, and lisinopril. She reports new-onset exertional chest pain that occurs when walking more than two blocks, which is relieved by rest. Her echocardiogram shows an ejection fraction of 40% with mild left ventricular dysfunction. She denies any symptoms of heart failure. Her blood pressure is 150/90 mmHg, and her heart rate is 68 bpm on examination. Which of the following is the most appropriate medication to add to this patient's regimen to manage her angina?

- A. Initiate short-acting nifedipine.
- B. Initiate amlodipine.
- C. Initiate diltiazem.
- D. Initiate verapamil.

The correct answer is B. Initiate amlodipine. This patient with a history of NSTEMI is experiencing exertional angina, indicating that her ischemic heart disease is not adequately controlled. Among the calcium channel blockers, amlodipine is a longer-acting dihydropyridine that has been shown to be safe in patients with heart failure, as evidenced by the PRAISE-2 trial. It is effective for the treatment of angina and can be used in patients with left ventricular dysfunction without the risk of exacerbating heart failure. Option A is incorrect because short-acting nifedipine, especially in moderate to high doses, has been associated with an increase in mortality post-myocardial infarction and should be avoided. Option C is incorrect because diltiazem, while a non-dihydropyridine calcium channel blocker that is less likely to cause reflex tachycardia, is not recommended in patients with clinical heart failure or moderate to severe left ventricular dysfunction due to the risk of worsening heart failure. Option D is incorrect for the same reason as option C; verapamil is contraindicated in patients with clinical heart failure or significant left ventricular dysfunction due to its negative inotropic effects. Short-acting and long-acting dihydropyridines, a type of calcium channel blockers, exhibit distinct characteristics and effects. Short-acting dihydropyridines like nifedipine act more rapidly but have been associated with potential adverse outcomes, especially in patients with coronary heart disease. On the other hand, long-acting dihydropyridines such as extended-release nifedipine and amlodipine are considered safer anti-hypertensive drugs due to reduced adverse events. Long-acting dihydropyridines are known for their vascular selectivity, promoting vasodilation without a significant direct effect on cardiac function. In contrast, non-dihydropyridines like verapamil and diltiazem have a greater impact on the heart but are less effective in vasodilation. Long-acting dihydropyridines have been used to treat conditions like hypertension by dilating arterial blood vessels effectively. They are particularly beneficial for individuals of Afro-Caribbean descent and older adults with high systolic blood pressure due to large blood vessel stiffness. Studies have shown that long-acting dihydropyridines, when used after acute myocardial infarction, are associated with lower rates of adverse outcomes compared to short-acting dihydropyridines. Long-acting dihydropyridine calcium channel blockers have demonstrated substantially lower rates of mortality and cardiac rehospitalization post-myocardial infarction, highlighting their potential benefits in managing cardiovascular conditions. Calcium channel blockers have been associated with varying outcomes postinfarction, with some instances showing increased ischemia and mortality rates, particularly with certain dihydropyridines like nifedipine, as well as diltiazem and verapamil in patients with clinical heart failure or moderate to severe left ventricular dysfunction. Studies have highlighted the potential risks of high doses of short-acting nifedipine leading to elevated mortality rates, although the implications for longer-acting dihydropyridines remain uncertain. Given these uncertainties and the lack of definitive positive impact on outcomes, calcium channel blockers are generally considered third-line anti-ischemic medications for postinfarction patients. It is advisable to exercise caution when prescribing calcium channel blockers, except for amlodipine, which has shown safety in patients with heart failure in the PRAISE-2 trial. The findings from PRAISE-1 and PRAISE-2 trials regarding amlodipine's safety in individuals with severe heart failure revealed a reduction in uncontrolled hypertension and chest pain/angina occurrences but an increase in peripheral edema and pulmonary edema cases among those receiving amlodipine treatment. The decrease in reports of chest pain and uncontrolled hypertension aligns with amlodipine's efficacy in managing angina and hypertension. While peripheral edema is a common side effect of amlodipine, pulmonary edema occurrences observed in both trials do not indicate an increased risk of exacerbating heart failure, heart failure hospitalization, or mortality in the amlodipine groups. This paradox suggests that pulmonary edema associated with amlodipine may result from its impact on widening pulmonary arterioles rather than directly affecting the heart's function. Notably, the PRAISE-2 trial demonstrated a lower incidence of strokes in participants treated with amlodipine, underscoring the potential benefits of antihypertensive medications in reducing stroke risk even in individuals without hypertension. These insights shed light on the complexities of calcium channel blocker use postinfarction and emphasize the importance of individualized treatment approaches based on patient characteristics and risk profiles.

> Packer M et al PRAISE-2 Study Group. Effect of amlodipine on the survival of patients with severe chronic heart failure due to a nonischemic cardiomyopathy: results of the PRAISE-2 study (prospective randomized amlodipine survival evaluation 2). JACC Heart Fail. 2013 Aug;1(4):308-314. PMID: 24621933.

3.17 Ivabradine The SIGNIFY Trial

Case 46

A 67-year-old male with a history of chronic stable angina, hypertension, and dyslipidemia presents to the clinic for a routine follow-up. He is currently on aspirin, simvastatin, lisinopril, and metoprolol. Despite adherence to his medication regimen, he reports persistent angina that occurs with minimal exertion, such as walking one to two blocks. He has no history of heart failure, and his ejection fraction was recently measured at 55%. His current blood pressure is 138/86 mmHg, and his heart rate is 68 bpm. An ECG performed in the clinic demonstrates normal sinus rhythm with no significant ST-T changes. He has no contraindications to additional antianginal therapy.
Which of the following is the most appropriate next step in managing this patient's angina?

- A. Initiate ivabradine to specifically lower heart rate and reduce angina frequency.
- B. Increase the dose of metoprolol to achieve better heart rate control.
- C. Initiate ranolazine to reduce angina frequency without affecting heart rate.
- D. Initiate amlodipine to provide additional antianginal efficacy.

The correct answer is C. Initiate ranolazine to reduce angina frequency without affecting heart rate. Ranolazine is an antianginal medication that works by inhibiting the late phase of the sodium current in the cardiac myocytes, thereby reducing intracellular calcium and myocardial oxygen demand. It is indicated for patients with chronic stable angina who continue to experience symptoms despite optimal therapy with other antianginals, such as beta-blockers. It does not affect heart rate or blood pressure, making it a suitable choice for this patient whose heart rate is already well-controlled. Option A is incorrect because ivabradine selectively blocks the If current in the sinoatrial node, leading to heart rate reduction. It is indicated for symptomatic chronic heart failure patients with reduced ejection fraction to decrease the risk of hospitalization for worsening heart failure. However, the SIGNIFY trial found potential harm in patients with significant angina without heart failure, making it a less appropriate choice for this patient. Option B is incorrect because the patient's heart rate is already within the target range on metoprolol, and further increasing the dose may lead to bradycardia without additional antianginal benefit. Option D is incorrect because, while amlodipine could be an option for additional antianginal effect, the patient's blood pressure is not elevated, and the primary goal is to control angina symptoms without further lowering the heart rate. Ranolazine would be a more appropriate choice given the patient's current heart rate and the lack of contraindications.

Grassi G. Evaluation of the SIGNIFY trial. Expert Opin Pharmacother. 2015;16(12):1861-4. PMID: 26153241

Fox K et al. SIGNIFY Investigators. Ivabradine in stable coronary artery disease without clinical heart failure. N Engl J Med. 2014 Sep 18;371(12):1091-9. PMID: 25176136

Case Note

Among patients who had stable coronary artery disease without clinical heart failure, the addition of ivabradine to standard background therapy to reduce the heart rate did not improve outcomes.

3.18 In-stent Restenosis (ISR) Management

Case 47

A 58-year-old male with a history of type 2 diabetes mellitus and prior percutaneous coronary intervention (PCI) with a bare metal stent placement in the left anterior descending (LAD) artery 8 months ago presents with recurrent exertional chest pain. He describes the pain as similar to that experienced prior to his initial stent placement, occurring after walking two blocks and relieved by rest. He is currently on aspirin, high-intensity statin therapy, metformin, and a beta-blocker. His blood pressure is 132/78 mmHg, heart rate is 72 bpm, and physical examination is unremarkable. A repeat coronary angiogram reveals in-stent restenosis in the LAD artery.

Which of the following is the most appropriate management for this patient's in-stent restenosis?

- A. Repeat PCI with placement of a drug-eluting stent in the LAD artery.
- B. Conservative management with optimization of medical therapy.
- C. Coronary artery bypass graft surgery (CABG).
- D. Percutaneous transluminal coronary angioplasty (PTCA) without stent placement.

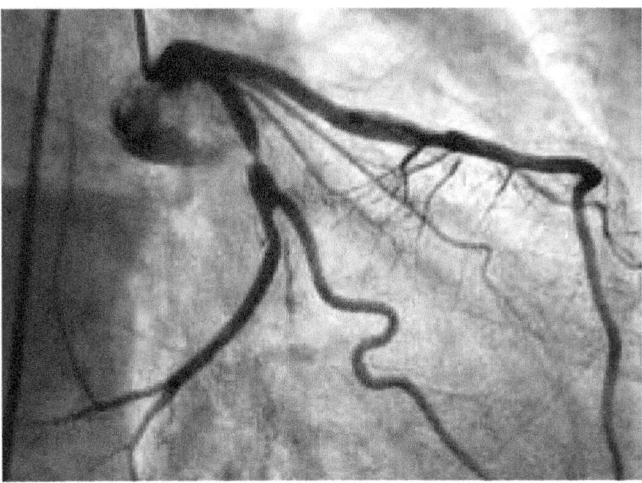

Figure 3.1: In-stent restenosis

The correct answer is A. Repeat PCI with placement of a drug-eluting stent in the LAD artery. In-stent restenosis (ISR) is a common complication following PCI, particularly with bare metal stents. The patient's recurrent symptoms and angiographic findings are indicative of ISR. The current standard of care for ISR is repeat PCI with the placement of a drug-eluting stent (DES), which releases antiproliferative agents that help reduce the rate of restenosis. DES has been shown to substantially reduce restenosis rates compared to bare metal stents, especially in patients with risk factors such as diabetes, small vessel diameter, and complex lesions. Option B is incorrect because conservative management with optimization of medical therapy alone is generally not sufficient for symptomatic ISR, especially in a patient who is already on appropriate medical therapy and has recurrent angina. Option C is incorrect because CABG is typically reserved for patients with more extensive coronary artery disease, multiple vessel involvement, or when PCI is not technically feasible or has failed repeatedly. There is no indication that this patient has such extensive disease. Option D is incorrect because PTCA alone without stent placement has a higher restenosis rate compared to repeat stenting, especially in the setting of ISR. The use of a DES in this scenario is preferred to reduce the likelihood of further restenosis. The standard approach for individuals experiencing acute myocardial infarction involves using stents during percutaneous coronary intervention (PCI). Randomized trials have shown that employing drug-eluting stents in STEMI patients can reduce the need for repeat interventions due to restenosis. Current-generation drug-eluting stents exhibit comparable or even lower rates of stent thrombosis when compared to bare metal stents. In cases where patients are unable to access or adhere to P2Y12 inhibitor therapy, bare metal stents may still be a viable option. For patients in cardiogenic shock, early catheterization and either percutaneous or surgical revascularization are recommended strategies that have been proven to reduce mortality rates. Research has indicated that the addition of abciximab, a Glycoprotein IIb/IIIa inhibitor, to heparin during primary PCI can reduce major thrombotic events and potentially lower mortality rates. The practice of administering a combination of medications (full- or reduced-dose fibrinolytic agents, with or without Glycoprotein IIb/IIIa inhibitors) followed by immediate PCI, known as "Facilitated" PCI, is not recommended. Patients should receive either primary PCI or fibrinolytic agents (with immediate rescue PCI for reperfusion failure), provided it can be promptly implemented as outlined in the ACC/AHA and European guidelines. Using drug-eluting stents (DES) over bare-metal stents (BMS) in ST-segment elevation myocardial infarction (STEMI) patients offers several advantages. DES have been shown to significantly reduce restenosis and target-vessel revascularization (TVR) rates compared to BMS in patients without acute coronary syndromes. While BMS can reduce TVR rates in STEMI patients, the benefits may not be as pronounced as with DES. However, concerns have arisen regarding a potential higher risk of stent thrombosis (ST) associated with DES, particularly in the setting of STEMI. Research indicates that DES provide a substantial reduction in restenosis and TVR rates, offering improved outcomes for STEMI patients undergoing percutaneous coronary intervention. Despite concerns about ST, the benefits of DES in reducing the need for repeat interventions and improving clinical outcomes outweigh the potential risks associated with these advanced stent technologies.

Alfonso Fet al. Management of in-stent restenosis. EuroIntervention. 2022 Jun 3;18(2):e103-e123. PMID: 35656726

3.19 Recommendation for Revascularization The FREEDOM Trial

Case 48

A 63-year-old female with a history of type 2 diabetes mellitus, hypertension, and recent non-ST elevation myocardial infarction (NSTEMI) is referred for evaluation of multivessel coronary artery disease. Coronary angiography revealed 70% stenosis in the proximal left anterior descending (LAD) artery, 75% stenosis in the first obtuse marginal branch of the left circumflex artery, and 80% stenosis in the mid-right coronary artery. Her diabetes is well-controlled with metformin and a GLP-1 agonist, and she has no history of renal insufficiency or prior revascularization procedures. Her left ventricular ejection fraction is 60%. She is currently on dual antiplatelet therapy, a high-intensity statin, and a beta-blocker. She wishes to discuss her revascularization options.
Which of the following is the most appropriate recommendation for revascularization in this patient?

- A. Elective percutaneous coronary intervention (PCI) with drug-eluting stents.
- B. Coronary artery bypass graft surgery (CABG).
- C. Medical management without revascularization.
- D. PCI with bare-metal stents.

The correct answer is B. Coronary artery bypass graft surgery (CABG). The FREEDOM trial demonstrated that in patients with diabetes and multivessel coronary disease, CABG is superior to PCI with drug-eluting stents with regard to major adverse cardiovascular events, including death, myocardial infarction (MI), and stroke at 5 years. This patient has diabetes and multivessel disease, which places her in a category where CABG has been shown to have better long-term outcomes compared to PCI. Additionally, the SYNTAX trial and other studies have shown that while mortality and infarction rates may be comparable in the short term, PCI is associated with a higher rate of repeat revascularization procedures. Option A is incorrect because, although PCI with drug-eluting stents is less invasive than CABG and may be considered in some patients with multivessel disease, in diabetic patients with multivessel disease, CABG has been shown to have better long-term outcomes. Option C is incorrect because the patient has symptomatic coronary artery disease with a recent NSTEMI, which typically warrants revascularization to improve outcomes, not just medical management. Option D is incorrect because the use of bare-metal stents would carry an even higher risk of restenosis and need for repeat revascularization compared to drug-eluting stents, and neither is preferred over CABG in this patient population. In diabetic patients with multivessel coronary artery disease, long-term outcomes favor coronary artery bypass grafting (CABG) over percutaneous coronary intervention (PCI). Studies have consistently shown that CABG is associated with improved long-term survival and reduced major adverse cardiovascular and cerebrovascular events (MACCEs) compared to PCI in this patient population. Specifically, diabetic individuals with multivessel disease undergoing PCI have been found to experience higher rates of all-cause mortality, MACCEs, myocardial infarction (MI), repeat revascularization, and cardiac death when compared to those undergoing CABG. However, it is important to note that the incidence of cerebrovascular accidents (CVA) was higher with CABG. Therefore, CABG remains the preferred management approach for eligible patients with diabetes and multivessel coronary artery disease due to its superior long-term outcomes over PCI. In diabetic patients with multivessel coronary artery disease, coronary artery bypass grafting (CABG) may present certain potential complications despite its overall benefits. Some complications that diabetic patients with multivessel disease undergoing CABG may face include a higher risk of postoperative arrhythmias, which is increased by 30% in diabetic individuals compared to non-diabetic patients. Additionally, while CABG has been associated with improved long-term outcomes and reduced major adverse cardiovascular and cerebrovascular events (MACCEs) compared to percutaneous coronary intervention (PCI), it is important to note that the incidence of cerebrovascular accidents (CVA) was found to be higher with CABG. Therefore, although CABG remains the preferred management approach for eligible patients with diabetes and multivessel coronary artery disease due to its superior long-term outcomes over PCI, the potential complications such as postoperative arrhythmias and a higher risk of CVA should be considered and monitored closely. The potential risks of cerebrovascular accidents (CVAs), also known as strokes, associated with coronary artery bypass grafting (CABG) in diabetic patients with multivessel coronary artery disease are significant. Stroke is one of the most devastating complications after CABG surgery, leading to permanent disability and a 3-6 fold increased risk of mortality.Diabetic patients, in particular, have a greater risk of stroke after CABG, especially those with a heavy atherosclerotic burden. The long-term risk for stroke after CABG is increased in patients with both type 1 and type 2 diabetes. Several factors contribute to the risk of stroke in these patients, including pre-existing cerebrovascular disease, atherosclerosis of the ascending aorta, and the presence of initial neurocognitive disorders.The presence of severe atherosclerosis of the ascending aorta is often an unexpected intra-operative finding during CABG and represents a challenge for the surgeon, potentially necessitating a change in the operative strategy. Furthermore, diabetes contributes to a 52% increase in the risk of all-cause mortality after CABG, and diabetic patients experience a 31% increase in major adverse cardio-cerebrovascular events (MACCEs) seven years after surgery compared to non-diabetic patients.This highlights the importance of careful risk assessment and management in diabetic patients undergoing CABG to minimize the risk of stroke and other adverse outcomes.

Farkouh ME et al. FREEDOM Follow-On Study Investigators. Long-Term Survival Following Multivessel Revascularization in Patients With Diabetes: The FREEDOM Follow-On Study. J Am Coll Cardiol. 2019 Feb 19;73(6):629-638. PMID: 30428398

> **Case Note**
>
> In patients with DM and MVD, coronary revascularization with CABG leads to lower all-cause mortality than with PCI-DES in long-term follow-up. (Comparison of Two Treatments for Multivessel Coronary Artery Disease in Individuals With Diabetes.

3.20 Cocaine-Induced Chest Pain: Managing ACS

> **Case 49**
>
> A 47-year-old male with no past medical history presents to the emergency department with acute onset of severe chest pain that started 1 hour ago while at a party. He admits to using cocaine shortly before the onset of symptoms. On examination, his blood pressure is 160/100 mmHg, heart rate is 110 bpm, and he appears anxious and diaphoretic. An ECG shown in Fig , Initial troponin I level is elevated. The patient is given aspirin, a beta-blocker, and nitroglycerin with partial relief of his chest pain.
> Which of the following is the most appropriate next step in the management of this patient?
>
> - A. Immediate coronary angiography with intent for percutaneous coronary intervention (PCI).
> - B. Intravenous benzodiazepines for sedation and symptomatic relief.
> - C. Administration of a thrombolytic agent.
> - D. High-dose statin therapy and observation.

ant.jpg 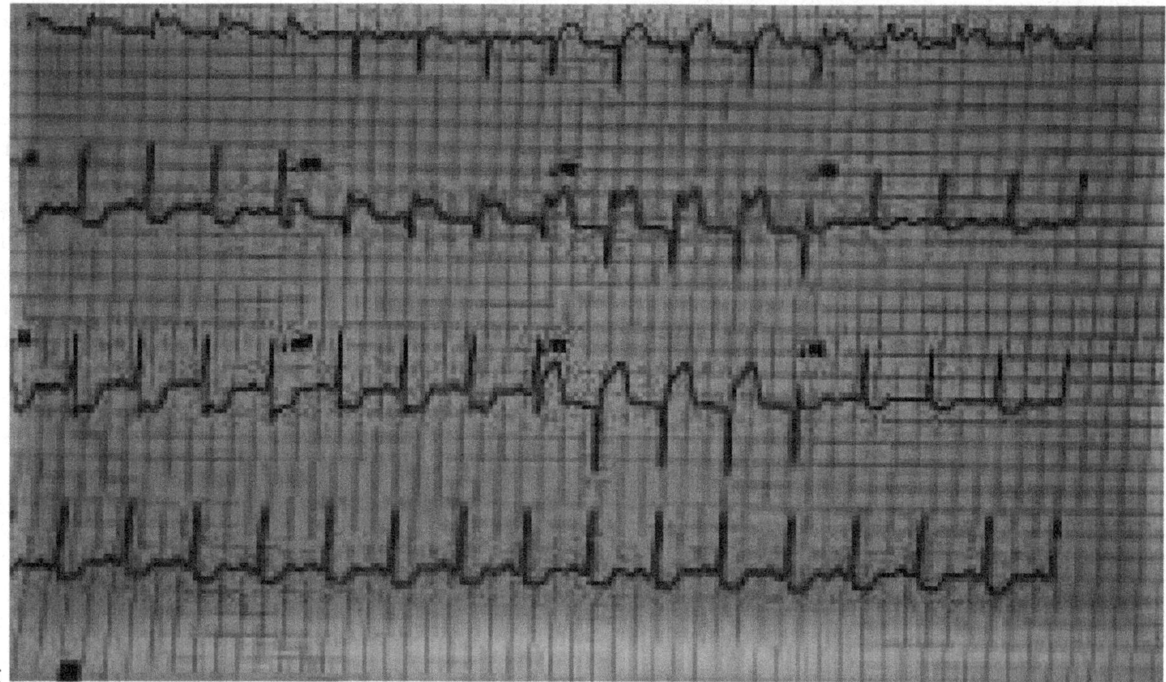

Figure 3.2: 47-year-old male

The correct answer is A. Immediate coronary angiography with intent for percutaneous coronary intervention (PCI). This patient is presenting with symptoms and signs consistent with an ST-elevation myocardial infarction (STEMI), likely induced by cocaine use. Cocaine can cause myocardial ischemia and infarction through coronary artery vasoconstriction and increased myocardial oxygen demand. The standard of care for STEMI is reperfusion therapy, preferably by PCI if it can be performed within the recommended time frame. Immediate coronary angiography will allow for direct visualization of the coronary anatomy and potential PCI to restore coronary blood flow. Option B is incorrect because, while benzodiazepines can be used to manage the agitation and hypertension associated with cocaine intoxication, they do not address the ongoing myocardial ischemia that requires reperfusion therapy. Option C is incorrect because thrombolytic therapy is generally contraindicated in cocaine-induced STEMI due to the increased risk of hemorrhagic complications, including intracranial hemorrhage, and because cocaine-induced STEMI is more often due to vasospasm rather than thrombosis. PCI is the preferred treatment if available. Option D is incorrect because, although high-dose statin therapy is part of the management of acute coronary syndromes, it is not the immediate treatment for ongoing STEMI. The priority is to restore coronary blood flow through reperfusion therapy. Cocaine can induce myocardial ischemia and infarction through coronary artery vasoconstriction or heightened myocardial energy demands, potentially accelerating atherosclerosis development and blood clot formation. Initial laboratory findings during presentation may appear normal, necessitating the use of cardiac myocyte necrosis markers such as myoglobin, CK-MB, troponin I, and troponin T to detect acute myocardial infarction (MI). High-sensitivity troponin stands out as the preferred biomarker for acute MI diagnosis. In cases of ST-segment elevation myocardial infarction (STEMI), initial markers are often within normal ranges as immediate reperfusion is prioritized. Conversely, abnormal CK-MB or troponin levels in patients without ST-segment elevation signal myocyte necrosis and MI presence. High-sensitivity troponin tests facilitate rapid heart attack assessment in emergency settings using 1- or 2-hour rule-out protocols. The universal MI definition involves elevated cardiac biomarkers exceeding the 99th percentile upper reference limit alongside evidence of myocardial ischemia indicated by ischemic symptoms, new ECG changes, new Q waves, or imaging revealing fresh loss of viable myocardium or wall motion abnormalities. Serum creatinine assessment is vital for risk evaluation, while estimated creatinine clearance guides appropriate dosing of specific antithrombotic medications like eptifibatide and enoxaparin. Cocaine exerts significant stress on the heart and vascular system, leading to various cardiovascular issues. The drug elevates blood pressure and heart rate, increasing the heart's workload and oxygen demands while constricting capillaries, reducing blood flow. This combination can result in immediate emergencies like heart attacks and long-term damage to the heart. The effects of cocaine on the heart include:

1. Coronary Artery Disease (CAD): Cocaine users are at risk of developing CAD, a condition that can lead to heart attacks, strokes, and sudden death.
2. Higher Blood Pressure: Cocaine significantly raises blood pressure, increasing the risk of cardiovascular problems and heart attacks.
3. Damage to the Heart's Structure: Cocaine use can physically damage the heart's structures, potentially leading to irregular heart rates and an increased risk of heart attack.
4. Heart Arrhythmias: Cocaine can cause irregular heart rates, affecting the heart's electrical system and potentially leading to life-threatening arrhythmias like ventricular tachycardia.
5. Congestive Heart Failure: Prolonged cocaine use can result in congestive heart failure, a condition where the heart muscle is unable to effectively pump blood throughout the body.
6. Long-term cocaine use can also impact the brain by constricting blood vessels, reducing oxygen levels, and causing serious issues like brain damage, aneurysms, strokes, seizures, and cognitive impairments. Seeking help for cocaine addiction is crucial to address these health risks effectively.

Agrawal PR et al Current strategies in the evaluation and management of cocaine-induced chest pain. Cardiol Rev. 2015 Nov-Dec;23(6):303-11. PMID: 25580707

3.21 Management of Recurrent Chest Pain with Normal Coronary Angiogram

Case 50

A 44-year-old woman presents to the clinic with recurrent episodes of chest pain that awaken her from sleep. The episodes are described as a constricting sensation over the precordium, lasting for 15 to 20 minutes and resolving spontaneously. She denies any precipitating factors such as exertion or stress. Her past medical history is unremarkable, and she takes no medications. She does not smoke and has no family history of coronary artery disease. An ECG during an episode shows transient ST-segment elevation in leads II, III, and aVF. Cardiac biomarkers are within normal limits. A subsequent coronary angiogram reveals no obstructive coronary artery disease.
Which of the following is the most appropriate management for preventing further episodes of this patient's chest pain?

- A. Initiate high-dose atorvastatin and daily aspirin.
- B. Begin treatment with a long-acting nitrate and a calcium channel blocker.
- C. Prescribe a beta-blocker with intrinsic sympathomimetic activity.
- D. Perform ergonovine provocation testing to confirm the diagnosis.

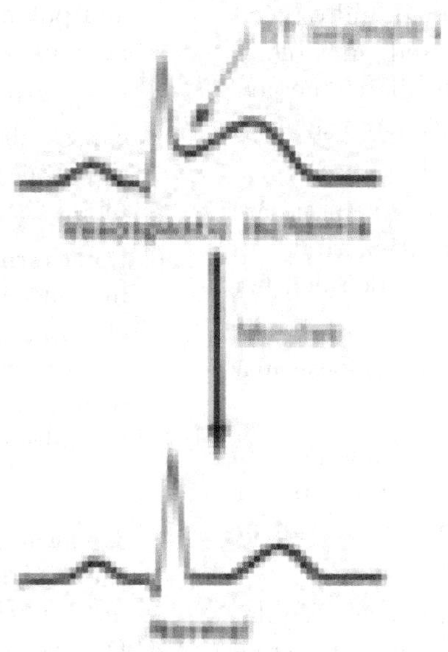

Figure 3.3: Prinzmetal (variant) angina)

The correct answer is B. Begin treatment with a long-acting nitrate and a calcium channel blocker. The patient's clinical presentation is consistent with Prinzmetal (variant) angina), which is characterized by episodic chest pain, often occurring at rest and sometimes awakening the patient from sleep, associated with transient ST-segment elevation on ECG. This condition is due to coronary artery vasospasm. Long-acting nitrates and calcium channel blockers are effective both for acute relief and prophylaxis of vasospastic episodes. These medications help prevent coronary artery spasm and are considered first-line therapy for Prinzmetal angina. Option A is incorrect because high-dose atorvastatin and daily aspirin are typically used in atherosclerotic coronary artery disease, which is not the primary issue in this patient, as her coronary angiogram did not show significant fixed stenoses. Option C is incorrect because beta-blockers can exacerbate coronary vasospasm by allowing unopposed alpha-1-mediated vasoconstriction, especially non-selective beta-blockers. Beta-blockers with intrinsic sympathomimetic activity are less likely to cause vasoconstriction but are still not the first-line treatment for Prinzmetal angina. Option D is incorrect because ergonovine provocation testing is not routinely recommended due to the risks involved, including the potential to induce severe and prolonged coronary spasm. It is typically reserved for cases where the diagnosis remains uncertain after noninvasive testing and should be performed in a controlled setting with close monitoring and ready access to vasodilator therapy. Patients presenting with chest pain and ST-segment elevation should undergo coronary arteriography to assess for fixed stenotic lesions, as their presence may signify an unstable phase of the disease necessitating aggressive medical therapy or revascularization. Even in the absence of significant lesions, there could be underlying endothelial disruption and plaque rupture. If coronary spasm is suspected, immediate measures should be taken to avoid triggers like cigarette smoking and cocaine. Episodes of coronary spasm typically respond well to nitrates, with both nitrates and calcium channel blockers (such as long-acting nifedipine, diltiazem, or amlodipine) proving effective for preventive management. Beta-blockers, by potentially allowing unopposed alpha-1-mediated vasoconstriction, have been associated with exacerbating coronary vasospasm. However, they may still have a role in treating patients with spasm related to fixed stenoses. Medications should be avoided or used with caution in individuals with coronary artery spasms:

1. Nonselective Beta-blockers: Drugs like propranolol can exacerbate coronary artery spasms and should be avoided
2. Aspirin: While low doses may be used cautiously, high doses of aspirin can inhibit prostacyclin production and may not be suitable for individuals with coronary artery spasms
3. Oral Sumatriptan: This medication used for acute migraines may be associated with coronary vasospasm and heart attacks, so its use should be avoided in individuals with known or suspected coronary artery spasms

4. Fluorouracil: Also known as 5-fluorouracil, this drug has been linked to inducing coronary artery spasms and should be avoided

de Luna AB et al. Prinzmetal angina: ECG changes and clinical considerations: a consensus paper. Ann Noninvasive Electrocardiol. 2014 Sep;19(5):442-53. PMID: 25262663

3.22 Management of Acute STEMI

Case 51

A 67-year-old man with a history of hypertension and hyperlipidemia presents to the emergency department with chest pain that started 2 hours ago. The pain is substernal, pressure-like, and radiates to his left arm. He also reports associated shortness of breath and diaphoresis. His blood pressure is 150/90 mmHg, heart rate is 85 bpm, and respiratory rate is 18 breaths per minute. Physical examination is unremarkable except for diaphoresis. An ECG shows ST-segment elevation in leads II, III, and aVF. He is given aspirin, a P2Y12 inhibitor, and sublingual nitroglycerin with partial relief of his chest pain. His initial troponin I level is within normal limits, and serum creatinine is 1.2 mg/dL (estimated GFR above 60 mL/min/1.73m2).
Which of the following is the most appropriate next step in the management of this patient?

- A. Repeat troponin measurement in 3 hours.
- B. Administer intravenous eptifibatide.
- C. Immediate coronary angiography with intent for percutaneous coronary intervention (PCI).
- D. Obtain a transthoracic echocardiogram to assess for wall motion abnormalities.

The correct answer is C. Immediate coronary angiography with intent for percutaneous coronary intervention (PCI). The patient is presenting with symptoms and ECG changes consistent with an ST-elevation myocardial infarction (STEMI). The universal definition of MI includes a rise of cardiac biomarkers with at least one value above the 99th percentile upper reference limit together with evidence of myocardial ischemia. However, in the acute setting of a STEMI, reperfusion therapy should not be delayed while waiting for cardiac biomarkers to become positive. Immediate coronary angiography is indicated to identify the occluded vessel and perform PCI to restore myocardial perfusion as quickly as possible, which is associated with improved outcomes. Option A is incorrect because, although serial troponin measurements are important for the diagnosis of myocardial infarction, they should not delay reperfusion therapy in a patient with a clear clinical presentation of STEMI. Option B is incorrect because, while eptifibatide is an antiplatelet agent used in the management of acute coronary syndromes, it is not the immediate priority in the management of STEMI where the primary goal is reperfusion, typically achieved through PCI. Option D is incorrect because, although an echocardiogram can provide information about wall motion abnormalities and overall cardiac function, it is not the immediate priority in the setting of STEMI where the focus is on rapid reperfusion. Primary percutaneous coronary intervention (PCI) involves immediate coronary angiography and stenting of the infarct-related artery, a superior approach to thrombolysis when performed by skilled operators in high-volume centers with rapid "door-to-balloon" times. Both US and European guidelines advocate for achieving door-to-balloon times within 90 minutes to optimize outcomes for patients with acute myocardial infarction (MI). Effective transfer systems have been shown in numerous studies to enhance patient outcomes. Timely transfer from non-PCI-capable hospitals to PCI-capable centers within 120 minutes can significantly improve results compared to fibrinolytic therapy, necessitating efficient systems for prompt identification, transfer, and PCI execution. Additionally, PCI carries a lower risk of hemorrhagic complications, such as intracranial hemorrhage, making it a preferred strategy for older patients and those unsuitable for fibrinolytic therapy. Primary percutaneous coronary intervention (PCI) and thrombolysis are both reperfusion therapies used in the treatment of acute myocardial infarction (MI). Here are the key differences between the two treatments based on the provided search results: Primary Percutaneous Coronary Intervention (PCI):

1. Effectiveness: Primary PCI is considered more effective than thrombolytic therapy, with a success rate of around 90% compared to 40-60% for throm-

bolysis.

2. Clinical Outcomes: Studies have shown that primary PCI is associated with better clinical outcomes, including reduced incidence of death, recurrent MI, and stroke at 6 weeks and 6 months after the index MI
3. Access Limitations: Primary PCI is often limited to hospitals with on-site cardiac surgery programs, which restricts access for many acute MI patients.

Thrombolysis:

1. Effectiveness: Thrombolytic therapy is less effective than primary PCI, with a lower success rate of around 40-60%
2. Mortality Benefit: In certain circumstances, such as in high-risk groups, thrombolysis may have a mortality benefit over primary PCI/
3. Time Factors: Thrombolysis can be a viable option within the first few hours of symptom onset, with comparable results to primary PCI during this early window.

In summary, while primary PCI is generally considered superior to thrombolytic therapy in terms of effectiveness and clinical outcomes, the choice between these treatments depends on factors like access to facilities and the patient's risk profile.

Partow-Navid R et al. Management of ST Elevation Myocardial Infarction (STEMI) in Different Settings. Int J Angiol. 2021 Mar;30(1):67-75. PMID: 34025097

Case Note

PCI is the preferred reperfusion strategy in STEMI if it can be performed within 90-120 minutes of first medical contact.

3.23 PLATO Trial and NSTEMI

Case 52

A 63-year-old woman with a history of hypertension and diabetes presents to the emergency department with chest discomfort and diaphoresis that started 3 hours ago while she was gardening. Her discomfort is relieved with sublingual nitroglycerin in the emergency department. Her initial ECG shows ST-segment depression in leads V4-V6 and her initial troponin I level is elevated. She is given aspirin, a high-dose statin, and a beta-blocker. Her blood pressure is 135/85 mmHg, heart rate is 78 bpm, and she is now asymptomatic. Given her presentation and initial management, which of the following is the most appropriate next step in the management of this patient's acute coronary syndrome?

- A. Administer a loading dose of clopidogrel and schedule for coronary angiography within 24 hours.
- B. Administer a loading dose of prasugrel and schedule for coronary angiography within 24 hours.
- C. Administer a loading dose of ticagrelor and schedule for coronary angiography within 24 hours.
- D. Withhold P2Y12 inhibitor therapy until coronary anatomy is defined via angiography.

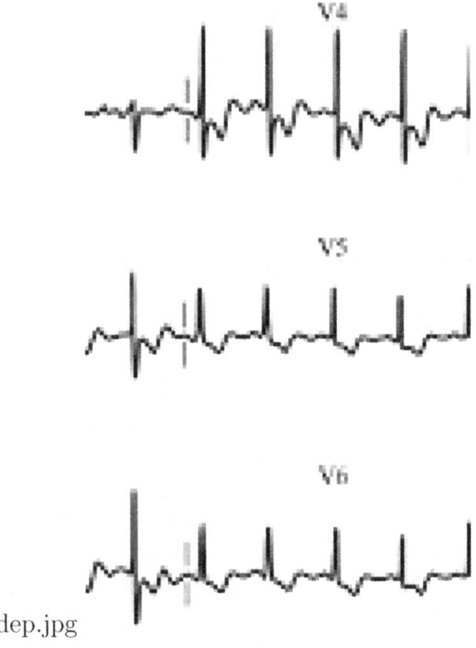

dep.jpg

Figure 3.4: A 63-year-old woman

The correct answer is C. Administer a loading dose of ticagrelor and schedule for coronary angiography within 24 hours. The patient is presenting with non-ST-segment elevation acute coronary syndrome (NSTE-ACS), as evidenced by her symptoms, ECG changes, and elevated troponin level. According to the ESC guidelines, ticagrelor is recommended for all patients at moderate to high risk for ACS (class I recommendation). The PLATO trial demonstrated that ticagrelor reduced cardiovascular death, MI, and stroke compared with clopidogrel, without a substantial increase in overall bleeding rates, although non-CABG-related bleeding was modestly higher. When using ticagrelor, low-dose aspirin is recommended to avoid the attenuation of its benefits observed with higher-dose aspirin. Option A is incorrect because, while clopidogrel is an option for patients who cannot receive ticagrelor or prasugrel, ticagrelor is preferred due to its more potent and consistent antiplatelet effect, as well as its mortality benefit demonstrated in the PLATO trial. Option B is incorrect because prasugrel is recommended for patients in whom PCI is planned and who are not at high risk for life-threatening bleeding. However, prasugrel is contraindicated in patients with a history of stroke or TIA, and caution is advised in patients who are elderly or have low body weight. Since the patient's history does not mention a prior stroke or TIA, and there is no information on her body weight or age, prasugrel could be considered, but ticagrelor remains the preferred agent due to its broader applicability and the class I recommendation for its use in moderate to high-risk ACS patients. Option D is incorrect because withholding P2Y12 inhibitor therapy until after coronary angiography may delay the provision of optimal antiplatelet therapy, which is crucial for reducing the risk of further ischemic events in NSTE-ACS.Initiating P2Y12 inhibitor therapy promptly is recommended unless contraindicated. Risk assessment is crucial in determining the appropriate management for patients with acute coronary syndrome (ACS), such as non-ST-segment elevation myocardial infarction (NSTEMI). High-risk ACS patients benefit most from treatments like glycoprotein IIb/IIIa inhibitors, LMWH heparin, and early invasive catheterization. According to ACC/AHA guidelines, high-risk patients typically require an early invasive strategy involving catheterization and revascularization. Those without high-risk features can undergo either an invasive or noninvasive approach, utilizing stress testing to detect residual ischemia or high risk. The ICTUS trial supports a strategy involving selective coronary angiography and revascularization for instability or inducible ischemia, even in troponin-positive patients (ACC/AHA class IIb recommendation). Bedside risk stratification tools include the GRACE Risk Score and the TIMI Risk Score. The GRACE Risk Score, applicable to patients with or without ST elevation, offers enhanced risk discrimination based on variables like age, Killip class, blood pressure, ST-segment deviation, cardiac arrest at presentation, serum creatinine, cardiac enzyme levels, and heart rate.

The TIMI Risk Score comprises seven factors such as age over 65, multiple cardiac risk factors, prior significant coronary stenosis, ST-segment deviation, recent anginal events, recent aspirin use, and elevated cardiac markers.

James SK et al.Ticagrelor versus clopidogrel in patients with acute coronary syndromes intended for non-invasive management: substudy from prospective randomised PLATelet inhibition and patient Outcomes (PLATO) trial. BMJ. 2011 Jun 17;342:d3527. PMID: 21685437

3.24 OASIS Trial and NSTEMI

Case 53

72-year-old man with a history of chronic kidney disease (stage III), hypertension, and previous transient ischemic attack (TIA) presents to the emergency department with chest pain and diaphoresis that began 6 hours ago. His medications include aspirin, atorvastatin, and lisinopril. On examination, his blood pressure is 140/85 mmHg, heart rate is 95 bpm, and he appears in moderate distress. An ECG shows ST-segment depression in leads II, III, and aVF. Initial troponin levels are elevated. He is diagnosed with non-ST-segment elevation myocardial infarction (NSTEMI) and is scheduled for early coronary angiography.
Given the patient's history and presentation, which of the following is the most appropriate anticoagulant therapy to initiate?

- A. Enoxaparin 1 mg/kg subcutaneously every 12 hours.
- B. Fondaparinux 2.5 mg subcutaneously once daily.
- C. Unfractionated heparin intravenous infusion.
- D. Bivalirudin intravenous infusion.

The correct answer is B. Fondaparinux 2.5 mg subcutaneously once daily. This patient with NSTEMI is at high risk for bleeding due to his age and history of chronic kidney disease. Fondaparinux, a factor Xa inhibitor, has been shown to be as effective as enoxaparin in preventing death, myocardial infarction, and refractory ischemia, with a significant reduction in major bleeding, as demonstrated in the OASIS-5 trial. This reduction in bleeding is particularly important in older adults and those at high risk for bleeding. Additionally, the patient's history of TIA suggests a need to minimize the risk of cerebral hemorrhage, which further supports the use of fondaparinux. If the patient undergoes coronary intervention, additional unfractionated heparin may be given during the procedure to prevent catheter-related thrombosis, as per the FUTURA trial recommendations. Option A is incorrect because enoxaparin, while effective in preventing recurrent ischemic events, may carry a higher bleeding risk compared to fondaparinux, especially in older patients and those with renal impairment. Option C is incorrect because unfractionated heparin requires close monitoring of anticoagulation status, which can be challenging in patients with chronic kidney disease, and it may also have a higher risk of bleeding compared to fondaparinux. Option D is incorrect because bivalirudin is a direct thrombin inhibitor that has been shown to be associated with less bleeding than heparin plus glycoprotein IIb/IIIa inhibitor. However, it does not have an FDA-approved indication for NSTEMI care outside of the setting of percutaneous coronary intervention (PCI), and the patient's history of TIA may increase the risk of cerebral hemorrhage with its use. The OASIS-5 trial (Fifth Organization to Assess Strategies in Ischemic Syndromes) was a randomized, double-blind, double-dummy trial comparing fondaparinux with enoxaparin in patients with unstable angina or non-ST-segment elevation myocardial infarction (NSTEMI). The trial included 20,078 patients and aimed to assess the efficacy and safety of fondaparinux, a factor Xa inhibitor, versus enoxaparin, a low molecular weight heparin (LMWH), in the management of acute coronary syndrome (ACS). The results of the OASIS-5 trial showed that fondaparinux was similar to enoxaparin for short-term efficacy in preventing death, myocardial infarction, and refractory ischemia. However, fondaparinux significantly reduced major bleeding by one-half and 30-day mortality by 17% compared to enoxaparin. This reduction in major bleeding was particularly important for older adults and those at high risk for bleeding, such as patients with renal impairment or a history of bleeding disorders. The trial also addressed the management of patients undergoing percutaneous coronary intervention (PCI). It was found that catheter thrombus was more common in patients receiving fondaparinux than in those receiving enoxaparin alone. However, this issue was largely prevented by using unfractionated heparin (UFH) at the time of PCI, without compromising the benefits of upstream fondaparinux. In conclusion, the OASIS-5 trial demonstrated that fondaparinux has a superior safety profile with a significant reduction in bleeding events compared to enoxaparin, while maintaining similar efficacy in preventing ischemic events in patients with ACS, making it a valuable anticoagulant option, especially in high-risk bleeding populations

Karthikeyan G et al. Fondaparinux in the treatment of acute coronary syndromes: evidence from OASIS 5 and 6. Expert Rev Cardiovasc Ther. 2009 Mar;7(3):241-9. PMID: 19296760.

3.25 PROVE-IT Trial and ACS

Case 54

A 58-year-old woman with no prior medical history presents to the emergency department with severe chest pain radiating to her left arm and jaw that started 1 hour ago. She is a smoker and has a family history of coronary artery disease. On examination, her blood pressure is 160/90 mmHg, heart rate is 110 bpm, and she is diaphoretic with cool extremities. An ECG shows ST-segment elevation in leads V2-V4. Initial troponin T is elevated. She is diagnosed with an ST-segment elevation myocardial infarction (STEMI) and undergoes primary percutaneous coronary intervention (PCI) with stent placement in the left anterior descending artery. Post-procedure, her chest pain has resolved, and her vital signs have stabilized. Based on the PROVE-IT trial findings and current guidelines, which of the following is the most appropriate lipid-lowering therapy to initiate in this patient?

- A. Atorvastatin 80 mg orally once daily.
- B. Pravastatin 40 mg orally once daily.
- C. Simvastatin 20 mg orally once daily.
- D. Wait for LDL cholesterol results before initiating statin therapy.

The correct answer is A. Atorvastatin 80 mg orally once daily. The PROVE-IT trial demonstrated that intensive lipid-lowering therapy with atorvastatin 80 mg daily improved outcomes in patients with acute coronary syndromes (ACS) compared to moderate lipid-lowering therapy with pravastatin 40 mg daily. The benefits of high-intensity statin therapy were observed as early as 3 months after initiation of therapy. Current guidelines recommend high-intensity statin therapy for all patients with ACS, regardless of baseline LDL cholesterol levels, to reduce the risk of subsequent cardiovascular events. Option B is incorrect because pravastatin 40 mg daily represents moderate-intensity statin therapy, which was shown to be less effective than high-intensity statin therapy in the PROVE-IT trial for patients with ACS. Option C is incorrect because simvastatin 20 mg daily is considered low-intensity statin therapy and is not adequate for the management of patients with ACS, who require high-intensity statin therapy according to current guidelines. Option D is incorrect because the initiation of high-intensity statin therapy should not be delayed until LDL cholesterol results are available. The benefit of statins in ACS is not solely dependent on the LDL cholesterol level but also on their pleiotropic effects, which include stabilization of atherosclerotic plaques, improvement of endothelial function, and reduction of inflammation. The PROVE-IT (Pravastatin or Atorvastatin Evaluation and Infection Therapy) trial was a landmark study designed to compare the efficacy of intensive versus moderate lipid-lowering therapy in patients who had recently experienced acute coronary syndromes (ACS). Specifically, the trial aimed to assess whether intensive lipid-lowering therapy with atorvastatin 80 mg daily would provide greater protection against death or major cardiovascular events compared to moderate lipid-lowering therapy with pravastatin 40 mg daily in this high-risk patient population. The findings from the PROVE-IT trial were significant and have had a profound impact on clinical practice. The trial demonstrated that intensive lipid-lowering therapy with atorvastatin 80 mg daily resulted in a 16% reduction in the primary endpoint, which was a composite of death from any cause, myocardial infarction, unstable angina requiring hospitalization, revascularization, or stroke, compared to moderate lipid-lowering therapy with pravastatin 40 mg daily. This benefit was observed as early as 30 days after initiation of therapy and was consistent across pre-specified subgroups. The trial's results challenged previous guidelines by suggesting that target low-density lipoprotein (LDL) cholesterol levels should be lower in patients following an ACS. The protective effect of intensive lipid-lowering was evident early on after therapy initiation and was consistent over the mean two-year follow-up period. The magnitude of improvement with intensive lipid-lowering over standard therapy was comparable to the benefit seen when comparing statins to placebo, highlighting the importance of aggressive lipid management in patients with ACS. In summary, the PROVE-IT trial established the superiority of high-dose atorvastatin over moderate-dose pravastatin in reducing the risk of subsequent cardiovascular events in patients with ACS, leading to the current recommendation for high-intensity statin therapy in this patient population regardless of baseline LDL cholesterol levels.

Murphy SA et al. Reduction in recurrent cardiovascular events with intensive lipid-lowering statin therapy compared with moderate lipid-lowering statin therapy after acute coronary syndromes from the PROVE IT-TIMI 22 J Am Coll Cardiol. 2009 Dec 15;54(25):2358-62. PMID: 20082923

3.26 Early Invasive Strategy VS Late Strategy

Case 55

A 67-year-old man with a history of hypertension and hyperlipidemia presents to the emergency department with intermittent episodes of chest pain at rest that began 12 hours ago. He reports that each episode lasts for about 10-15 minutes. He has taken aspirin 325 mg at home with no relief. His current medications include lisinopril and atorvastatin. On examination, his blood pressure is 150/90 mmHg, heart rate is 88 bpm, and he is currently pain-free. An ECG shows ST-segment depression in leads II, III, and aVF. His initial troponin I level is elevated at 0.5 ng/mL (normal under 0.03 ng/mL). Echocardiography reveals an ejection fraction of 45% with no wall motion abnormalities.
Based on the ACC/AHA guidelines, which of the following is the most appropriate next step in the management of this patient?

- A. Continue medical management and observe.
- B. Schedule a stress test to be performed during this admission.
- C. Proceed with an early invasive strategy with cardiac catheterization.
- D. Discharge with outpatient follow-up and stress testing within 72 hours.

The correct answer is C. Proceed with an early invasive strategy with cardiac catheterization According to the ACC/AHA guidelines for managing Acute Coronary Syndromes (ACS), an early invasive strategy is indicated in patients with high-risk features. This patient has several high-risk features that warrant an early invasive approach: recurrent angina at rest (chest pain or discomfort), elevated troponin levels, and ST-segment depression on ECG. These features suggest ongoing ischemia and an increased risk of adverse cardiac events, making early cardiac catheterization and potential revascularization the most appropriate management strategy. Option A is incorrect because medical management alone is not sufficient for a patient with high-risk features of unstable angina or non-ST-elevation myocardial infarction (NSTEMI). Option B is incorrect because a stress test is not the appropriate next step for a patient with high-risk features who should undergo an early invasive strategy. Stress testing is more appropriate for patients with low to intermediate risk features who are stable. Option D is incorrect because discharging the patient with outpatient follow-up and stress testing within 72 hours does not address the immediate high-risk features that this patient presents with. This approach would be more appropriate for a patient with low-risk features and a stable presentation. In the case of patients with a high-risk and unstable condition who undergo percutaneous coronary intervention (PCI), it is advisable to contemplate the administration of an intravenous glycoprotein IIb/IIIa antagonist. Examples of such antagonists include tirofiban, which can be administered at a loading dose of 25 g/kg/min followed by a maintenance dose of 0.15 g/kg/min, or eptifibatide at a dosage of 180 g/kg. The recommended dosage for Nitroglycerin as an anti-ischemic therapy is 0.3-0.6 mg administered sublingually or through buccal spray. If the patient continues to experience chest discomfort even after receiving three doses of Nitroglycerin administered at 5-minute intervals, it is advisable to contemplate the administration of intravenous Nitroglycerin. The suggested heart rate for the administration of beta blockers as a form of anti-ischemic therapy is within the range of 50-60 beats per minute. The patient should be admitted to a unit where continuous electrocardiogram (ECG) monitoring can be conducted. Initially, it is recommended that the patient remain at bed rest. In addition, the administration of morphine sulfate intravenously at a dosage of 2-5 mg every 5-30 minutes may be considered for chest discomfort that is unresponsive to other treatments. Furthermore, the inclusion of a high dose of HMG-CoA reductase inhibitor and the consideration of an ACE inhibitor should also be considered. The immediate invasive strategy for managing patients with non-ST segment elevation acute coronary syndrome (NSTE-ACS) encompasses individuals who exhibit refractory angina, indications of heart failure or the development or exacerbation of mitral regurgitation, hemodynamic instability, recurrent angina or ischemia during periods of rest or with minimal exertion despite intensive medical treatment, and sustained episodes of ventricular tachycardia or ventricular fibrillation. The management of patients with non-ST-segment elevation acute coronary syndrome (NSTE-ACS) typically involves an early invasive strategy. This strategy is recommended for patients who do not meet the criteria for an immediate invasive approach but have certain indicators, such as a GRACE risk score greater than 140, a temporal change in troponin levels, or the presence of new or presumably new ST segment depression. The delayed invasive strategy for managing patients with non-ST-segment elevation acute coronary syndrome (NSTE-ACS) encompasses individuals who do not meet the aforementioned criteria but have additional factors such as diabetes mellitus, renal insufficiency (estimated glomerular filtration rate under 60 mL/min per 1.73 m^2), reduced left ventricular systolic function (ejection fraction under 0.40), early postinfarction angina, a history of percutaneous coronary intervention within the past 6 months, prior coronary artery bypass graft surgery, or a GRACE risk score between 109 and 140 or a TIMI risk score of 2 or higher. The preferred approach for patients with low-risk scores and non-ST segment elevation acute coronary syndrome (NSTE-ACS) is the ischemia-guided strategy. This strategy encompasses low-risk score patients, such as those with a TIMI score of 0 or 1 and a GRACE score of less than 109. It also includes low-risk, troponin-negative female patients, as well as situations where patient or clinician preference is the determining factor in the absence of high-risk characteristics. The principles governing the long-term management of unstable angina encompass several key factors. These include emphasizing the significance of smoking cessation, attaining an optimal weight, adhering to a diet low in saturated and trans fats, engaging in regular exercise, and effectively controlling blood pressure, lipid levels, and diabetic conditions. The principles can be further strengthened through the promotion of patient participation in a cardiac rehabilitation program. To effectively manage unstable angina over an extended period, it is recommended to maintain a regimen consisting of several medications. These include aspirin at a dosage of 75-100 mg per day, a P2Y12 receptor antagonist such as clopidogrel, prasugrel, or ticagrelor for a minimum duration of one year, a beta blocker, a high-dose statin such as atorvastatin at 80 mg daily (with the option to add ezetimibe at a dosage of 10 mg daily if necessary to achieve a low-density lipoprotein level below 70 mg/dL), and an ACE inhibitor or angiotensin receptor blocker. The latter is particularly important for individuals who are hypertensive, diabetic, or have a reduced left ventricular ejection fraction. It is advised to continue these medications for long-term management of unstable angina.

Bae S et al. Early Invasive Strategy Based on the Time of Symptom Onset of Non-ST-Segment Elevation Myocardial Infarction. JACC Cardiovasc Interv. 2023 Jan 9;16(1):64-75.PMID: 36599589

Case Note

In this case, the patient has multiple high-risk features, including:

- Elevated troponin levels
- ST-segment depression on ECG
- Reduced left ventricular ejection fraction (45

The presence of these high-risk features indicates a higher risk for adverse events, and an early invasive strategy with cardiac catheterization is recommended .

Table 3.4: Indications for Catheterization and Percutaneous Coronary Intervention NSTEMI

Class	Indications	Details
I	Early invasive strategy for high-risk indicators	Recurrent angina/ischemia at rest or with low-level activity, Elevated troponin, ST-segment depression, Recurrent ischemia with evidence of HF, High-risk stress test result, EF ¡ 40%, Hemodynamic instability, Sustained ventricular tachycardia, PCI within 6 months, Prior CABG
I (without high-risk indicators)	Early conservative or early invasive strategy	In the absence of high-risk indicators
IIa	Early invasive strategy for repeated ACS presentations despite therapy	For patients with repeated presentations for ACS despite therapy
III	Avoidance of revascularization	Extensive comorbidities in patients in whom benefits of revascularization are not likely to outweigh the risks
Potential False Positive	Low likelihood of ACS	Acute chest pain with low likelihood of ACS

3.27 Silent Myocardial Infarction

Case 56

A 74-year-old woman with a history of type 2 diabetes mellitus and hypertension presents to the clinic for a routine follow-up. She mentions she has been feeling generally unwell with episodes of nausea and shortness of breath, particularly when walking her dog, which she attributes to her age. She denies any chest pain. Her current medications include metformin, lisinopril, and amlodipine. On examination, her blood pressure is 145/85 mmHg, heart rate is 78 bpm, and she has no respiratory distress at rest. An ECG performed in the clinic shows Q waves in leads II, III, and aVF with T wave inversions in the same leads. Her last ECG 6 months ago was normal.
Based on the clinical scenario, which of the following is the most appropriate next step in the management of this patient?

- A. Reassure the patient and continue current management.
- B. Initiate high-dose statin therapy and schedule a stress test.
- C. Refer for immediate cardiac catheterization.
- D. Obtain cardiac biomarkers and a transthoracic echocardiogram.

wave.jpg

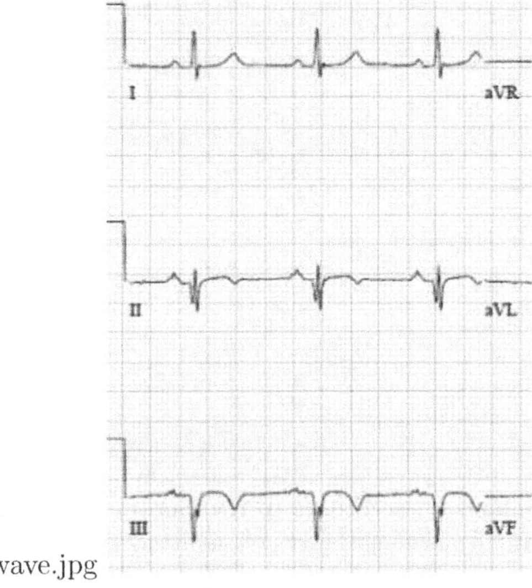

Figure 3.5: A 74-year-old woman

The correct answer is D. Obtain cardiac biomarkers and a transthoracic echocardiogram. The patient's ECG changes are suggestive of a possible silent myocardial infarction, which is not uncommon in older patients, women, and those with diabetes mellitus. These patients often present without the classic symptom of chest pain. The new Q waves and T wave inversions in the inferior leads on ECG are concerning for an infarction that may have gone unnoticed by the patient. The next step is to obtain cardiac biomarkers to assess for recent myocardial damage and a transthoracic echocardiogram to evaluate for wall motion abnormalities, which can confirm the diagnosis and assess the extent of cardiac involvement. Option A is incorrect because the new ECG changes are significant and warrant further investigation, despite the absence of chest pain. Option B is incorrect because, although initiating high-dose statin therapy may be part of the long-term management for this patient, it is not the immediate next step before confirming the diagnosis and extent of myocardial infarction. Option C is incorrect because immediate cardiac catheterization may be indicated after confirming an acute myocardial infarction with cardiac biomarkers and echocardiogram, especially if there is evidence of ongoing ischemia or complications. However, it is not the first step before confirming the diagnosis. Option D is the most appropriate next step because it involves both confirming the diagnosis of myocardial infarction with biomarkers and assessing cardiac function with an echocardiogram, which is crucial for guiding further management. The diagnostic criteria for acute myocardial infarction (AMI) are based on a combination of clinical findings, including cardiac biomarkers, electrocardiogram (ECG) changes, and symptoms. The universally accepted criteria include:

1. Cardiac Troponins: Elevation of cardiac troponins in peripheral blood is mandatory to establish a diagnosis of myocardial infarction. Troponins are highly sensitive and specific biomarkers of myocardial injury and are considered the gold standard for detecting myocardial necrosis.
2. ECG Changes: The presence of ST elevations, ST depressions, T-wave inversions, and pathological Q-waves on the ECG can be indicative of myocardial ischemia and infarction. These changes help localize the area of the heart that is affected and the extent of the ischemia.
3. Symptoms: Patients may present with typical ischemic chest pain, or they may experience dyspnea, nausea, unexplained weakness, or a combination of these symptoms. While symptoms are important, the diagnosis of AMI does not solely rely on them, especially since some patients, such as those with diabetes or the elderly, may have a silent or atypical presentation.

Kolesova MV et al Silent Myocardial Infarction: A Case Report. Cureus. 2023 Aug 22;15(8):e43906. PMID: 37638270

Case Note

The classification of myocardial infarction according to the European Society of Cardiology (ESC), American College of Cardiology (ACC), and American Heart Association (AHA) includes several types of MI: Type 1: Spontaneous myocardial infarction related to atherosclerotic plaque rupture with resulting intraluminal thrombus.

- Type 2: Myocardial infarction secondary to an ischemic imbalance, such as coronary endothelial dysfunction, coronary artery spasm, or conditions leading to increased oxygen demand or decreased supply.
- Type 3: Myocardial infarction resulting in death when biomarker values are unavailable.
- Type 4a: Myocardial infarction related to percutaneous coronary intervention (PCI).
- Type 4b: Myocardial infarction related to stent thrombosis.

In addition to these criteria, the diagnosis of MI can be supported by imaging evidence of new loss of viable myocardium or new regional wall motion abnormality in the context of a clinical presentation consistent with myocardial ischemia.

3.28 Suspicion of Reinfarction Case

Case 57

A 63-year-old man with a history of coronary artery disease and a previous myocardial infarction (MI) one week ago presents to the emergency department with severe chest pain that started 2 hours ago. The pain is similar to his previous MI, described as a heavy pressure in the center of his chest, radiating to his left arm. He is diaphoretic and appears in distress. His current medications include aspirin, clopidogrel, atorvastatin, and metoprolol. On examination, his blood pressure is 140/85 mmHg, heart rate is 95 bpm, and he has an S3 gallop. An ECG shows ST-segment elevation in leads II, III, and aVF. His initial troponin I level is elevated at 0.8 ng/mL normal < 0.03 ng/mL, which is unchanged from his levels 24 hours ago.
Based on the clinical scenario, which of the following is the most appropriate next step in the management of this patient?

- A. Administer fibrinolytic therapy immediately.
- B. Repeat troponin I levels in 3-4 hours to assess for a rising trend.
- C. Obtain CK-MB levels and compare them to previous values.
- D. Proceed with urgent coronary angiography.

The correct answer is C. Obtain CK-MB levels and compare them to previous values. In a patient with a recent myocardial infarction, troponin levels may remain elevated for several days to a week or longer, which limits their utility in diagnosing a new, early reinfarction. CK-MB levels, on the other hand, typically return to normal within 24 hours after an MI. Therefore, if there is a suspicion of reinfarction, as in this patient who presents with symptoms and ECG changes consistent with a new infarction, measuring CK-MB levels can be helpful. If the CK-MB has normalized since the last MI and is now elevated again, this would suggest a new myocardial injury. Option A is incorrect because fibrinolytic therapy is generally contraindicated in patients who have had recent surgery, trauma, or other risks for bleeding, and it is not the first-line treatment when coronary angiography and potential percutaneous coronary intervention (PCI) are available. Option B is incorrect because troponin levels may not show a rising trend in the early hours of reinfarction due to their prolonged elevation after an initial MI. Option D is incorrect as the immediate next step because, although urgent coronary angiography may be indicated, it is important to first establish biochemical evidence of reinfarction, especially when the troponin levels have not changed. If CK-MB is elevated, indicating a new MI, urgent angiography would then be the appropriate management. CK-MB (Creatine Kinase-MB) and troponins are both biomarkers used to diagnose myocardial infarction (MI), but they have different characteristics in terms of timing and specificity for cardiac muscle injury. CK-MB:

1. Rises within 4-6 hours after the onset of MI, peaks at about 24 hours, and returns to normal within 48-72 hours.
2. Because CK-MB clears from the bloodstream relatively quickly, it can be useful for diagnosing reinfarction that occurs shortly after an initial MI.
3. Less specific than troponin as it can be elevated in conditions involving skeletal muscle damage.

Troponins (Troponin I and Troponin T):

1. Rise within 3-12 hours after the onset of MI, peak at 24-48 hours, and can remain elevated for 1-2 weeks.
2. Highly specific for cardiac muscle injury and are considered the gold standard for MI diagnosis.
3. Because of their prolonged elevation after an MI, troponins are not as useful for diagnosing early reinfarction.
4. Troponins are also used for risk stratification and prognosis in patients with acute coronary syndromes.

In summary, while both CK-MB and troponins are used to diagnose MI, troponins are more specific to cardiac tissue and remain elevated longer, making them more useful for late presentations of MI. CK-MB, with its shorter duration of elevation, can be helpful in diagnosing a new MI that occurs soon after an initial event

White HD et al Reinfarction after percutaneous coronary intervention or medical management using the universal definition in patients with total occlusion after myocardial infarction: results from long-term follow-up of the Occluded Artery Trial (OAT) cohort. Am Heart J. 2012 Apr;163(4):563-71. PMID: 22520521

Reddy K et al Recent advances in the diagnosis and treatment of acute myocardial infarction. World J Cardiol. 2015 May 26;7(5):243-76.PMID: 26015857

3.29 Fibrinolytic Therapy VS PCI

Case 58

A 68-year-old man with a history of controlled hypertension presents to the emergency department with severe chest pain that started 2 hours ago. The pain is described as a crushing sensation behind the sternum, radiating to his left arm. He is diaphoretic and appears anxious. His blood pressure on presentation is 190/115 mmHg, heart rate is 88 bpm, and he is in sinus rhythm. An ECG shows ST-segment elevation of 0.2 mV in leads V2 through V4. His past medical history is significant for a transient ischemic attack (TIA) 9 months ago, from which he fully recovered. His medications include hydrochlorothiazide and amlodipine.
Based on the clinical scenario, which of the following is the most appropriate next step in the management of this patient?

- A. Administer fibrinolytic therapy after controlling blood pressure.
- B. Perform immediate coronary angiography with the intent to perform primary percutaneous coronary intervention (PCI).
- C. Administer intravenous nitroglycerin and reassess the ECG in 30 minutes.
- D. Treat with beta-blockers and schedule a stress test for the next day.

The correct answer is B. Perform immediate coronary angiography with the intent to perform primary percutaneous coronary intervention (PCI). The patient is presenting with symptoms and ECG findings consistent with an ST-elevation myocardial infarction (STEMI). Given the patient's history of a TIA within the past year, fibrinolytic therapy is relatively contraindicated due to the increased risk of intracranial hemorrhage. Additionally, his blood pressure is significantly elevated, which is another relative contraindication to fibrinolytic therapy. Primary PCI is the preferred treatment for STEMI when it can be performed in a timely manner by experienced operators, as it is associated with better outcomes compared to fibrinolytic therapy, including a lower risk of intracranial hemorrhage and a higher rate of artery patency. Option A is incorrect because, although controlling blood pressure is necessary, the patient's recent TIA makes fibrinolytic therapy a less safe option compared to primary PCI. Option C is incorrect because, while intravenous nitroglycerin can help with chest pain and ischemia, it does not address the underlying cause of the STEMI and the need for immediate reperfusion therapy. Option D is incorrect because beta-blockers are not the initial treatment for STEMI, and scheduling a stress test for the next day is inappropriate given the acute nature of the patient's presentation and the need for immediate reperfusion. Following the placement of drug-eluting or bare metal stents in acute coronary syndrome (ACS) patients, a standard recommendation is dual antiplatelet therapy for one year, irrespective of stent type. Extending dual antiplatelet therapy beyond one year, as studied in Dual Antiplatelet Therapy (DAPT) trials for up to 30 months, demonstrated reduced incidences of death, myocardial infarction (MI), and stroke in patients with drug-eluting stents. However, this prolonged therapy also showed an increased risk of bleeding and potential mortality elevation. Prolonged use of clopidogrel post drug-eluting stent placement should be individualized based on thrombotic and bleeding risks. For elective or stable percutaneous coronary intervention (PCI) cases unrelated to ACS, the recommended duration of dual antiplatelet therapy is a minimum of 1 month for bare metal stents and at least 3 months for drug-eluting stents. These recommendations are informed by stent studies' therapy durations and the understanding of endothelialization timing post bare metal and drug-eluting stent implantation. In situations where PCI is inaccessible or the time from initial medical contact to PCI exceeds 120 minutes without contraindications, intravenous fibrinolysis is a viable treatment option for ST-segment elevation myocardial infarction (STEMI) patients. Optimal door-to-needle time for fibrinolysis should ideally be under 30 minutes to maximize its benefits. Complications associated with fibrinolysis include bleeding, reperfusion arrhythmias, and allergic reactions, particularly with streptokinase use. In cases where chest pain or ST elevation persists beyond 90 minutes post-fibrinolysis, consideration should be given to referral for rescue PCI. Additionally, coronary angiography post-fibrinolysis is advisable for individuals experiencing recurrent angina or displaying high-risk features like significant ST elevation, signs of heart failure, or decreased systolic blood pressure. Regarding non-ST segment elevation myocardial infarction (NSTEMI), fibrinolytic therapy is not recommended as part of initial management. Different management strategies are employed for individuals diagnosed with NSTEMI compared to those with ST-segment elevation myocardial infarction. The potential complications of prolonged use of clopidogrel post drug-eluting stent placement primarily involve an increased risk of bleeding complications. Studies, including the Dual Antiplatelet Therapy (DAPT) trials, have explored the outcomes of extending dual antiplatelet therapy (DAPT) with aspirin and clopidogrel beyond the standard recommendation of one year after coronary stenting.

1. Increased Bleeding Risk: Extending clopidogrel therapy beyond six months after stent placement does not significantly reduce death or ischemic events but increases the risk of bleeding complications.
2. This finding is consistent across various studies, indicating that while prolonged DAPT can reduce incidences of myocardial infarction (MI), death, and stroke, it also poses a significant risk of major bleeding.
3. No Significant Reduction in Ischemic Events with Prolonged Therapy: The benefits of reducing ischemic events such as death, MI, and stroke do not significantly outweigh the increased bleeding risk associated with prolonged clopidogrel use beyond the standard duration.
4. Some studies have found that long-term DAPT might not significantly affect the reduction in the risk of death from any cause, MI, or stroke, and is not associated with minor or major bleeding events.
5. Individualized Therapy Based on Risk Assessment: Given the increased risk of bleeding, the decision to extend clopidogrel therapy beyond the recommended duration should be individualized, taking into account both thrombotic and bleeding risks.
6. Patients with a higher risk of ischemic events might benefit from prolonged therapy, but this must be carefully weighed against their risk of bleeding.
7. Consideration of Alternative Antiplatelet Agents: The results and recommendations might vary if alternative P2Y12 inhibitors, such as prasugrel or ticagrelor, are used instead of clopidogrel. These agents have different efficacy and safety profiles, which could influence the optimal duration of DAPT.

In summary, while prolonged use of clopidogrel post drug-eluting stent placement can reduce the risk of certain ischemic events, it significantly increases the risk of bleeding. The decision to extend DAPT beyond the standard duration should be made on an individual basis, considering the patient's specific risk factors for both thrombotic and bleeding events

Armstrong PWet al. Fibrinolysis or primary PCI in ST-segment elevation myocardial infarction. N Engl J Med. 2013 Apr 11;368(15):1379-87 PMID: 23473396

Case 58B

A 58-year-old woman with no significant past medical history presents to the emergency department 45 minutes after the onset of severe chest pain, described as a squeezing sensation across her chest with radiation to her left arm. She is diaphoretic and appears anxious. Her blood pressure is 130/80 mmHg, heart rate is 110 bpm, and she is in sinus rhythm. An ECG shows ST-segment elevation of 0.2 mV in leads V1 through V4. The nearest PCI-capable facility is 90 minutes away, and there is no helicopter transport available. The emergency department is equipped with fibrinolytic agents and has the capability to administer them.
Based on the clinical scenario, which of the following is the most appropriate next step in the management of this patient?

- A. Administer alteplase as soon as possible.
- B. Administer tenecteplase as a single bolus immediately.
- C. Transfer the patient to the nearest PCI-capable facility for primary PCI.
- D. Administer a reduced-dose thrombolytic with a platelet glycoprotein IIb/IIIa inhibitor.

Table 3.5: Summary of Fibrinolytic Therapy

Category	Details
Benefit	Reduces mortality and limits infarct size in patients with STEMI or with left bundle branch block. b. The greatest benefit occurs if treatment is initiated within the first 3 hours after the onset of presentation when up to a 50% reduction in mortality rate can be achieved. c. Survival benefit is greatest in patients with large infarctions. d. Primary PCI of the infarct-related artery is superior to thrombolysis when done by experienced operators with rapid time from first medical contact to intervention.
Contraindications	Major bleeding complications occur in 0.5–5% of patients, the most serious of which is intracranial hemorrhage. b. The major risk factors for intracranial bleeding are age 75 years or older, hypertension at presentation, low body weight, and the use of fibrin-specific fibrinolytic agents. c. Absolute contraindications include previous hemorrhagic stroke, other strokes or cerebrovascular events within 1 year, known intracranial neoplasm, recent head trauma, active internal bleeding, or suspected aortic dissection. d. Relative contraindications include BP greater than 180/110 mm Hg at presentation, known bleeding diathesis, trauma within 2–4 weeks, major surgery within 3 weeks, current use of anticoagulants, and prior allergic reaction or exposure to streptokinase or anistreplase within 2 years.
Fibrinolytic agents	Four fibrinolytic agents are available for acute MI. b. Most patients in the United States are treated with alteplase, reteplase, or tenecteplase. c. The principal objective should be to administer a thrombolytic agent within 30 minutes of presentation. d. After completion of the fibrinolytic infusion, aspirin and anticoagulation should be continued until revascularization or for the duration of the hospital stay. e. Anticoagulation with LMWH (enoxaparin or fondaparinux) is preferable to unfractionated heparin. f. In the EXTRACT trial, enoxaparin significantly reduced death and MI at day 30, at the expense of a modest increase in bleeding.

The correct answer is B. Administer tenecteplase as a single bolus immediately. The patient is presenting with an acute ST-elevation myocardial infarction (STEMI), and immediate reperfusion therapy is indicated. Given that the nearest PCI-capable facility is 90 minutes away and there is no helicopter transport available, fibrinolytic therapy is the most appropriate choice to achieve timely reperfusion. Tenecteplase has the advantage of being administered as a single bolus, which can reduce time to treatment, an important factor given the time-dependent nature of STEMI treatment. The goal is to administer thrombolytic therapy within 30 minutes of presentation to the emergency department. Option A is incorrect because, although alteplase is an effective fibrinolytic agent, it requires a more complex administration protocol compared to tenecteplase, which may delay treatment. Option C is incorrect because the delay in transfer to a PCI-capable facility would exceed the recommended time frame for optimal reperfusion therapy. Fibrinolytic therapy should be initiated when primary PCI cannot be performed within 120 minutes of first medical contact. Option D is incorrect because the combination of reduced-dose thrombolytic with a platelet glycoprotein IIb/IIIa inhibitor does not reduce mortality and is associated with increased bleeding complications. The priority in this scenario is to administer the most effective and timely reperfusion therapy available. Certain contraindications make fibrinolytic therapy unsafe, including a history of hemorrhagic stroke, recent cerebrovascular events, intracranial neoplasm, recent head trauma, active internal bleeding, or suspected aortic dissection. Specific conditions like high blood pressure, recent trauma or surgery, bleeding disorders, and other medical situations may also preclude the use of certain treatments.In the United States, the primary fibrinolytic agents for acute myocardial infarction (MI) are alteplase, reteplase, or tenecteplase. While there are slight variations in effectiveness among them, the priority is prompt treatment of suitable candidates. The key objective is to administer a thrombolytic agent within 30 minutes of presentation or during transport. The single-bolus administration of tenecteplase offers an attractive option for expedited treatment. Combining a reduced-dose thrombolytic with a platelet glycoprotein IIb/IIIa inhibitor does not reduce mortality rates but may increase bleeding risks slightly. Post-fibrinolytic infusion, aspirin (81–325 mg/day) and anticoagulation should be continued until revascularization or throughout the hospital stay (up to 8 days). Low-molecular-weight heparin (enoxaparin or fondaparinux) is preferred over unfractionated heparin for anticoagulation purposes. The recommended time frame for administering a thrombolytic agent in acute myocardial infarction (AMI) is as soon as possible, ideally within the first 30 minutes after arriving at the hospital for treatment, often referred to as "door-to-needle time". This rapid administration is crucial because the efficacy of thrombolytic therapy in restoring blood flow and minimizing heart muscle damage decreases as the time from symptom onset to treatment increases. For ST-segment elevation myocardial infarction (STEMI) patients, thrombolytic therapy is recommended when primary percutaneous coronary intervention (PCI) is not immediately available and if the anticipated delay from hospital admission to PCI is expected to be greater than 120 minutes. The goal is to administer the thrombolytic agent within 30 minutes of first medical contact. Outcomes are better if thrombolytic therapy is administered within 12 hours after the heart attack starts, but the benefits are greatest when treatment is initiated within the first few hours. The STREAM trial also supports prehospital administration of thrombolytics when the transport time to a PCI-capable facility is extended.

3.30 Post-PCI ACE Treatment

Case 59

A 72-year-old man with a history of hypertension and hyperlipidemia is admitted to the hospital following a large anterior ST-elevation myocardial infarction (STEMI). He was treated with primary percutaneous coronary intervention (PCI) to the left anterior descending artery within 90 minutes of symptom onset. His post-procedural course has been uneventful, and he is now 24 hours post-PCI. His blood pressure is 125/75 mmHg, heart rate is 68 bpm, and he is in sinus rhythm. His current medications include aspirin, ticagrelor, atorvastatin, and metoprolol. An echocardiogram shows a left ventricular ejection fraction (LVEF) of 35% with anterior wall hypokinesis. He has no signs of heart failure or hypotension.
Based on the clinical scenario, which of the following is the most appropriate next step in the management of this patient?

- A. Start an ACE inhibitor immediately.
- B. Perform a repeat echocardiogram in 48 hours before deciding on ACE inhibitor therapy.
- C. Initiate ACE inhibitor therapy only if symptoms of heart failure develop.
- D. Withhold ACE inhibitor therapy due to the patient's age and risk of renal complications.

Table 3.6: STEMI Treatment Drugs

Beta-Adrenergic Blocking Agents	Trials have shown modest short-term benefit from beta-blockers started during the first 24 hours after acute MI if there are no contraindications. Aggressive beta-blockade can increase shock, with overall harm in patients with HF. Early beta-blockade should be avoided in patients with any degree of HF, evidence of low-output state, increased risk of cardiogenic shock, or other relative contraindications to beta-blockade. Carvedilol was shown to be beneficial in the CAPRICORN trial following the acute phase of large MI.
Nitrates	Nitroglycerin is the agent of choice for continued or recurrent ischemic pain and is useful in lowering BP or relieving pulmonary congestion. Routine nitrate administration is not recommended, since no improvement in outcome has been observed in the ISIS-4 or GISSI-3 trials. Nitrates should be avoided in patients who received phosphodiesterase inhibitors in the prior 24 hours.
ACE Inhibitors	A series of trials have shown both short- and long-term improvement in survival with ACE inhibitor therapy. The benefits are greatest in patients with an EF of 40% or less, large infarctions, or clinical evidence of HF. ACE inhibitor treatment should be commenced early in patients without hypotension, especially patients with large or anterior MI. It is reasonable to use ACE inhibitors for all patients following STEMI who do not have contraindications.
Angiotensin Receptor Blockers	The VALIANT trial showed that valsartan is equivalent to captopril in reducing mortality. Valsartan should be used for all patients with ACE inhibitor intolerance. The combination of captopril and valsartan was no better than either agent alone and resulted in more side effects.
Aldosterone Antagonists	The RALES trial showed that spironolactone can reduce the mortality rate of patients with advanced HF. The EPHESUS trial showed a 15% relative risk reduction in mortality with eplerenone for patients post-MI with LV dysfunction and either clinical HF or diabetes. Kidney dysfunction or hyperkalemia are contraindications, and patients must be monitored carefully for development of hyperkalemia.
Calcium Channel Blockers	There are no studies to support the routine use of calcium channel blockers in most patients with acute MI. They have the potential to exacerbate ischemia and cause death from reflex tachycardia or myocardial depression. Long-acting calcium channel blockers should generally be reserved for management of hypertension or ischemia as second- or third-line medications after beta-blockers and nitrates.

The correct answer is A. Start an ACE inhibitor immediately. The patient has a reduced left ventricular ejection fraction (LVEF) of 35% following a large anterior STEMI, which places him at increased risk for adverse outcomes, including heart failure and mortality. Multiple trials, including SAVE, AIRE, SMILE, TRACE, and others, have demonstrated that ACE inhibitors improve survival in patients with reduced ejection fraction and clinical evidence of heart failure after myocardial infarction. Given that the patient is stable, without hypotension, and has no contraindications to ACE inhibitor therapy, it is appropriate to start this medication early to improve long-term survival. Option B is incorrect because the current echocardiogram already shows a reduced LVEF, which is an indication for ACE inhibitor therapy. Delaying the initiation of ACE inhibitor therapy to perform a repeat echocardiogram is not supported by evidence and could deny the patient the early benefits of the medication. Option C is incorrect because ACE inhibitor therapy has been shown to improve outcomes even in the absence of clinical heart failure symptoms, particularly in patients with reduced ejection fraction post-MI. Option D is incorrect because, while age and renal function are important considerations when prescribing ACE inhibitors, they are not contraindications in the absence of renal failure or other specific risks. The benefits of ACE inhibitors in this setting outweigh the potential risks, and renal function can be monitored after initiation of therapy. The contraindications for ACE inhibitor therapy in patients with reduced ejection fraction post-myocardial infarction (MI) include:

1. Hypersensitivity Reactions: ACE inhibitors are contraindicated in patients with a history of hypersensitivity to any component of the drug, including those who have experienced angioedema related to previous treatment with an ACE inhibitor, idiopathic or hereditary angioedema, or those currently using aliskiren in patients with diabetes mellitus.
2. Pregnancy: ACE inhibitors are contraindicated during pregnancy due to teratogenic effects such as decreased fetal renal function, anuria, renal failure, skull hypoplasia, and death.

Relative Contraindications:

1. Abnormal Renal Function: ACE inhibitors can cause elevation of potassium and worsen renal function. Patients with abnormal but stable renal function require close monitoring on an ACE inhibitor, and if renal function starts to decline, the ACE inhibitor should be discontinued immediately.
2. Aortic Valve Stenosis: Patients with aortic valve stenosis should not receive ACE inhibitors due to the risk of severe hypotension caused by afterload reduction.
3. Hypovolemia: ACE inhibitors can worsen dehydration and hypovolemia, so they should not be used in patients with these conditions.

Monitoring:

- Monitoring renal function, including Blood Urea Nitrogen (BUN) and serum creatinine, is essential when patients are on ACE inhibitor therapy

Ann SH et al. Comparison between angiotensin-converting enzyme inhibitor and angiotensin receptor blocker after percutaneous coronary intervention. Int J Cardiol. 2020 May 1;306:35-41. PMID: 31727411

Case Note

A series of trials have shown both short- and long-term improvement in survival with ACE inhibitor therapy. The benefits are greatest in patients with an EF of 40% or less, large infarctions, or clinical evidence of HF. ACE inhibitor treatment should be commenced early in patients without hypotension, especially patients with large or anterior MI. It is reasonable to use ACE inhibitors for all patients following STEMI who do not have contraindications.

3.31 Role of Beta Blockers in ACS

Case 60

A 63-year-old woman with a history of type 2 diabetes mellitus and previous myocardial infarction is admitted to the hospital with a new, non-ST-elevation myocardial infarction (NSTEMI). She is hemodynamically stable with a blood pressure of 140/85 mmHg and a heart rate of 78 bpm. She is currently on aspirin, clopidogrel, and atorvastatin. Her initial troponin I level is elevated at 0.5 ng/mL (normal under 0.04 ng/mL), and her ECG shows T-wave inversions in the anterior leads without ST-segment changes. She has no signs of heart failure or respiratory distress, and her lungs are clear on auscultation. Her current medications do not include a beta-blocker.

Based on the clinical scenario, which of the following is the most appropriate next step in the management of this patient?

- A. Start intravenous metoprolol immediately.
- B. Initiate oral metoprolol at a low dose and titrate as tolerated.
- C. Withhold beta-blocker therapy due to the risk of cardiogenic shock.
- D. Administer carvedilol only if left ventricular systolic dysfunction is confirmed on echocardiography.

The correct answer is B. Initiate oral metoprolol at a low dose and titrate as tolerated. The patient is hemodynamically stable following an NSTEMI with no signs of heart failure or low-output state. Beta-blockers have been shown to provide a mortality benefit when started early after myocardial infarction, including NSTEMI, in patients without contraindications. Starting oral metoprolol at a low dose and titrating as tolerated can help reduce myocardial oxygen demand and prevent recurrent ischemia. The patient's stable condition without contraindications suggests that it is safe to initiate beta-blocker therapy. Option A is incorrect because there is no indication for intravenous beta-blocker therapy in this stable patient. Intravenous administration is typically reserved for patients with ongoing ischemia or hypertension who require rapid control of symptoms. Option C is incorrect because the patient is not at increased risk of cardiogenic shock; she is hemodynamically stable and has no signs of heart failure. Withholding beta-blocker therapy in this patient would deny her the potential benefits of this class of medication post-MI. Option D is incorrect because the benefit of beta-blockers post-MI is not solely contingent on the presence of left ventricular systolic dysfunction. While carvedilol has demonstrated benefits in patients with systolic dysfunction, it is not mandatory to confirm this through echocardiography before commencing beta-blocker therapy in an eligible patient. Research has shown a modest improvement in short-term outcomes when beta-blockers are initiated within 24 hours of an acute myocardial infarction (MI), with a recommended dosage of metoprolol at 25–50 mg orally twice daily in the absence of contraindications. Aggressive beta-blockade can potentially exacerbate shock and overall harm in heart failure patients. Therefore, it is advisable to avoid early initiation of beta-blockers in individuals with heart failure, signs of low cardiac output, high risk of cardiogenic shock, or other conditions unsuitable for beta-blockade. Carvedilol, as evidenced in the CAPRICORN trial following a significant MI, should be initiated at 6.25 mg twice daily and titrated up to 25 mg twice daily. The potential risks of beta-blocker therapy in heart failure patients include:

Hypotension: Beta-blockers can cause a significant reduction in blood pressure, which may lead to symptomatic hypotension, particularly in patients who are volume-depleted or taking other blood pressure-lowering medications.

1. Bradycardia: These medications can slow the heart rate, potentially leading to bradycardia, which can be symptomatic and may require intervention if it becomes severe.
2. Dizziness: Patients may experience dizziness as a result of the blood pressure-lowering effects of beta-blockers, which can increase the risk of falls, particularly in the elderly.
3. Fatigue: Beta-blockers can cause fatigue, which may affect a patient's quality of life and ability to perform daily activities.

Despite these potential risks, beta-blocker therapy is associated with significant benefits in patients with heart failure, including reductions in all-cause mortality, heart failure hospitalizations, and worsening heart failure. The absolute increases in risk for adverse effects such as hypotension, dizziness, and bradycardia are relatively small, and overall fewer patients are withdrawn from beta-blocker therapy than from placebo. Therefore, the benefits of beta-blockers generally outweigh the risks in patients with heart failure, provided there are no contraindications to their use.

Peck KY et al. Role of beta blockers following percutaneous coronary intervention for acute coronary syndrome. Heart. 2021 May;107(9):728-733.PMID: 32887736

3.32 The EPHESUS Trial and LV Dysfunction

Case 61

A 66-year-old man with a history of coronary artery disease and a previous myocardial infarction is seen in the clinic for routine follow-up. He reports increasing fatigue and shortness of breath on exertion over the past few months. His current medications include aspirin, lisinopril, metoprolol, and atorvastatin. Physical examination reveals an S3 heart sound and mild bilateral ankle edema. His blood pressure is 130/80 mmHg, and his heart rate is 72 bpm in sinus rhythm. Laboratory tests show a serum potassium of 4.5 mEq/L and a serum creatinine of 1.1 mg/dL. An echocardiogram reveals a left ventricular ejection fraction (LVEF) of 35% with no valvular abnormalities. He has no history of diabetes mellitus.
Based on the clinical scenario, which of the following is the most appropriate next step in the management of this patient?

- A. Start spironolactone 25 mg daily.
- B. Increase the dose of lisinopril to improve LVEF.
- C. Initiate eplerenone 25 mg daily, with close monitoring of serum potassium and renal function.
- D. Refer the patient for implantable cardioverter-defibrillator (ICD) therapy evaluation.

The correct answer is C. Initiate eplerenone 25 mg daily, with close monitoring of serum potassium and renal function. The patient has clinical signs of heart failure (HF) with reduced ejection fraction (LVEF of 35%) and is already on standard therapy including an ACE inhibitor and a beta-blocker. The RALES trial showed benefits of spironolactone in patients with advanced HF, and the EPHESUS trial showed a mortality benefit with eplerenone in patients post-MI with LV dysfunction and either clinical HF or diabetes. While the patient does not have diabetes, he does have clinical HF with LV dysfunction, making him a candidate for an aldosterone antagonist. Eplerenone is preferred over spironolactone due to its more selective action and lower risk of endocrine side effects. Close monitoring of serum potassium and renal function is necessary due to the risk of hyperkalemia, especially when used in conjunction with an ACE inhibitor. Option A is incorrect because while spironolactone could be considered, eplerenone is often preferred due to its selectivity and better side effect profile. Option B is incorrect because there is no indication that increasing the dose of lisinopril will provide additional benefit in terms of mortality or hospitalization for HF, and the patient is already on standard therapy for HF. Option D is incorrect because while an ICD may be indicated for primary prevention of sudden cardiac death in patients with HF and reduced ejection fraction, the immediate next step in management should focus on optimizing medical therapy, which includes the addition of an aldosterone antagonist. Aldosterone antagonists, also known as mineralocorticoid receptor antagonists (MRAs), work by blocking the action of aldosterone, a hormone produced by the adrenal glands that is involved in regulating blood pressure and fluid balance. In heart failure patients, aldosterone can contribute to the pathology of the disease by causing coronary inflammation, cardiac hypertrophy, myocardial fibrosis, ventricular arrhythmias, and ischemic and necrotic lesions.

The mechanism of action of aldosterone antagonists in heart failure includes:

1. Diuretic Effect: By blocking aldosterone receptors, these drugs prevent the reabsorption of sodium and water by the kidneys, leading to increased excretion of water and salt in the urine. This helps to reduce the volume overload that is common in heart failure.
2. Potassium-Sparing: Aldosterone antagonists pre-

vent the excretion of potassium, which is often lost in urine when other diuretics are used. This helps to maintain normal potassium levels in the body, which is important for heart function.

3. Anti-Fibrotic and Anti-Hypertrophic Effects: Aldosterone promotes myocardial fibrosis and hypertrophy, which can worsen heart failure. By antagonizing aldosterone, these drugs can help to prevent or reverse these harmful effects on the heart muscle.

4. Improvement in Heart Function: By reducing myocardial fibrosis and ventricular remodeling, aldosterone antagonists can improve the functional capacity and symptoms of heart failure.

5. Reduction in Mortality and Hospitalization: Clinical trials such as the RALES and EPHESUS have shown that aldosterone antagonists can significantly reduce mortality and hospitalizations for patients with heart failure.

The two main aldosterone antagonists used in clinical practice are spironolactone and eplerenone. Spironolactone is a non-selective aldosterone antagonist, while eplerenone is more selective for the aldosterone receptor, which may lead to fewer side effects. It is important to monitor for hyperkalemia and renal function when using these medications, especially in conjunction with other drugs that affect the renin-angiotensin-aldosterone system (RAAS), such as ACE inhibitors

Iqbal J et al. Effect of eplerenone in percutaneous coronary intervention-treated post-myocardial infarction patients with left ventricular systolic dysfunction: a subanalysis of the EPHESUS trial. Eur J Heart Fail. 2014 Jun;16(6):685-91. PMID: 24706498

3.33 The AUGUSTUS Trial Post PCI Treatment

Case 62

A 70-year-old man with a history of chronic atrial fibrillation (CHADS2 score of 3) and recent percutaneous coronary intervention (PCI) with placement of a drug-eluting stent (DES) in the left anterior descending artery is seen for follow-up in the clinic. He was discharged on aspirin 81 mg daily, clopidogrel 75 mg daily, and warfarin with a target INR of 2.0-3.0. His other medical problems include hypertension and chronic kidney disease stage III. He has no history of gastrointestinal bleeding. His current medications also include lisinopril, metoprolol, and atorvastatin. His blood pressure is 135/85 mmHg, heart rate is irregularly irregular at 78 bpm, and his current INR is 2.4. He reports no bleeding or bruising.
Based on the clinical scenario and the current guidelines, which of the following is the most appropriate management of this patient's antithrombotic therapy?

- A. Continue current regimen of warfarin, aspirin, and clopidogrel.
- B. Discontinue aspirin and continue warfarin and clopidogrel.
- C. Switch warfarin to a direct oral anticoagulant (DOAC) and continue aspirin and clopidogrel.
- D. Switch warfarin to a DOAC and discontinue aspirin.

The correct answer is B. Discontinue aspirin and continue warfarin and clopidogrel. The patient has atrial fibrillation with a high CHADS2 score indicating a clear indication for anticoagulation with warfarin. He also has a recent DES placement, which necessitates the use of dual antiplatelet therapy (DAPT) with aspirin and clopidogrel. However, the risk of bleeding with triple therapy (warfarin, aspirin, and clopidogrel) is significant. Based on the consensus statements and trial evidence, such as from the AUGUSTUS trial, it is reasonable to discontinue aspirin after a short duration post-PCI, especially in a patient without a history of gastrointestinal bleeding. This approach balances the risk of stent thrombosis with the high risk of bleeding associated with triple therapy. Option A is incorrect because continuing triple therapy increases the risk of bleeding without a significant reduction in thrombotic events, as evidenced by the PIONEER and AUGUSTUS trials. Option C is incorrect because while switching to a DOAC may reduce bleeding risk compared to warfarin, continuing triple therapy even with a DOAC still poses a higher bleeding risk than dual therapy. Option D is incorrect because although switching to a DOAC may be reasonable, the AUGUSTUS trial suggests that discontinuing aspirin after a short duration post-PCI is beneficial in reducing bleeding events without a significant increase in stent thrombosis. Therefore, the patient should remain on anticoagulation and a single antiplatelet agent (clopidogrel). The AUGUSTUS trial was a multicenter, randomized clinical trial that used a 2x2 factorial design to compare the safety and efficacy of antithrombotic therapy in patients with atrial fibrillation who had a recent acute coronary syndrome (ACS) or percutaneous coronary intervention (PCI). The trial specifically compared the use of apixaban, a non-vitamin K oral anticoagulant (NOAC), with vitamin K antagonists (VKAs) like warfarin, and also compared the use of aspirin with placebo. The key findings of the AUGUSTUS trial were:

1. Patients receiving apixaban experienced significantly lower rates of bleeding compared to those receiving VKAs. The primary safety outcome, which was International Society on Thrombosis and Haemostasis (ISTH) major or clinically relevant nonmajor bleeding, occurred in 10.5% of patients on apixaban versus 14.7% on VKAs (p under 0.0001).
2. The addition of aspirin resulted in greater bleeding without any difference in efficacy. The primary safety outcome for aspirin versus placebo was 16.1% versus 9.0%, respectively (p under 0.0001).
3. Secondary outcomes included death or hospitalization, with patients on apixaban having lower rates compared to those on VKAs. Specifically, death or hospitalization occurred in 23.5% of patients on apixaban versus 27.4% on VKAs (HR 0.83, 95% CI 0.74-0.93; p = 0.002).
4. The trial also found a lower risk of stroke in patients taking apixaban compared to those on VKAs
5. The AUGUSTUS trial suggested that discontinuing aspirin after a short duration post-PCI could be beneficial in reducing bleeding events without a significant increase in stent thrombosis.

Overall, the AUGUSTUS trial contributed to the understanding of antithrombotic therapy in a complex patient population with atrial fibrillation and recent ACS or PCI, indicating that an apixaban-based strategy without aspirin could reduce bleeding risks without significantly increasing ischemic events

Lopes R et al Antithrombotic Therapy after Acute Coronary Syndrome or PCI in Atrial Fibrillation. N Engl J Med. 2019 Apr 18;380(16):1509-1524.PMID: 30883055

Case Note

In patients with atrial fibrillation and a recent acute coronary syndrome or PCI treated with a P2Y12 inhibitor, an antithrombotic regimen that included apixaban, without aspirin, resulted in less bleeding and fewer hospitalizations without significant differences in the incidence of ischemic events than regimens that included a vitamin K antagonist, aspirin, or both.

3.34 Rescue PCI After Failed Fibrinolysis?

Case 63

A 58-year-old man presents to the emergency department with chest pain that started 2 hours ago. He has a history of hypertension and hyperlipidemia. His initial ECG shows ST-segment elevation in leads II, III, and aVF. He is given aspirin, clopidogrel, and intravenous fibrinolytic therapy because the nearest PCI-capable hospital is 90 minutes away. Two hours after fibrinolysis, his chest pain has resolved, but repeat ECG shows only 30% resolution of the initial ST-segment elevation. His blood pressure is 130/80 mmHg, heart rate is 70 bpm, and he is in sinus rhythm. He has no rales on lung auscultation, and there are no additional heart sounds. His serum troponins were elevated at presentation and have not been rechecked yet.
Based on the clinical scenario, which of the following is the most appropriate next step in the management of this patient?

- A. Repeat fibrinolytic therapy.
- B. Arrange for immediate transfer to a PCI-capable hospital for rescue angioplasty.
- C. Perform stress testing to evaluate for residual ischemia.
- D. Continue medical management with observation in the coronary care unit.

The correct answer is B. Arrange for immediate transfer to a PCI-capable hospital for rescue angioplasty. The patient has evidence of failed reperfusion given the lack of at least 50% resolution of ST-segment elevation after fibrinolytic therapy. In this scenario, rescue PCI is indicated to reduce the composite risk of death, reinfarction, stroke, or severe heart failure. The patient is within the window of time (3–24 hours after fibrinolytic therapy) where PCI has been shown to improve outcomes, and he is currently stable, making transfer feasible. Option A is incorrect because repeat fibrinolytic therapy is not recommended due to the increased risk of bleeding and lack of evidence for benefit after failed initial fibrinolysis. Option C is incorrect because stress testing in the acute setting of failed reperfusion is not appropriate and delays definitive care. The patient needs immediate revascularization, not non-invasive testing. Option D is incorrect because continuing medical management alone in the setting of failed fibrinolysis is associated with worse outcomes compared to rescue PCI. Observation without plans for revascularization would not be appropriate care for this patient. The group that underwent immediate or early percutaneous coronary intervention (PCI) following fibrinolysis experienced a higher incidence of major bleeding episodes compared to the group that received primary PCI alone. The STREAM Investigative Team primarily influenced the early PCI group, showing a greater occurrence of serious bleeding events than other groups. To address the elevated risk of intracranial hemorrhage in patients aged 75 and older, the dose of tenecteplase was halved. Following this adjustment, no instances of cerebral hemorrhage were observed in the elderly cohort. Excluding this trial would lead to similar rates of serious bleeding events as seen in the primary PCI alone group. There was no significant difference in major bleeding events between ischemia-guided or delayed PCI strategies. Regardless of whether immediate, early, or delayed PCI follows fibrinolysis, the fibrinolytic process may contribute to a heightened risk of severe bleeding. Therefore, a reduced dosage of fibrinolytic agents is advisable for patients aged 75 years and older.

Holmes DR Jr et al. Rescue percutaneous coronary intervention after failed fibrinolytic therapy: have expectations been met? Am Heart J. 2006 Apr;151(4):779-85. PMID: 16569532 Armstrong PW et al STREAM Investigative Team. Fibrinolysis or primary PCI in ST-segment elevation myocardial infarction. N Engl J Med. 2013 Apr 11;368(15):1379-87. PMID: 23473396

Case Note

Rescue PCI was associated with significantly lower risk of long-term adverse outcomes for patients with STEMI who failed fibrinolytic therapy.

3.35 Arrhythmias After Acute Myocardial Infarction

Case 64

A 63-year-old woman is admitted to the coronary care unit following an acute myocardial infarction (MI). On the second day of admission, she develops palpitations and light-headedness. Her blood pressure is 110/70 mmHg, and her heart rate is 160 bpm. The ECG shows atrial fibrillation with a rapid ventricular response without evidence of ST-segment changes. Her echocardiogram shows an ejection fraction of 40% with no significant valvular disease. She is currently on aspirin, clopidogrel, and a statin. She has no history of chronic obstructive pulmonary disease or asthma. Her serum electrolytes are within normal limits, and there is no evidence of hypoxia.
Based on the clinical scenario, which of the following is the most appropriate next step in the management of this patient's atrial fibrillation?

- A. Administer intravenous metoprolol.
- B. Administer intravenous diltiazem.
- C. Proceed with immediate electrical cardioversion.
- D. Administer intravenous amiodarone.

The correct answer is A. Administer intravenous metoprolol. The patient has developed atrial fibrillation with a rapid ventricular response following an MI. Given that her blood pressure is stable, and she has preserved cardiac function (ejection fraction of 40%), intravenous beta-blockers are the treatment of choice for rate control and potential rhythm control. Metoprolol can be administered intravenously in this setting to rapidly control the heart rate. Option B is incorrect because while intravenous diltiazem is an alternative for rate control in atrial fibrillation, it is less preferable in the setting of acute MI due to its negative inotropic effects, which can exacerbate any underlying myocardial dysfunction. Option C is incorrect because electrical cardioversion is typically reserved for hemodynamically unstable patients or those with evidence of heart failure, ischemia, or hypotension, which this patient does not have. Option D is incorrect because while amiodarone can be used for rhythm control in atrial fibrillation, the first step in this stable patient should be rate control with a beta-blocker. Amiodarone would be considered if beta-blockers are contraindicated or if rhythm control is specifically indicated due to hemodynamic compromise or failure of rate control. Sinus tachycardia is a common occurrence that can be triggered by increased adrenergic activity or hemodynamic challenges stemming from hypovolemia or cardiac pump failure. Beta-blockers are not recommended in cases of the latter. Supraventricular premature beats are frequently observed and may indicate the onset of atrial fibrillation. Address electrolyte imbalances, hypoxia, and discontinue causative medications, particularly aminophylline. Atrial fibrillation should be promptly managed by either rate control or rhythm conversion. Intravenous beta-blockers like metoprolol (2.5–5 mg IV every 2–5 minutes, max 15 mg over 10 minutes) or short-acting esmolol (50–200 mcg/kg/min) are preferred if cardiac function permits. In cases where beta-blockers are unsuitable or ineffective, intravenous diltiazem at a rate of 5-15 mg/hour can be administered. Electrical cardioversion, typically starting at 100 joules, may be necessary for atrial fibrillation in the presence of complications such as hypotension, heart failure, or ischemia; however, recurrence of the arrhythmia is common. Intravenous amiodarone can be given with an initial bolus of 150 mg followed by a continuous infusion of 15-30 mg/hour, or a rapid oral loading dose of 400 mg three times daily to aid in restoring or maintaining sinus rhythm for cardioversion. Arrhythmias following myocardial infarction (MI) are a significant clinical concern that requires prompt identification and intervention. While the incidence of arrhythmias post-MI has decreased in the reperfusion era, their occurrence can lead to increased morbidity and mortality. Arrhythmias are more prevalent in individuals who do not receive timely reperfusion, particularly those with reduced left ventricular ejection fraction (LVEF).

Frampton J et al Arrhythmias After Acute Myocardial Infarction. Yale J Biol Med. 2023 Mar 31;96(1):83-94. PMID: 37009192

Case 64B

A 56-year-old man with a history of hypertension and smoking is admitted to the coronary care unit following an ST-elevation myocardial infarction (STEMI). He underwent successful primary percutaneous coronary intervention (PCI) to the right coronary artery 4 hours ago. His post-procedure course has been uneventful until he suddenly complains of palpitations. His blood pressure is 110/68 mmHg, and he appears alert and oriented. The telemetry monitor shows a wide-complex tachycardia at a rate of 170 bpm without hemodynamic compromise. The ECG confirms sustained ventricular tachycardia (VT). His serum potassium and magnesium levels are within normal limits.
Based on the clinical scenario, which of the following is the most appropriate next step in the management of this patient's ventricular tachycardia?

- A. Administer intravenous lidocaine 1 mg/kg bolus.
- B. Perform immediate electrical cardioversion.
- C. Start an intravenous amiodarone infusion.
- D. Observe and monitor the rhythm without intervention.

sus.jpg 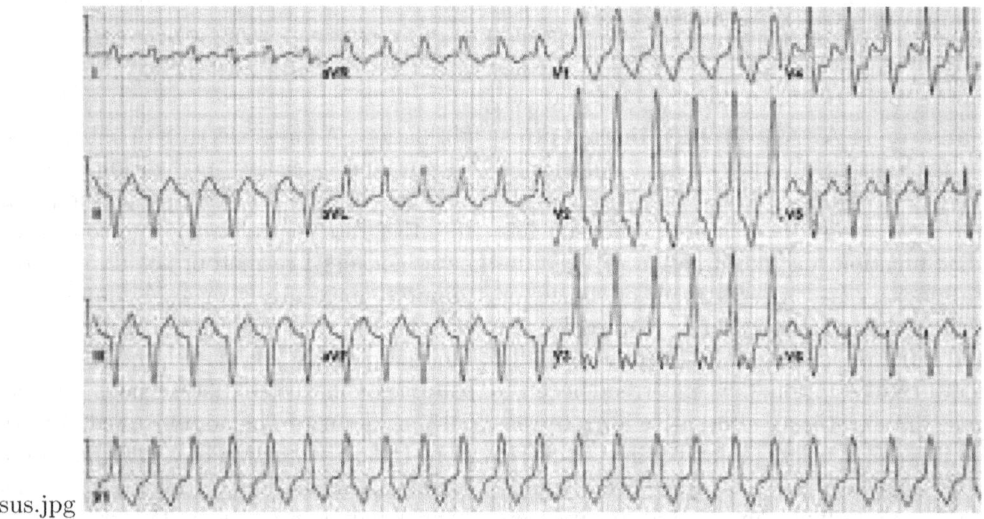

Figure 3.6: VT

The correct answer is A. Administer intravenous lidocaine 1 mg/kg bolus. The patient has developed sustained ventricular tachycardia post-STEMI. He is hemodynamically stable, which allows for a trial of medical management before considering electrical cardioversion. Lidocaine is a class 1B antiarrhythmic that is effective for the treatment of ventricular arrhythmias, especially in the acute setting of myocardial infarction. A bolus of 1 mg/kg can be administered quickly and is the recommended first-line treatment in this scenario. Option B is incorrect because immediate electrical cardioversion is the treatment of choice for hemodynamically unstable patients with VT. This patient is stable, so it is appropriate to attempt pharmacologic therapy first. Option C is incorrect because while intravenous amiodarone is an alternative treatment for VT, it is generally considered after lidocaine if lidocaine is ineffective or contraindicated. In this case, there is no contraindication to lidocaine, and it should be tried first. Option D is incorrect because sustained VT post-MI is a life-threatening arrhythmia that requires intervention. Observation without intervention could lead to hemodynamic compromise or degeneration into ventricular fibrillation. Contraindications for the use of lidocaine in the treatment of ventricular arrhythmias include:

1. Hypersensitivity to lidocaine or amide-type local anesthetics: Patients with a known history of hypersensitivity reactions to lidocaine or other amide-type local anesthetics should not receive lidocaine.

2. Adams-Stokes syndrome, SA/AV/intraventricular heart block in the absence of an artificial pacemaker: Lidocaine should not be used in patients with these conditions unless a pacemaker is present, as it can exacerbate conduction issues.
3. Congestive heart failure (CHF), cardiogenic shock, second and third-degree heart block (if no pacemaker is present), Wolff-Parkinson-White Syndrome: These conditions are listed as contraindications due to the potential for lidocaine to worsen cardiac conduction and precipitate arrhythmias.
4. Severe hepatic impairment: Since lidocaine is primarily metabolized in the liver, patients with severe liver disease may have an increased risk of lidocaine toxicity.
5. Concomitant use with certain drugs: Lidocaine should be used with caution or is contraindicated with drugs that affect hepatic enzyme metabolism, such as those that inhibit CYP3A4 or CYP1A2, due to the potential for increased lidocaine levels and toxicity.
6. Digitalis toxicity accompanied by supraventricular arrhythmias: Caution is advised when using lidocaine in patients with digitalis toxicity, as it may exacerbate arrhythmias.
7. Electrolyte imbalances: Patients with significant electrolyte derangements may be at higher risk for lidocaine toxicity.
8. Pseudocholinesterase deficiency: This condition can increase the risk of lidocaine toxicity.

Case 64C

A 72-year-old man with a history of coronary artery disease presents with chest pain and is diagnosed with an acute anterior wall myocardial infarction. He undergoes successful revascularization with PCI to the left anterior descending artery. On the second day of his hospitalization, he suddenly develops dizziness and near-syncope. His blood pressure is 95/60 mmHg, and his heart rate is 38 bpm. The telemetry monitor shows a regular rhythm with a wide QRS complex. An ECG confirms the presence of complete heart block with a wide-complex escape rhythm. His medications include aspirin, ticagrelor, a beta-blocker, an ACE inhibitor, and a statin. There is no evidence of acute ischemia on the ECG, and his chest pain has resolved.
Based on the clinical scenario, which of the following is the most appropriate next step in the management of this patient's conduction disturbance?

- A. Administer intravenous atropine 1 mg.
- B. Observe and continue current medical therapy.
- C. Insert a temporary transvenous pacemaker.
- D. Schedule for permanent pacemaker implantation.

degree.jpg

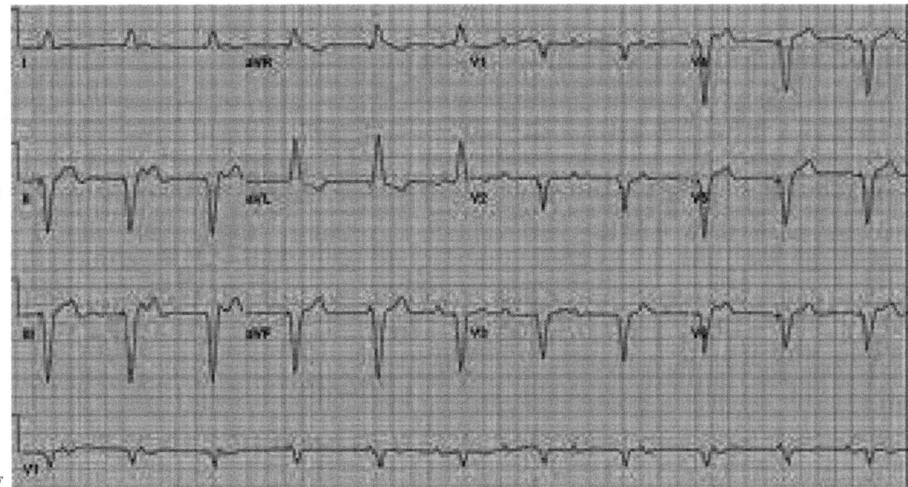

Figure 3.7: A 72-year-old man

The correct answer is C. Insert a temporary transvenous pacemaker. The patient has developed complete heart block with a wide-complex escape rhythm following an anterior wall myocardial infarction. This type of block is usually infranodal, indicating extensive damage to the His-Purkinje system. The escape rhythm is often unreliable and can lead to hemodynamic compromise, as evidenced by the patient's dizziness, near-syncope, and hypotension. Immediate temporary pacing is indicated to ensure a reliable heart rate and to prevent further episodes of syncope or progression to asystole. Option A is incorrect because while intravenous atropine can be used to increase the heart rate in cases of AV block, it is often ineffective in infranodal block or complete heart block, especially with a wide QRS complex, which suggests significant damage to the conduction system. Option B is incorrect because observation and continuation of current medical therapy without addressing the complete heart block could lead to further hemodynamic instability and is not an appropriate management strategy for this patient. Option D is incorrect as the immediate next step because while the patient may eventually require a permanent pacemaker, the first priority is to stabilize the heart rate and rhythm acutely with a temporary pacemaker. The decision for permanent pacing can be made later once the patient's condition has stabilized and the transient nature of the block has been assessed. Nodal and infranodal atrioventricular (AV) blocks are types of heart block that refer to the location within the heart's electrical conduction system where the blockage occurs. Nodal AV Block

- Location: Occurs within the AV node.
- ECG Characteristics: Usually results in a narrow QRS complex because the blockage is at the level of the AV node, and the ventricles are typically activated normally through the His-Purkinje system.
- Response to Medication: Nodal blocks can often be improved with medications that increase heart rate or enhance AV nodal conduction, such as atropine or isoproterenol.
- Vagal Maneuvers: Vagal maneuvers, which increase vagal tone, can exacerbate nodal blocks.

Infranodal AV Block

- Location: Occurs within the His-Purkinje system, which includes the bundle of His or the bundle branches.
- ECG Characteristics: Often displays a wide QRS complex because the blockage is below the AV node, affecting the normal activation of the ventricles.
- Response to Medication: Infranodal blocks can worsen with medications that increase heart rate or enhance AV nodal conduction, as these interventions may not improve conduction through the damaged His-Purkinje system
- Vagal Maneuvers: Vagal maneuvers may improve infranodal blocks, as they do not affect the infranodal conduction system as much as they do the AV node

3.36 Acute LV failure Post-Myocardial Infarction

Case 65

A 68-year-old man with a history of diabetes mellitus and previous myocardial infarction is admitted to the hospital with severe chest pain. He is diagnosed with an acute inferior wall myocardial infarction and undergoes successful revascularization with PCI. On the third day of hospitalization, he develops acute onset of dyspnea, a cough productive of frothy sputum, and is noted to be hypoxic with an oxygen saturation of 88% on room air. Physical examination reveals an elevated jugular venous pressure, bilateral rales halfway up both lung fields, and a third heart sound (S3). His blood pressure is 145/90 mmHg, and his heart rate is 102 bpm. Chest X-ray shows pulmonary edema. The patient is already receiving supplemental oxygen via nasal cannula. Based on the clinical scenario, which of the following is the most appropriate next step in the management of this patient's acute left ventricular (LV) failure?

- A. Administer intravenous furosemide 40 mg.
- B. Administer sublingual isosorbide dinitrate 5 mg.
- C. Start intravenous sodium nitroprusside infusion.
- D. Start intravenous dobutamine infusion.

The correct answer is A. Administer intravenous furosemide 40 mg. The patient is presenting with signs and symptoms of acute pulmonary edema secondary to LV failure post-myocardial infarction. The initial management should focus on improving symptoms and oxygenation, as well as reducing preload and afterload. Intravenous diuretics such as furosemide are the first-line treatment in this setting because they provide rapid relief of pulmonary congestion through diuresis and venodilation. The patient's blood pressure is adequate to tolerate the preload reduction without significant risk of hypotension. Option B is incorrect because while sublingual isosorbide dinitrate is a vasodilator that can help reduce preload, the patient's acute pulmonary edema with hypoxia requires more aggressive initial management with intravenous diuretics to rapidly remove fluid from the lungs. Option C is incorrect because sodium nitroprusside is a potent vasodilator that can rapidly decrease both preload and afterload, but it is typically reserved for cases of acute LV failure with severe hypertension or when there is a need for rapid titration of afterload reduction in an intensive care setting with invasive hemodynamic monitoring. The patient's blood pressure, although on the higher side, does not necessitate this aggressive approach at this time. Option D is incorrect because inotropic agents like dobutamine are generally avoided unless there is evidence of low cardiac output with hypotension (cardiogenic shock). In this patient, the blood pressure is preserved, and the use of inotropes could increase myocardial oxygen demand and potentially worsen ischemia. Answer The primary management of congestive heart failure (CHF) typically involves the intravenous administration of diuretics, like furosemide, at a dose of 40 mg. Inhaled oxygen and vasodilators, particularly nitrates, are recommended. Nitrates can be given orally, topically, or intravenously unless the patient exhibits hypotension with a systolic blood pressure below 100 mmHg. The therapeutic benefit of Digitalis in acute myocardial infarction is generally limited. In the setting of acute myocardial infarction (MI), a pulmonary capillary wedge (PCW) pressure between 15 and 20 mmHg is considered appropriate. When PCW pressure exceeds 20 mmHg without hypotension, treatment involves diuretics alongside vasodilator therapy. Intravenous nitroglycerin should be initiated at 10 g/min, or alternatively, nitroprusside can be started at 0.5 g/kg per min. Dosages should be adjusted to optimize blood pressure, PCW pressure, and systemic vascular resistance (SVR).

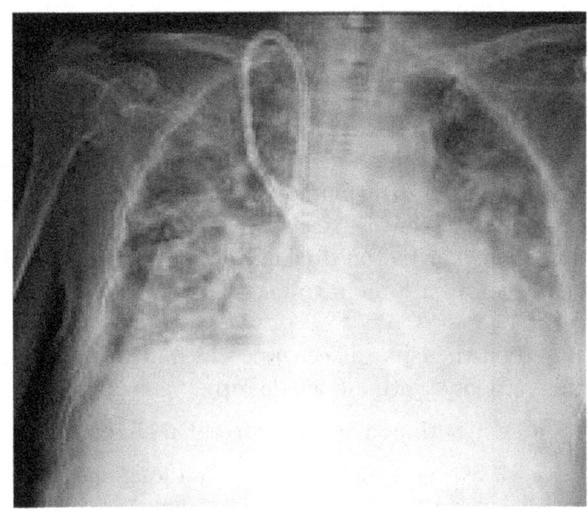

Figure 3.8: A 68-year-old man

For CHF management involving diuretics, vasodilators, and inotropic therapy, invasive hemodynamic monitoring techniques like the Swan-Ganz pulmonary artery catheter and arterial line can be beneficial, especially in patients with concurrent hypotension. CHF can result from systolic dysfunction, characterized by impaired heart pumping ability, increased left ventricular (LV) diastolic stiffness, or acute mechanical complications. If PCW pressure exceeds 20 mmHg and the patient is hypotensive, evaluation for ventricular septal defect (VSD) or acute mitral regurgitation is recommended. In such scenarios, consider initiating dobutamine at 1-2 g/kg per minute and titrate up to a maximum of 10 g/kg per minute cautiously due to potential side effects like drug-induced tachycardia or ventricular ectopy. After stabilizing on parenteral vasodilator therapy, transition to oral therapy typically involves an angiotensin-converting enzyme (ACE) inhibitor or angiotensin receptor blocker (ARB). Long-term aldosterone antagonist use like spironolactone (25-50 mg daily) or eplerenone (25-50 mg daily) should be considered if LVEF is under or 40% or in the presence of symptomatic heart failure or diabetes; however, caution is advised in cases of renal insufficiency or hyperkalemia.

Bahit MC et al. Post-Myocardial Infarction Heart Failure. JACC Heart Fail. 2018 Mar;6(3):179-186. PMID: 29496021.

3.37 Long-Term Antithrombotic Therapy after ACS

Case 66

A 63-year-old woman with a history of hyperlipidemia and smoking is brought to the emergency department with chest pain lasting for 2 hours. Her electrocardiogram (ECG) shows ST-segment elevations in leads II, III, and aVF. She is diagnosed with an acute ST-elevation myocardial infarction (STEMI) and is taken to the cardiac catheterization lab for primary percutaneous coronary intervention (PCI). During the procedure, a drug-eluting stent is successfully placed in the right coronary artery. Her post-procedure course is uneventful, and she is started on dual antiplatelet therapy with aspirin and ticagrelor. On the second day, she mentions that she often forgets to take her medications and is worried about the possibility of missing doses in the future.
Based on the clinical scenario, which of the following is the most appropriate next step in the management of this patient's antiplatelet therapy?

- A. Continue with the current regimen of aspirin and ticagrelor.
- B. Switch from ticagrelor to a long-acting P2Y12 inhibitor.
- C. Replace ticagrelor with a daily regimen of a glycoprotein IIb/IIIa inhibitor.
- D. Substitute ticagrelor with a bare metal stent and a shorter duration of P2Y12 inhibitor therapy.

Table 3.7: Long-Term Antithrombotic Therapy after ACS

Aspirin	Discharge on aspirin, 81–325 mg/day, is a key quality indicator of MI care. Highly effective, inexpensive, and well-tolerated.
P2Y12 Inhibitor	Should also be received by patients who received a coronary stent. Patients who require warfarin anticoagulation present a challenge, as the combination of aspirin, clopidogrel, and warfarin has a high risk of bleeding.
Warfarin	"Triple therapy" should be limited to patients with a clear indication for warfarin. Should be used for the shortest period of time. Used with strategies to reduce risk of bleeding and with consideration of a lower target anticoagulation intensity during the period of concomitant treatment with aspirin and P2Y12 therapy.
Rivaroxaban/Clopidogrel	The PIONEER trial studied three treatment regimens for patients with atrial fibrillation who had coronary stent placement. There was less bleeding in the patients who received rivaroxaban plus clopidogrel than in those who received "triple therapy".
Dabigatran/Clopidogrel	Dual therapy with dabigatran and clopidogrel was shown to be beneficial for bleeding compared to triple therapy, with similar rates of thrombotic cardiovascular events. However, MI and stent thrombosis occurred more often with the 110-mg dose of dabigatran than with clopidogrel alone.
Apixaban/Warfarin	The AUGUSTUS trial found that apixaban resulted in 31% less major and clinically relevant nonmajor bleeding than warfarin for patients with atrial fibrillation and coronary stents or ACSs or both. Avoiding aspirin, after an average of 6 days after the PCI, resulted in less bleeding and a nonsignificant increase in stent thrombosis.

The correct answer is A. Continue with the current regimen of aspirin and ticagrelor. After the placement of a drug-eluting stent, dual antiplatelet therapy (DAPT) with aspirin and a P2Y12 inhibitor is recommended to prevent stent thrombosis, a potentially life-threatening complication. Ticagrelor is a potent P2Y12 inhibitor with a twice-daily dosing regimen. Despite the patient's concern about forgetting to take her medications, it is important to emphasize the necessity of adherence to DAPT and to implement strategies to improve compliance, such as medication reminders, before considering a change in therapy. There is no long-acting P2Y12 inhibitor available that would allow less frequent dosing. Option B is incorrect because there is no long-acting P2Y12 inhibitor available that would provide a once-daily dosing option. All currently available P2Y12 inhibitors require at least once-daily dosing. Option C is incorrect because glycoprotein IIb/IIIa inhibitors are not used for long-term antiplatelet therapy following stent placement. They are used acutely during PCI to reduce major thrombotic events but are not suitable for chronic maintenance therapy due to their route of administration (intravenous) and risk profile. Option D is incorrect because the patient has already had a drug-eluting stent placed, and it is not standard practice to replace a stent once it has been implanted. Additionally, the duration of DAPT should not be shortened based on the patient's concerns about medication adherence without a compelling reason, such as a high risk of bleeding. The focus should be on improving adherence to the prescribed regimen. The recommended duration of dual antiplatelet therapy (DAPT) after stent placement varies depending on the patient's risk factors for bleeding and ischemic events, as well as the clinical presentation at the time of percutaneous coronary intervention (PCI). The guidelines have evolved over time, with a shift from a one-size-fits-all approach to a more individualized strategy that balances the risks of bleeding and ischemia.

1. For patients with acute coronary syndrome (ACS) treated with a drug-eluting stent (DES), at least 12 months of DAPT is recommended. However, for those at high bleeding risk, a shorter duration of 6 months can be considered.
2. In patients with stable ischemic heart disease (SIHD) treated with a DES, at least 6 months of DAPT with clopidogrel is recommended, but just 3 months can be considered for those at high bleeding risk, or even just 1 month if 3 months of DAPT poses safety concerns.
3. Recent trials have explored even shorter durations of DAPT. The STOP-DAPT trial, for example, investigated the efficacy and safety of one-month DAPT followed by clopidogrel monotherapy and concluded that it decreases the risk of ischemic and bleeding events, suggesting non-inferiority to 12-month DAPT.
4. For patients with chronic coronary syndrome, a DAPT duration of 6 months is recommended, with the possibility of shortening to at least 1 month in high bleeding risk (HBR) patients.
5. In the case of patients with STEMI treated with DAPT in conjunction with fibrinolytic therapy, P2Y12 inhibitor therapy (clopidogrel) should be continued for a minimum of 14 days and ideally at least 12 months.

It is important to note that the duration of DAPT may be influenced by the type of stent used, the patient's bleeding risk, and whether the patient has ACS or SIHD. The decision should be made on a case-by-case basis, taking into account the individual patient's risk factors and clinical scenario

3.38 Cardiogenic Shock Post MI

Case 67

A 56-year-old man with a past medical history of hypertension and a recent myocardial infarction treated with thrombolytic therapy presents with sudden onset of hypotension, with a blood pressure of 85/50 mmHg, heart rate of 110 bpm, and cool, clammy skin. He is alert but anxious. His jugular venous pressure is elevated, and heart sounds are distant. Breath sounds are clear, and there is no peripheral edema. His urine output has been low over the past hour. An echocardiogram reveals no pericardial effusion, normal right ventricular size and function, and a left ventricular ejection fraction of 35% with anterior wall hypokinesis. Intravenous fluids have been initiated, and the patient has received a total of 300 mL of normal saline with no improvement in blood pressure.
Based on the clinical scenario, which of the following is the most appropriate next step in the management of this patient's condition?

- A. Continue aggressive fluid resuscitation with normal saline.
- B. Initiate intravenous norepinephrine infusion.
- C. Insert an intra-aortic balloon pump (IABP).
- D. Perform immediate coronary angiography and consider revascularization.

The correct answer is B. Initiate intravenous norepinephrine infusion. The patient is presenting with signs and symptoms consistent with cardiogenic shock, characterized by hypotension and evidence of poor end-organ perfusion (low urinary output, cool extremities) following a recent myocardial infarction. The absence of pericardial effusion and normal right ventricular function on echocardiography make acute tamponade or right ventricular infarction unlikely. The patient has not responded to initial fluid resuscitation, suggesting that the shock state is not solely due to hypovolemia. Norepinephrine is the preferred vasopressor in cardiogenic shock as it elevates systemic vascular resistance, enhances coronary and cerebral perfusion pressure, and does not significantly increase heart rate. It is favored over dopamine due to its superior safety profile and better outcomes supported by limited evidence from randomized clinical trials. Option A is deemed inappropriate because the patient has already undergone fluid resuscitation without blood pressure improvement, and further aggressive fluid administration could worsen pulmonary congestion without addressing the underlying cardiogenic shock. Option C is considered incorrect as per the IABP-SHOCK II trial, which did not demonstrate a mortality benefit with intra-aortic balloon pump (IABP) use in cardiogenic shock compared to standard care. Therefore, IABP is not the primary treatment unless there are mechanical complications of myocardial infarction present. Option D is not the immediate next step because although emergent cardiac catheterization and potential revascularization are crucial in managing cardiogenic shock, the patient first requires hemodynamic stabilization with vasopressors. Once stabilized, angiography should be performed to assess the need for revascularization. n cardiogenic shock, norepinephrine is recommended as the primary vasopressor based on meta-analyses showing reduced mortality rates. Dobutamine, a beta-adrenergic agonist, enhances contractility and reduces afterload. It is indicated for patients with low cardiac output and high pulmonary capillary wedge pressure (PCWP) without hypotension. If there is impaired myocardial function (reduced cardiac output and elevated PCWP) or signs of hypoperfusion despite adequate volume resuscitation and a satisfactory mean arterial pressure (MAP), dobutamine can be added to a vasopressor regimen. Initiate with an initial intravenous infusion rate of 0.1–0.5 mcg/kg/min, which can be adjusted based on hemodynamic response within a range of 2–20 mcg/kg/min. After 48 hours, tachyphylaxis may occur due to beta-adrenergic receptor downregulation. Milrinone, a phosphodiesterase inhibitor, can be used as an alternative to dobutamine.

Samsky MD et al Cardiogenic Shock After Acute Myocardial Infarction: A Review. JAMA. 2021 Nov 9;326(18):1840-1850.PMID: 34751704

Case Note

A 2021 study on cardiogenic shock patients showed no significant difference in mortality rates between milrinone and dobutamine treatments. Amrinone is another phosphodiesterase inhibitor that can be considered. These medications elevate cyclic AMP levels and enhance cardiac contractility by bypassing beta-adrenergic receptors, with both causing vasodilation as a side effect.

3.39 Papillary Muscle Rupture Post MI

Case 68

72-year-old man with a history of coronary artery disease and a recent inferior myocardial infarction (MI) 5 days ago presents with acute dyspnea, orthopnea, and a new loud holosystolic murmur heard best at the left lower sternal border. He is tachypneic with a respiratory rate of 28 breaths per minute, blood pressure of 90/60 mmHg, and heart rate of 112 bpm. The patient is afebrile. Oxygen saturation is 88% on room air. Physical examination reveals jugular venous distension, bilateral pulmonary crackles, and a palpable thrill at the left lower sternal border. The patient is placed on supplemental oxygen, and a bedside echocardiogram shows a flail posterior mitral leaflet with severe mitral regurgitation and a left ventricular ejection fraction of 40%. There is no evidence of ventricular septal defect (VSD) on color Doppler imaging. The patient is given intravenous furosemide with mild improvement in respiratory distress.
Based on the clinical scenario, which of the following is the most appropriate next step in the management of this patient's condition?

- A. Continue medical management with diuretics and afterload reduction.
- B. Initiate intra-aortic balloon counterpulsation (IABC) and consult cardiothoracic surgery for urgent repair.
- C. Administer intravenous glycoprotein IIb/IIIa inhibitors and prepare for percutaneous coronary intervention (PCI).
- D. Perform immediate coronary angiography to assess for recurrent myocardial infarction.

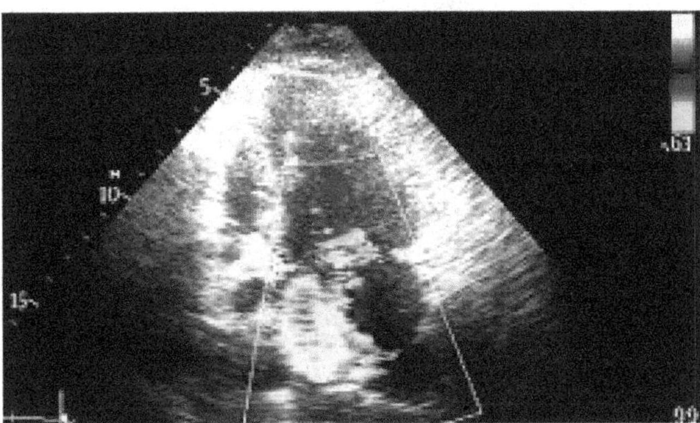

Figure 3.9: Papillary muscle rupture

The correct answer is B. Initiate intra-aortic balloon counterpulsation (IABC) and consult cardiothoracic surgery for urgent repair. The patient presents with signs and symptoms of acute severe mitral regurgitation due to papillary muscle rupture following an inferior MI. This is a mechanical complication of MI and is characterized by the sudden onset of a loud holosystolic murmur, pulmonary edema, and hypotension. The use of IABC can help to stabilize the patient hemodynamically by reducing left ventricular afterload and improving coronary perfusion, thereby decreasing the degree of mitral regurgitation and enhancing forward flow. Urgent surgical intervention is indicated as the definitive treatment for papillary muscle rupture, as medical management alone is associated with a high mortality rate. Option A is incorrect because while medical management with diuretics and afterload reduction can provide temporary symptomatic relief, it is not sufficient as definitive treatment for papillary muscle rupture, which typically requires surgical repair due to the risk of rapid hemodynamic deterioration. Option C is incorrect because glycoprotein IIb/IIIa inhibitors and PCI are not the treatments of choice for mechanical complications of MI such as papillary muscle rupture. These interventions are more appropriate for addressing ongoing ischemia or thrombotic complications. Option D is incorrect because while coronary angiography is important in the assessment of recurrent MI, the immediate concern is the mechanical complication of papillary muscle rupture, which requires urgent surgical repair. Coronary angiography may be performed as part of the preoperative evaluation but should not delay the initiation of IABC and surgical consultation.

Harari R et al. Papillary muscle rupture following acute myocardial infarction: Anatomic, echocardiographic, and surgical insights. Echocardiography. 2017 Nov;34(11):1702-1707. PMID: 29082549

3.40 Left Ventricular Free Wall Rupture Post MI

Case 69

A 68-year-old woman with a history of hypertension and a recent anterior myocardial infarction (MI) 4 days ago is brought to the emergency department with sudden onset of chest pain and dyspnea. On examination, she is hypotensive with a blood pressure of 85/50 mmHg, tachycardic with a heart rate of 118 bpm, and tachypneic with a respiratory rate of 26 breaths per minute. She appears distressed, with pale, cool skin. Auscultation of the heart reveals muffled heart sounds, and there is jugular venous distension. The electrocardiogram shows persistent ST-segment elevations in the anterior leads with new Q waves. A bedside echocardiogram demonstrates a large pericardial effusion with diastolic collapse of the right ventricle consistent with cardiac tamponade. There is also evidence of a contained rupture of the left ventricular free wall with a narrow-neck connection to a pseudoaneurysm.
Based on the clinical scenario, which of the following is the most appropriate next step in the management of this patient's condition?

- A. Immediate pericardiocentesis to relieve tamponade.
- B. Urgent coronary angiography to assess for ongoing ischemia.
- C. Administration of intravenous thrombolytics to address residual thrombus.
- D. Emergency consultation with cardiothoracic surgery for repair of the left ventricular free wall rupture.

The correct answer is D. Emergency consultation with cardiothoracic surgery for repair of the left ventricular free wall rupture. The patient presents with clinical signs of cardiac tamponade, which is a life-threatening condition, and evidence of a contained left ventricular free wall rupture that has led to the formation of a pseudoaneurysm. While pericardiocentesis can provide temporary relief in the setting of tamponade, the underlying issue of the myocardial rupture with pseudoaneurysm formation requires surgical intervention. The narrow-neck connection to the left ventricle (LV) suggests that the rupture is contained, but there is a high risk of delayed rupture, which can be fatal. Therefore, emergency surgical repair is the definitive treatment and should be pursued immediately. Option A is incorrect because, although pericardiocentesis can relieve tamponade, it does not address the underlying mechanical complication of LV free wall rupture. Without surgical repair, the patient remains at high risk for complete rupture and death. Option B is incorrect because, while coronary angiography is important in the assessment of ongoing ischemia, it is not the immediate priority in the setting of a contained LV free wall rupture with tamponade. The patient requires surgical intervention to prevent catastrophic rupture. Option C is incorrect because the administration of intravenous thrombolytics could exacerbate the myocardial rupture and is contraindicated in the setting of a known mechanical complication post-MI. Left ventricular free wall rupture (LVFWR) is a critical and potentially life-threatening complication that can occur following an acute myocardial infarction (AMI). Immediate medical attention and often surgical intervention are necessary to prevent mortality. This report consolidates insights from recent studies and clinical experiences related to the surgical management of LVFWR. LVFWR is observed in up to 2% of AMI patients, typically manifesting between one and seven days post-infarction, although delayed occurrences have been documented up to a month or later. There are two distinct types of LVFWR: blow-out and oozing, with the blow-out variant associated with a higher early mortality rate compared to the oozing type. Patients presenting with recent myocardial infarction symptoms such as severe chest pain, vomiting, hemodynamic instability, arrhythmias, syncope, and signs of cardiac tamponade should undergo evaluation for LVFWR. Bedside echocardiography, whether transthoracic or transesophageal, is the preferred diagnostic modality. Timely surgical repair is the preferred treatment approach for LVFWR, with various techniques available including infarctectomy, direct suturing, patch repair, and sutureless repair. Sutureless repair methods, particularly utilizing tissue adhesive materials, have garnered attention due to their reduced trauma to the infarcted area and the potential for performing the procedure without cardiopulmonary bypass (CPB). Sutureless repair employing a collagen patch represents a straightforward, rapid, and reproducible option, especially suited for the oozing type of LVFWR. TachoComb/TachoSil, a tissue adhesive material, has shown a tendency towards decreased in-hospital mortality compared to traditional suture repair methods, particularly for the oozing subtype. However, sutureless repair is not recommended for blow-out LVFWR cases, emphasizing the importance of careful patient selection. Despite notable perioperative mortality rates that can reach up to 50%, survivors of LVFWR surgery can achieve long-term survival with preserved left ventricular function and favorable functional outcomes. A study from a single center reported an in-hospital mortality rate of 28.6%, with low cardiac output syndrome identified as the primary cause of postoperative mortality. Among survivors, the 3-year and 12-year overall survival rates were reported at 82.5% and 55.2%, respectively. Advanced age, concurrent ventricular septal rupture (VSR), and cardiac arrest at presentation were recognized as independent risk factors for unfavorable early outcomes. A pseudoaneurysm, also known as a false aneurysm, occurs when there is a leakage of arterial blood from an artery into the surrounding tissue, creating a cavity that maintains a persistent communication with the originating artery. This condition can arise from various causes, including arterial puncture during medical procedures like cardiac catheterization, trauma, surgical complications, or infections. Treatment for a pseudoaneurysm depends on its size, location, and cause, as well as the patient's symptoms and overall health. Small pseudoaneurysms may resolve on their own and can be managed conservatively with regular medical checkups and ultrasound monitoring. Larger or symptomatic pseudoaneurysms typically require intervention to prevent complications such as hemorrhage.

Antunes MJ. Left ventricular free wall rupture: A real nightmare. J Card Surg. 2021 Sep;36(9):3334-3336.PMID: 34101916

Matteucci M et al/Surgical repair of left ventricular free-wall rupture complicating acute myocardial infarction: a single-center 30 years of experience. Front Cardiovasc Med. 2024 Jan 10;10:1348981.PMID: 38268854

3.41 ≫Postinfarction Management

Case 70

A 64-year-old man with a history of type 2 diabetes mellitus presents to the emergency department with chest pain that started 2 hours ago. An electrocardiogram (ECG) confirms a diagnosis of ST-elevation myocardial infarction (STEMI). He is treated with aspirin, ticagrelor, and undergoes successful primary percutaneous coronary intervention (PCI) with stent placement in the left anterior descending artery. His post-procedural course is complicated by transient hypotension, which responds to intravenous fluids. An echocardiogram shows a left ventricular ejection fraction (LVEF) of 35% with anterior wall hypokinesis. He is started on a beta-blocker, high-intensity statin, and an ACE inhibitor. On hospital day 3, he remains asymptomatic with no recurrent chest pain, but he has not yet undergone any form of stress testing.
Which of the following is the most appropriate next step in the management of this patient?

- A. Discharge the patient with a plan to perform an outpatient stress test in 3–6 weeks.
- B. Perform a submaximal exercise stress test prior to discharge.
- C. Initiate aldosterone blockade therapy.
- D. Schedule an immediate cardiac catheterization.

The correct answer is C. Initiate aldosterone blockade therapy. According to the clinical scenario, the patient has an LVEF of 35% and a history of diabetes mellitus, which are both indications for aldosterone blockade therapy in the setting of STEMI. This is based on evidence that aldosterone blockade in such patients can reduce mortality and morbidity. The patient has already undergone successful revascularization with PCI and is hemodynamically stable, making immediate repeat cardiac catheterization unnecessary. Option A is incorrect because the patient has already undergone revascularization, and the current guidelines recommend risk stratification with non-invasive stress testing before discharge or within the early weeks post-MI in patients who have not been revascularized or if there is a concern for residual ischemia. This patient has been revascularized and is asymptomatic, so an outpatient stress test can be scheduled as part of his follow-up care but is not urgent before discharge. Option B is incorrect because submaximal exercise stress testing prior to discharge is generally recommended for patients who have not undergone cardiac catheterization. This patient has already had a successful PCI, and there is no indication of recurrent ischemia at this time. Option D is incorrect because the patient has already undergone successful PCI, and there is no clinical indication of recurrent ischemia or other complications that would necessitate an immediate repeat cardiac catheterization. Post-myocardial infarction care should commence with the identification and modification of risk factors. Managing hyperlipidemia and cessation of smoking are crucial in preventing further cardiac events and mortality. Initiation of statin therapy prior to hospital discharge reduces the risk of recurrent atherothrombotic episodes. Additionally, controlling blood pressure, participating in cardiac rehabilitation, and engaging in regular exercise are recommended practices. These interventions not only offer significant psychological benefits but also contribute to a more favorable recovery outlook. Beta-blockers play a vital role in improving survival rates by reducing the incidence of sudden death in high-risk patient populations. While their efficacy may be limited in individuals without comorbidities, mild heart attacks, or normal stress test results, various beta-blockers have demonstrated benefits. Studies have shown that titrating carvedilol to 25 mg orally twice daily can reduce mortality in patients with left ventricular dysfunction receiving contemporary treatment. Beta-blockers with intrinsic sympathomimetic activity have shown advantages in post-myocardial infarction patients. Patients who experience substantial myocardial damage often develop progressive left ventricular enlargement and impaired function, leading to heart failure and reduced long-term survival. For those with ejection fractions below 40%, prolonged use of ACE inhibitors (or ARBs) helps prevent left ventricular dilatation, delays heart failure onset, and increases life expectancy. Clinical trials like HOPE have demonstrated a 20% reduction in mortality rates, nonfatal myocardial infarction, and stroke with ramipril treatment in patients with coronary or peripheral vascular disease without confirmed LV systolic dysfunction. Therefore, considering ACE inhibitor therapy is advisable across a broader spectrum of patients, especially those with diabetes and even mild systolic hypertension due to the significant benefits observed. Antiplatelet medications such as aspirin (75–100 mg daily after the initial dose) and P2Y12 inhibitor therapy for one year are recommended for their beneficial effects. Prasugrel offers greater reduction in thrombotic events compared to clopidogrel but carries a higher bleeding risk and is not recommended for individuals with a history of stroke. Ticagrelor presents advantages over clopidogrel. Calcium channel blockers do not improve overall prognoses and should not be prescribed solely for secondary prevention. Non-beta-blocker antiarrhythmic medications have not shown effectiveness except in patients with symptomatic arrhythmias. Amiodarone is preferred for individuals experiencing symptomatic post-myocardial infarction supraventricular arrhythmias as it did not improve survival but also did not cause harm unlike other medications in this context. Implantable defibrillators enhance survival in patients with post-infarction left ventricular dysfunction and heart failure. However, the DINAMIT study did not show an advantage in implanting defibrillators within 40 days after an acute myocardial infarction.

Dorian Pet al. Mechanisms underlying the lack of effect of implantable cardioverter-defibrillator therapy on mortality in high-risk patients with recent myocardial infarction: insights from the Defibrillation in Acute Myocardial Infarction Trial (DINAMIT). Circulation. 2010 Dec 21;122(25):2645-52. PMID: 21135366

Case 70B

A 58-year-old man with a recent history of myocardial infarction (MI) two weeks ago is seen for a follow-up visit. He has a history of hypertension and hyperlipidemia. He quit smoking immediately after his MI. His current medications include aspirin 81 mg daily, ticagrelor 90 mg twice daily, lisinopril 10 mg daily, metoprolol tartrate 50 mg twice daily, and atorvastatin 80 mg at bedtime. His blood pressure is 132/84 mmHg, and his heart rate is 68 bpm. His post-MI echocardiogram showed an ejection fraction of 45% with mild inferior wall hypokinesis. He has no chest pain, dyspnea, or palpitations. He is interested in measures to prevent another cardiac event.
Which of the following is the most appropriate recommendation to add to this patient's current regimen for secondary prevention of MI?

- A. Initiate amiodarone therapy.
- B. Prescribe a calcium channel blocker.
- C. Enroll the patient in a cardiac rehabilitation program.
- D. Implant an automatic implantable cardioverter-defibrillator (AICD).

The correct answer is C. Enroll the patient in a cardiac rehabilitation program. Cardiac rehabilitation programs are a key component of secondary prevention after MI. They provide structured exercise, education on heart-healthy living, and counseling to reduce stress, which can help improve the patient's prognosis and quality of life. This patient has stable vital signs, is on appropriate medical therapy, and has no symptoms suggestive of arrhythmias or heart failure that would require additional pharmacologic or device intervention at this time. Option A is incorrect because amiodarone is an antiarrhythmic medication that is not indicated for routine use in post-MI patients without symptomatic arrhythmias. It is used for individuals with symptomatic postinfarction supraventricular arrhythmias, which this patient does not have. Option B is incorrect because calcium channel blockers have not been shown to improve prognosis in post-MI patients when used solely for secondary prevention. They are typically used for blood pressure control or angina relief, neither of which is an issue for this patient. Option D is incorrect because the DINAMIT trial found no benefit to implanting defibrillators in the early period following acute MI. AICDs are considered for secondary prevention in patients with an ejection fraction of 35% or less and symptomatic heart failure despite optimal medical therapy, or for primary prevention in certain high-risk patients, which does not apply to this patient.

Case 70C

A 63-year-old man with type 2 diabetes mellitus presents to the hospital with an acute anterior ST-elevation myocardial infarction (STEMI). He undergoes successful primary percutaneous coronary intervention (PCI) with stent placement in the proximal left anterior descending (LAD) artery. Post-procedure, his chest pain resolves, and his ECG shows resolution of ST elevations. A subsequent coronary angiogram reveals a 70% stenosis in the left main coronary artery and 80% stenosis in the proximal right coronary artery (RCA). His left ventricular ejection fraction (LVEF) is 40%. He is currently stable on dual antiplatelet therapy with aspirin and ticagrelor, a high-intensity statin, a beta-blocker, and an ACE inhibitor.
Which of the following is the most appropriate next step in the management of this patient's coronary artery disease?

- A. Continue medical therapy and plan for elective coronary artery bypass grafting (CABG) in 12 months.
- B. Perform PCI on the left main coronary artery and RCA lesions during the same hospitalization.
- C. Schedule elective CABG within the next few days, ensuring minimal interruption of P2Y12 inhibitor therapy.
- D. Discharge the patient with a plan to reassess the noninfarct-related lesions in 3 months.

The correct answer is C. Schedule elective CABG within the next few days, ensuring minimal interruption of P2Y12 inhibitor therapy. The patient has significant left main and multivessel coronary artery disease, which are both indications for CABG, especially in the presence of diabetes mellitus and left ventricular dysfunction. The timing of CABG should take into account the recent stent placement and the need to continue dual antiplatelet therapy to prevent stent thrombosis. However, the presence of a significant left main lesion represents a high risk for future events and warrants revascularization sooner rather than later. The decision to proceed with CABG should involve a heart team approach, including a cardiologist and a cardiothoracic surgeon, to determine the optimal timing and strategy for surgery, balancing the risks of stent thrombosis with the benefits of complete revascularization. Option A is incorrect because waiting 12 months to address significant left main and multivessel disease in a diabetic patient with reduced LVEF is not appropriate given the high risk of adverse events associated with these lesions. Option B is incorrect because PCI of the left main coronary artery, especially when associated with multivessel disease, is generally less favorable compared to CABG in diabetic patients. The complexity of the disease in this patient makes CABG a more suitable option for complete and durable revascularization. Option D is incorrect because discharging the patient without addressing the significant left main and multivessel disease would leave the patient at high risk for future cardiac events. Reassessment in 3 months would not be appropriate given the current findings and the patient's risk profile.

Case 70D

A 72-year-old woman with a history of chronic kidney disease (stage III), diabetes mellitus, and hypertension is evaluated for progressive exertional angina despite optimal medical therapy. She had a myocardial infarction 5 years ago, treated with percutaneous coronary intervention (PCI) to the right coronary artery. A recent coronary angiography revealed triple-vessel disease with significant stenosis in the left main coronary artery, left anterior descending artery, and circumflex artery. Her left ventricular ejection fraction (LVEF) is 30%. She is currently taking aspirin, a high-intensity statin, a beta-blocker, and an ACE inhibitor.
Given the patient's comorbidities and complex coronary anatomy, which of the following is the most appropriate management strategy?

- A. Schedule elective coronary artery bypass grafting (CABG) with careful perioperative management.
- B. Perform PCI on the left main coronary artery and staged PCI on the remaining vessels.
- C. Continue aggressive medical management with optimization of antianginal medications.
- D. Refer for a minimally invasive direct coronary artery bypass (MIDCAB) procedure.

The correct answer is A. Schedule elective coronary artery bypass grafting (CABG) with careful perioperative management. This patient has significant left main and triple-vessel disease, which are indications for CABG, especially given her diabetes mellitus and reduced LVEF. Although she has multiple comorbidities that increase her surgical risk, CABG is still the preferred method of revascularization in patients with diabetes and extensive coronary artery disease because it has been shown to improve survival compared to PCI. Careful perioperative management is crucial due to her age, chronic kidney disease, and poor LV function, which all contribute to a higher operative risk. Option B is incorrect because PCI, while less invasive, is generally less favorable compared to CABG in patients with diabetes and extensive multivessel disease, particularly when the left main coronary artery is involved. Option C is incorrect because the patient has progressive symptoms despite optimal medical therapy, indicating that revascularization is necessary to improve symptoms and potentially prognosis. Option D is incorrect because MIDCAB is a less invasive surgical option but is typically not suitable for patients requiring multiple grafts, as in the case of this patient with triple-vessel disease. Additionally, MIDCAB does not have established long-term durability compared to traditional CABG.

3.42 Management of Right Ventricular Infarction

Case 71

A 68-year-old male with a history of hypertension and smoking presents to the emergency department with severe chest pain of 2 hours' duration. His blood pressure is 90/60 mmHg, heart rate is 110 beats per minute, and respiratory rate is 18 breaths per minute. Physical examination reveals elevated jugular venous pressure (JVP), clear lung fields, and no peripheral edema. The ECG shows ST-segment elevation in the inferior leads (II, III, aVF) and ST-segment elevation in the right-sided chest lead (V4R). The initial troponin I level is elevated. The patient receives aspirin, a loading dose of clopidogrel, and heparin. An echocardiogram shows hypokinesis of the right ventricular (RV) wall with preserved left ventricular function.
What is the most appropriate next step in the management of this patient?

- A) Administer intravenous furosemide to relieve JVP elevation.
- B) Infuse 500 mL of 0.9% saline over 2 hours to improve LV filling.
- C) Give sublingual nitroglycerin to lower the blood pressure and reduce myocardial oxygen demand.
- D) Start an intravenous infusion of a beta-blocker to decrease heart rate and improve myocardial oxygenation.

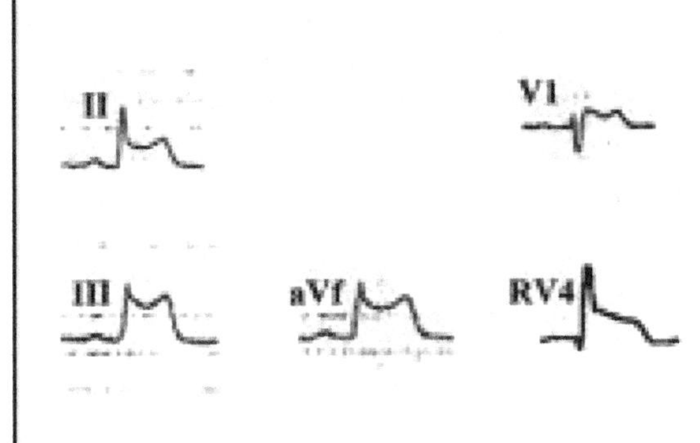

Figure 3.10: ECG RVMI

Correct Answer: B) Infuse 500 mL of 0.9% saline over 2 hours to improve LV filling. This patient presents with clinical and ECG findings suggestive of a right ventricular (RV) infarction, which is a complication of inferior wall myocardial infarction. The key features of RV infarction include hypotension, elevated JVP, and clear lungs, as the RV dysfunction leads to decreased left ventricular (LV) filling and cardiac output without causing pulmonary congestion. Administering intravenous furosemide [A] is contraindicated in the setting of RV infarction because it would decrease intravascular volume, potentially exacerbating hypotension and reducing preload, which is critical for maintaining cardiac output when the RV is compromised. Sublingual nitroglycerin [C] is also contraindicated as it causes venodilation, which can further decrease venous return to the heart and worsen hypotension in the setting of RV infarction. Starting an intravenous infusion of a beta-blocker [D] to decrease heart rate could be detrimental in acute RV infarction because beta-blockers can decrease inotropy and lead to further reduction in cardiac output. Additionally, the patient's heart rate is likely elevated due to compensatory mechanisms in response to hypotension and should not be suppressed without careful consideration of the hemodynamic status. The correct management [B] for RV infarction is to improve LV filling by increasing preload, which can be achieved by fluid loading. The administration of 500 mL of 0.9% saline over 2 hours is recommended to enhance preload and improve cardiac output. Inotropic support may be necessary if the patient does not respond to fluid resuscitation, but it should be used judiciously and typically after adequate fluid loading has been attempted. In summary, the most appropriate next step in the management of this patient with RV infarction is to infuse 500 mL of 0.9% saline over 2 hours to improve LV filling [B]. This approach addresses the pathophysiology of RV infarction by increasing preload to support the compromised RV and improve overall cardiac output.

Namana et al. Right ventricular infarction. Cardiovasc Revasc Med. 2018 Jan;19(1 Pt A):43-50. PMID: 28822687

Case Note

Right ventricular infarction is a condition that should be suspected in all patients with inferior ST-elevation myocardial infarction (STEMI). The diagnostic criteria for right ventricular infarction in patients with inferior STEMI include:

- ST elevation in V1
- ST elevation in V1 and ST depression in V2 (this is highly specific for RV infarction)
- Isoelectric ST segment in V1 with marked ST depression in V2
- ST elevation in III larger then II

The diagnosis is confirmed by the presence of ST elevation in the right-sided leads (V3R-V6R). V1 is the only standard ECG lead that directly looks at the right ventricle. Lead III is more rightward facing than lead II and hence more sensitive to the injury current produced by the right ventricle.

1. Right ventricular infarction complicates up to 40% of inferior STEMIs. Isolated right ventricular infarction is extremely uncommon. It's important to note that ST elevation in the right-sided leads is a transient phenomenon, lasting less than 10 hours in 50% of patients with RV infarction.
2. In the context of an acute myocardial infarction, clinicians first need to determine if the occlusion is strictly a left ventricular (LV) infarction or if it is also jeopardizing the right ventricular (RV) free wall and septum. With RV infarction, the ECG may show an acute anterior Q-wave pattern (leads V1 through V3) as well as a right-sided Q pattern (leads V3R through V6R).
3. Approximately 25% to 50% of cases of inferior wall myocardial infarction are associated with a right ventricular myocardial infarction (RVMI). The presence of RVMI is associated with a 2.6-fold increased risk of mortality as well as an increase in ventricular arrhythmias, high-grade atrioventricular block, and mechanical complications. The hemodynamic syndrome associated with RVMI includes hypotension, elevated venous pressures, and shock without evidence of congestive heart failure.
4. All patients with chest pain should receive a 12-lead ECG early in the patient encounter. When the patient is suffering acute inferior STEMI, a right-sided 12-lead ECG can help to identify right ventricular infarction. Be careful with nitroglycerin in the setting of right ventricular infarction.

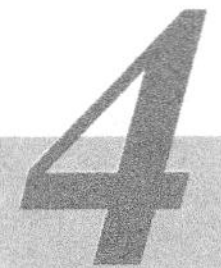

CONGENITAL HEART DISEASE

4.1 Case of Blood Pressure Discrepancy Between The Arms

Case 72

A 18-year-old male presents to your clinic for a routine physical examination before starting a new school year. He has no significant past medical history and denies any symptoms. On examination, you note a blood pressure of 165/90 mm Hg in the right arm and 140/85 mm Hg in the left arm. His heart sounds are normal with no murmurs, rubs, or gallops. However, you note a significant delay in the femoral pulse compared to the radial pulse. Given this patient's history and physical examination findings, which of the following is the most likely diagnosis?

- A) Aortic dissection.
- B) Takayasu arteritis.
- C) Coarctation of the aorta.
- D) Peripheral artery disease.

Answer: C. Coarctation of the aorta. This patient's blood pressure discrepancy between the arms and the delay in the femoral pulse compared to the radial pulse suggest a diagnosis of coarctation of the aorta. Coarctation of the aorta is a congenital condition characterized by a narrowing of the aorta, which can lead to hypertension and reduced blood flow to the lower body. It is often asymptomatic and may be discovered incidentally during a routine physical examination, as in this case. The other options are less likely given the patient's age and lack of symptoms suggestive of these conditions. The treatment for coarctation of the aorta (CoA) is aimed at relieving the obstruction in the aorta to restore normal blood flow to the lower part of the body and to reduce the risk of complications. The choice of treatment depends on the severity of the condition, the age of the patient, and the presence of other heart defects or health issues. Here are the main treatment options:

Surgery is often the gold standard for treating CoA, especially in cases of severe obstruction. There are several surgical techniques available:

1. Resection and End-to-End Anastomosis: This involves removing the narrowed section of the aorta and then reconnecting the two ends.
2. Patch Aortoplasty: A patch is sewn into the area of the coarctation to widen the narrowed section.
3. Left Subclavian Flap Aortoplasty: Part of the left

subclavian artery is used to enlarge the narrowed area.

4. Tubular Bypass Grafts: A tube graft is used to bypass the narrowed section of the aorta.

In some cases, particularly in older children and adults, a less invasive procedure called balloon angioplasty may be used. This involves inserting a catheter with a balloon at its tip into the narrowed area and then inflating the balloon to widen the aorta. Sometimes, a stent is placed to keep the aorta open. Medications may be prescribed to manage symptoms or complications before and after surgical or catheter-based interventions. For example, drugs to control high blood pressure are commonly used. After treatment, whether surgical or catheter-based, lifelong monitoring is necessary to watch for potential complications such as re-narrowing of the aorta (re-coarctation), high blood pressure, or aortic aneurysm. Regular health checkups with a cardiologist are essential to manage these risks.

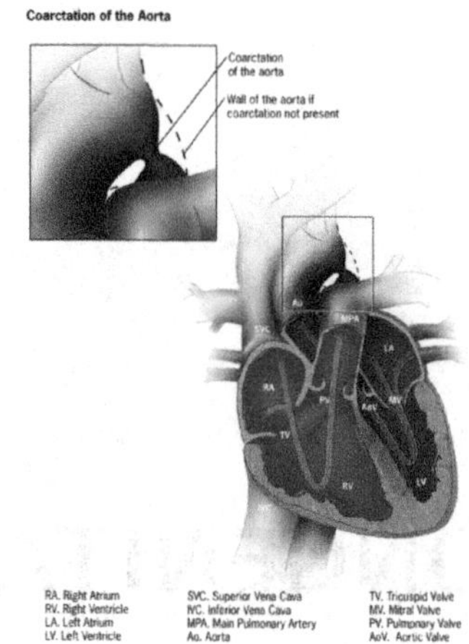

Figure 4.1: Coarctation of the aorta

Case 72B

A 30-year-old female with a history of hypertension presents with a blood pressure of 180/100 mmHg in the upper extremities and 140/80 mmHg in the lower extremities. She reports intermittent claudication and headaches. On physical examination, there is a systolic murmur best heard over the left scapular area, and diminished femoral pulses compared to brachial pulses. An echocardiogram reveals a 60% narrowing of the descending thoracic aorta at the suspected site of coarctation with a peak gradient of 35 mm Hg across the stenosis. Collateral blood vessels are noted on imaging. The patient is currently asymptomatic from a cardiac perspective and is planning to start a family within the next year.
What is the most appropriate next step in the management of this patient's coarctation of the aorta?

- A) Initiate medical management with antihypertensive medications and plan for close follow-up.
- B) Refer for percutaneous endovascular stenting with a covered stent.
- C) Schedule for surgical resection of the coarctation site with end-to-end anastomosis.
- D) Continue observation and reassess if the patient becomes symptomatic.

Correct Answer: B) Refer for percutaneous endovascular stenting with a covered stent. This patient presents with findings consistent with severe coarctation of the aorta, including a significant pressure gradient (above 20 mm Hg), collateral vessel formation, and a narrowing of the descending thoracic aorta by more than 50%. Given these findings, intervention is indicated to prevent the long-term complications associated with severe coarctation, such as hypertension, aortic rupture, infective endarteritis, cerebral hemorrhage, and aortic dissection. Initiating medical management with antihypertensive medications alone [[A]] is not sufficient in this case because it does not address the underlying anatomical abnormality and the patient's desire to become pregnant, which could be complicated by the coarctation. Surgical resection with end-to-end anastomosis [[C]] is a traditional treatment for coarctation of the aorta, but it carries a higher risk of complications, including a 1-4% mortality rate and the risk of spinal cord injury. This option is typically considered when percutaneous intervention is not feasible. Continuing observation [[D]] is not appropriate in this patient due to the severity of the coarctation, the presence of symptoms related to the coarctation (headaches and claudication), and the patient's future pregnancy plans, which could be adversely affected by the coarctation. The best option for this patient is percutaneous endovascular stenting with a covered stent [[B]]. This approach is less invasive than surgery and has been shown to be advantageous over bare metal stents. Covered stents are FDA-approved and are associated with lower risks of complications such as aneurysm formation at the site of the coarctation. Given that most adult coarctation repairs are now performed percutaneously and the patient's desire for pregnancy, this option would likely provide the best outcome with the least amount of risk. Cardiac failure commonly manifests in infants and older individuals who have not received treatment, particularly in cases of severe coarctation. Patients exhibiting a peak gradient above 20 mm Hg should be evaluated for intervention, especially if collateral blood vessels are present. According to ESC guidelines, severe coarctation is defined by stenosis severity exceeding 50%. Untreated individuals with severe coarctation face significant risks such as hypertension, aortic rupture, infective endarteritis, or cerebral hemorrhage before the age of 50, with a higher incidence of aortic dissection. Severe coarctation can also pose challenges during pregnancy due to compromised placental blood flow support. Surgical removal of the coarctation site carries a mortality rate of 1–4% and a risk of spinal cord injury. Endovascular stenting is the preferred percutaneous intervention, with covered stents (self-expanding or balloon-expandable) offering more benefits than bare metal stents when feasible anatomically. These stents have received FDA approval and are typically the preferred approach for adult patients undergoing coarctation repair. Surgical removal with end-to-end anastomosis is recommended when percutaneous intervention is not feasible. Despite surgical interventions, a significant percentage of patients (25–50%) may still experience hypertension in the years following treatment due to lasting effects on various physiological systems. The method of repair (balloon dilatation, stenting, or surgical resection) may influence the development of hypertension. Regular monitoring is essential to detect any recurrence of coarctation stenosis post-treatment. In conclusion, for a patient with severe aortic coarctation and plans for future pregnancy, the most appropriate course of action is referral for percutaneous endovascular stenting using a covered stent. This intervention addresses the anatomical abnormality, reduces the risk of long-term complications, and is the preferred approach for adults with suitable anatomy for the procedure.

Tanous D et al Covered stents in the management of coarctation of the aorta in the adult: initial results and 1-year angiographic and hemodynamic follow-up. Int J Cardiol. 2010 Apr 30;140(3):287-95. PMID: 19100637

,

4.2 Progressive Dyspnea in a Patient with History of Pulmonic Stenosis

Case 73

A 34-year-old woman with a history of moderate pulmonic stenosis diagnosed in childhood presents to the clinic for a routine follow-up. She reports increasing dyspnea on exertion over the past six months. She denies chest pain, syncope, or palpitations. On physical examination, a systolic ejection murmur is heard best at the left upper sternal border, and it radiates to the back. An echocardiogram reveals a peak gradient of 68 mm Hg across the pulmonic valve and right ventricular hypertrophy. The right ventricular systolic pressure is estimated at 85 mm Hg. There is no evidence of right-to-left shunting, and the pulmonic valve is domed with preserved mobility. The patient has no history of endocarditis.
Which of the following is the most appropriate next step in the management of this patient?

- A. Initiate beta-blocker therapy to reduce right ventricular afterload.
- B. Perform percutaneous balloon valvuloplasty.
- C. Schedule surgical commissurotomy.
- D. Continue with routine follow-up and reassess in one year.

The correct answer is B. Perform percutaneous balloon valvuloplasty. According to the AHA/ACC and ESC guidelines, definitive indications for intervention in pulmonic stenosis include symptomatic patients and those with a resting peak gradient greater than 64 mm Hg or a mean gradient greater than 35 mm Hg, regardless of symptoms. This patient is symptomatic with dyspnea on exertion and has a peak gradient of 68 mm Hg, which meets the criteria for intervention. Percutaneous balloon valvuloplasty is highly successful, especially in patients with domed valves, and is the treatment of choice. Option A is incorrect because beta-blocker therapy is not the primary treatment for moderate to severe pulmonic stenosis and would not address the mechanical obstruction caused by the stenotic valve. Option C is incorrect because surgical commissurotomy is generally reserved for cases where percutaneous balloon valvuloplasty is not feasible or has failed, or when there is significant pulmonic regurgitation or a dysplastic valve. Option D is incorrect because the patient is symptomatic with a significant gradient across the pulmonic valve, which warrants intervention rather than routine follow-up without treatment.

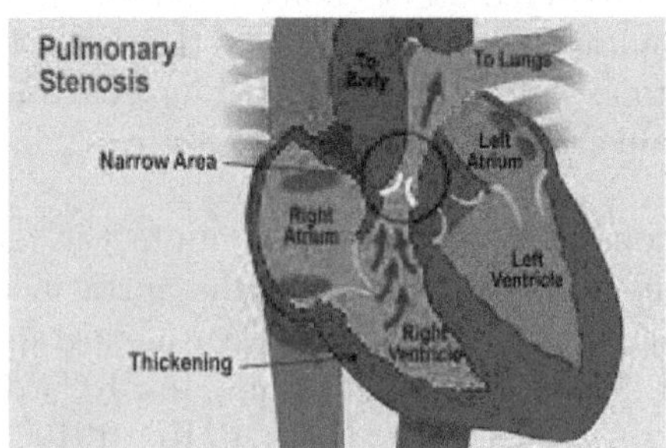

Figure 4.2: PS

Individuals with mild pulmonic stenosis can lead a normal life without requiring treatment. While mild narrowing may not manifest symptoms in childhood and adolescence, signs typically emerge with age. It is important to monitor the progression of stenosis as it may worsen over time in some patients, underscoring the necessity of regular follow-up. Severe stenosis rarely leads to sudden death but can result in right heart failure in individuals as young as their 20s and 30s. Exercising during pregnancy is generally well-tolerated unless there is severe stenosis. Both the American Heart Association/American College of Cardiology (AHA/ACC) guidelines and the European Society of Cardiology (ESC) guidelines generally concur, although the ESC suggests that severe pulmonic stenosis should be considered if the right ventricular systolic pressure exceeds 80 mm Hg. Class I indications for intervention encompass all symptomatic patients and those with a resting peak-to-peak gradient exceeding 64 mm Hg or a mean gradient exceeding 35 mm Hg, irrespective of symptoms. Symptoms may include cyanosis due to right-to-left shunting through a patent foramen ovale (PFO) or atrial septal defect (ASD). Percutaneous balloon valvuloplasty is highly effective for patients with domed valves and is the preferred treatment option. In cases of severe pulmonary valve regurgitation or dysplasia, surgical commissurotomy or pulmonary valve replacement with a bioprosthetic valve or homograft may be required. Obstruction in the pulmonary outflow tract resulting from RV to PA conduit obstruction or homograft pulmonary valve stenosis can be alleviated with a percutaneously implanted pulmonary valve. Both the Medtronic Melody valve and the Edwards SAPIEN XT valve have received FDA approval for this purpose. Typically, these valves are positioned by initially placing a stent in the pulmonary artery (PA), followed by inserting the transcatheter device into the stent. It is essential to assess the potential impact of the new catheter valve on the coronary artery by temporarily inflating a balloon before deploying the device, as it could lead to compression. Percutaneous pulmonary valve replacement is FDA-approved for individuals with conduit stenosis or those who have undergone the Ross procedure. While valve replacements have been conducted off-label for patients with native pulmonary valve disease, such as those who have undergone tetralogy of Fallot repair (provided the PA root size allows for valve seating), careful evaluation and consideration are necessary.

Friedman SH et al. Progressive Dyspnea in a Woman with Congenital Heart Disease and Pulmonary Arterial Hypertension. Ann Am Thorac Soc. 2022 Jul;19(7):1221-1225.PMID: 35772094

Case Note

Endocarditis prophylaxis is not required for native valves following valvuloplasty unless there has been previous pulmonary valve endocarditis, which is rare. It should be used if surgical or percutaneous valve replacement has occurred. There seems to be an increased incidence of pulmonary valve endocarditis after percutaneous pulmonary valve replacement with the Melody valve, which is under close observation by the FDA.

4.3 Managing Cryptogenic Stroke in a Patient with Patent Foramen Ovale

Case 74

A 43-year-old man with a history of cryptogenic stroke one year ago presents for evaluation. He has no significant past medical history except for the previous stroke, for which no clear etiology was identified despite a comprehensive workup. His neurological deficits have since resolved completely. A transthoracic echocardiogram with bubble study shows the presence of a patent foramen ovale (PFO) with a small left-to-right shunt at rest, which becomes a moderate right-to-left shunt with Valsalva maneuver. There is no atrial septal aneurysm. His right heart structures are not enlarged, and pulmonary artery pressures are normal. He is currently on aspirin therapy.

Given the patient's history and current findings, which of the following is the most appropriate management strategy?

- A. Initiate anticoagulation with warfarin.
- B. Refer for percutaneous PFO closure.
- C. Continue aspirin therapy and add a statin.
- D. Schedule for surgical PFO closure.

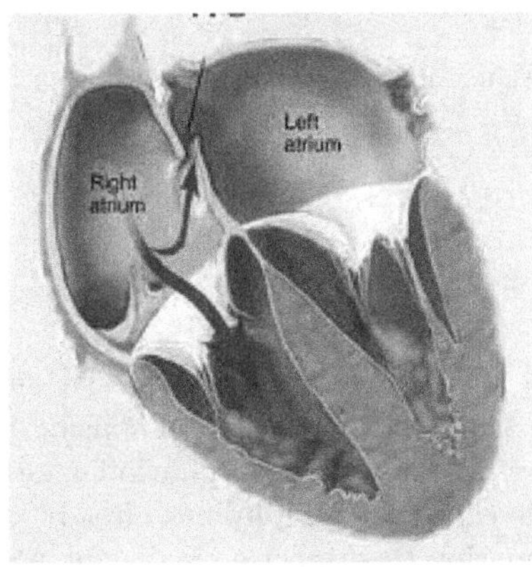

Figure 4.3: PFO

The correct answer is B. Refer for percutaneous PFO closure. In patients younger than 55 years with cryptogenic stroke and a PFO with no other identifiable cause, percutaneous PFO closure should be considered. This recommendation is supported by data showing a reduction in recurrent stroke in patients with PFO who undergo closure compared to those receiving medical treatment alone. The presence of a moderate right-to-left shunt with Valsalva maneuver in the setting of a previous cryptogenic stroke makes this patient a candidate for closure despite the absence of an atrial septal aneurysm. Option A is incorrect because anticoagulation with warfarin is generally considered in patients with a clear thromboembolic source or high-risk features for thromboembolism, which are not present in this case. Option C is incorrect because while continuing aspirin therapy is a reasonable option, the patient has already had a cryptogenic stroke, and the presence of a PFO with a shunt suggests that PFO closure may provide additional benefit in preventing recurrent strokes. Option D is incorrect because surgical closure is more invasive and generally reserved for cases where percutaneous closure is not feasible or has failed, or when there are additional intracardiac repairs that need to be addressed. Patent foramen ovale (PFO) is typically associated with minimal shunting, resulting in patients being asymptomatic with a normal heart size. However, PFOs can predispose individuals to paradoxical emboli and may be a potential cause of cryptogenic strokes in patients under 55 years old. Exercise can induce shunting if there is right heart enlargement or stiffness. Interestingly, the risk of recurrent paradoxical emboli remains low regardless of PFO closure status, reducing the urgency of addressing these defects in cryptogenic stroke cases. The benefits of PFO closure for cryptogenic stroke or transient ischemic attack (TIA) have been complicated by the identification of frequent episodes of paroxysmal atrial fibrillation through 30-day monitoring in these patients, suggesting that atrial fibrillation may be a significant risk factor for stroke/TIA in some cases. Occasionally, a non-pathological PFO may result in cyanosis, especially when right atrial pressure is elevated due to pulmonary or right ventricular hypertension or severe tricuspid regurgitation. Patients experiencing hypoxemia, particularly during standing or exercise, should contemplate PFO closure if no other cause is identified and there is evident right-to-left shunting through the PFO. The efficacy of surgical or percutaneous PFO closure compared to anticoagulation with warfarin, direct oral anticoagulants (DOACs), or aspirin for individuals with cryptogenic stroke or TIA remains uncertain. Individuals under 55 years old presenting with cryptogenic stroke/TIA and solely a PFO should be evaluated for potential PFO closure.

Abdelghani M et al. Management of Patients with Patent Foramen Ovale and Cryptogenic Stroke: An Update. Cardiology. 2019;143(1):62-72. PMID: 31307049

4.4 Managing Exertional Dyspnea in a Patient with Suspected ASD

Case 75

A 35-year-old woman presents to the cardiology clinic with complaints of increasing shortness of breath on exertion over the past six months. She has no significant past medical history and takes no medications. On physical examination, there is a moderately loud systolic ejection murmur in the second and third interspaces parasternally, and S2 is widely split and does not vary with respiration. An electrocardiogram (ECG) shows right axis deviation and incomplete right bundle branch block. A chest radiograph reveals enlarged pulmonary arteries and increased pulmonary vascularity. Transthoracic echocardiography demonstrates right atrial and right ventricular enlargement with a suspected secundum atrial septal defect (ASD). A saline contrast study confirms the presence of a significant left-to-right shunt.
Which of the following is the most appropriate next step in the management of this patient?

- A) Initiate medical management with diuretics and beta-blockers.
- B) Perform a transesophageal echocardiography (TEE) to further assess the ASD.
- C) Schedule the patient for elective surgical closure of the ASD.
- D) Conduct a cardiac catheterization to assess pulmonary artery pressures and pulmonary vascular resistance (PVR).

Correct Answer: D) Conduct a cardiac catheterization to assess pulmonary artery pressures and pulmonary vascular resistance (PVR). The patient presents with symptoms and signs suggestive of an atrial septal defect (ASD) with a significant left-to-right shunt, as evidenced by the echocardiographic findings and the presence of a systolic ejection murmur, fixed splitting of S2, and changes on ECG and chest radiography. Before considering closure of the ASD, it is essential to assess the hemodynamic significance of the shunt and the pulmonary vasculature. Cardiac catheterization is the gold standard for measuring pulmonary artery pressures and pulmonary vascular resistance (PVR). This information is crucial because the presence of elevated PVR can affect the decision to close the ASD. If PVR is significantly elevated, closure of the ASD may lead to right heart failure or could be contraindicated altogether. Medical management with diuretics and beta-blockers may be part of the treatment for heart failure symptoms but does not address the underlying structural issue and is not the next step before confirming hemodynamic significance. Transesophageal echocardiography (TEE) is helpful when transthoracic echocardiography quality is not optimal or when further anatomical details of the ASD are needed, particularly when considering percutaneous closure. However, the scenario suggests that the transthoracic echocardiography has already provided sufficient information to suspect a significant ASD. Scheduling the patient for elective surgical closure of the ASD may be premature without first assessing the pulmonary pressures and PVR. Surgical or percutaneous closure is generally indicated for patients with a significant left-to-right shunt, right atrial and ventricular enlargement, and symptoms, but only after confirming that the pulmonary vasculature can handle the increased flow post-closure. In summary, cardiac catheterization to assess pulmonary artery pressures and PVR is the most appropriate next step in the management of this patient with an ASD and symptoms of exertional dyspnea. This assessment will guide the decision-making process regarding the potential closure of the ASD.

Zarambaitė E et al. The Treatment Strategy for the Atrial Septal Defect in the Presence of Severe Pulmonary Hypertension. Medicina (Kaunas). 2022 Jul 2;58(7):892. PMID: 35888611

Case Note

Cardiac catheterization is the gold standard for measuring pulmonary artery pressures and pulmonary vascular resistance (PVR).

4.5 Addressing Worsening Dyspnea in a Patient with Large VSD

Case 75

A 32-year-old woman with a known large ventricular septal defect (VSD) presents with worsening dyspnea on exertion and fatigue over the past 6 months. She has a history of well-controlled systemic hypertension and no prior surgeries. On physical examination, she has a loud holosystolic murmur best heard at the left lower sternal border. There is no cyanosis or clubbing, and her oxygen saturation is 97% on room air. An echocardiogram shows a large VSD with a left-to-right shunt, a Qp:Qs ratio of 2.3, and mild pulmonary hypertension with a pulmonary artery systolic pressure of 45 mm Hg. The right ventricle is mildly dilated but with normal function. There is no evidence of Eisenmenger syndrome.
Which of the following is the most appropriate next step in the management of this patient?

- A. Initiate therapy with a pulmonary hypertension medication such as sildenafil.
- B. Refer for surgical closure of the VSD.
- C. Continue with medical management and reassess in 6 months.
- D. Place an inferior vena cava (IVC) filter to prevent paradoxical embolism.

The correct answer is B. Refer for surgical closure of the VSD. This patient has a large VSD with a significant left-to-right shunt (Qp:Qs ratio above 2), which is causing symptoms of heart failure (dyspnea on exertion and fatigue) and has led to pulmonary hypertension and right ventricular dilation. Surgical closure of the VSD is indicated to prevent further progression of her symptoms, potential right heart failure, and further increase in pulmonary pressures. The presence of mild pulmonary hypertension does not preclude surgery, and the absence of Eisenmenger syndrome makes her a suitable candidate for surgical repair. Option A is incorrect because while medications for pulmonary hypertension may help alleviate symptoms, they do not address the underlying issue of the left-to-right shunt and may not prevent the progression of heart failure or pulmonary hypertension. Option C is incorrect because the patient is symptomatic with evidence of a significant shunt and mild pulmonary hypertension, which warrants intervention rather than watchful waiting. Option D is incorrect because there is no evidence of a right-to-left shunt, and the patient does not have Eisenmenger syndrome or other risk factors for paradoxical embolism that would necessitate an IVC filter. Individuals with a small VSD typically have a regular life span, with a slight chance of developing infective endocarditis. Antibiotic prophylaxis after dental work is recommended only when the VSD is residual from a prior patch closure or when there is associated pulmonary hypertension and cyanosis. Individuals with significant VSD shunts may develop heart failure at a young age, and living past 40 years old without treatment is rare. n asymptomatic patients with small shunts (pulmonary to systemic flow ratio less than 1.5), surgery or intervention is typically unnecessary. RV infundibular stenosis or pulmonary valve stenosis can provide protection to the pulmonary circuit, allowing some adult patients with a large ventricular septal defect (VSD) to be considered for surgery if there is no pulmonary hypertension present. Surgical closure of a VSD is generally safe, except in cases of severe Eisenmenger physiology. While there are approved devices for nonsurgical closure of muscular VSDs and promising outcomes with devices for membranous VSDs, a notable complication is conduction disturbance. Percutaneous devices are sanctioned for closing VSDs associated with acute myocardial infarction (MI), but results in this high-risk patient group have not been as favorable. In acute MI scenarios, devices have been utilized intraoperatively to create a stable base for sewing a pericardial patch across the ventricular septum, given the often extensive necrosis and complex pathways involved. A described percutaneous technique involves sewing together the two sides of the device using a subxiphoid approach. Medications used to manage pulmonary hypertension stemming from a VSD are akin to those for idiopathic pulmonary hypertension and can effectively alleviate symptoms and reduce cyanosis. It is crucial to employ filters on intravenous lines for patients with a right-to-left shunt to prevent contamination or air embolism entry into the bloodstream.

Morray BH. Ventricular Septal Defect Closure Devices, Techniques, and Outcomes. Interv Cardiol Clin. 2019 Jan;8(1):1-10. PMID: 30449417

4.6 Routine Follow-Up for a Patient with Repaired Tetralogy of Fallot

Case 76

A 34-year-old male with a history of repaired Tetralogy of Fallot in early childhood presents to the clinic for a routine follow-up. He reports increasing shortness of breath on exertion and occasional palpitations. His physical examination reveals a grade 3/6 holosystolic murmur at the left lower sternal border and a single second heart sound. An ECG shows right bundle branch block with no evidence of arrhythmia. A transthoracic echocardiogram demonstrates a dilated right ventricle (RV) with moderate pulmonary regurgitation and a residual ventricular septal defect (VSD) with a left-to-right shunt. Cardiac MRI confirms the presence of severe RV dilation and quantifies RV end-diastolic volume at 160 mL/m^2 (normal under 85 mL/m2) and RV ejection fraction at 40% (normal above 50
What is the most appropriate next step in the management of this patient?

- A) Medical management with beta-blockers and diuretics.
- B) Electrophysiological study to evaluate for inducible ventricular arrhythmias.
- C) Surgical pulmonary valve replacement and VSD closure.
- D) Continue current management and reassess in one year.

Correct Answer: C) Surgical pulmonary valve replacement and VSD closure. This patient with a history of repaired Tetralogy of Fallot is presenting with symptoms of exercise intolerance and palpitations, which are concerning for worsening right ventricular function and potential arrhythmias. The echocardiogram and cardiac MRI findings of severe RV dilation and moderate pulmonary regurgitation with a residual VSD are indicative of significant hemodynamic sequelae that are likely contributing to his symptoms. Medical management with beta-blockers and diuretics [[A]] may provide symptomatic relief but does not address the underlying mechanical issues of pulmonary regurgitation and the residual VSD, which are contributing to RV volume overload and dilation. An electrophysiological study [[B]] may be indicated if there was evidence of sustained arrhythmias on ECG or Holter monitoring, or if the patient had syncope suggestive of arrhythmogenic etiology. However, in this scenario, there is no mention of documented arrhythmias, and the patient's symptoms can be explained by the structural abnormalities identified. Continuing current management and reassessment in one year [[D]] would not be appropriate given the patient's symptoms and the evidence of RV decompensation. Delaying intervention could lead to further deterioration of RV function and increase the risk of irreversible RV failure and arrhythmias. The most appropriate next step is surgical pulmonary valve replacement and VSD closure [[C]]. This intervention is indicated to relieve the RV volume overload caused by the pulmonary regurgitation and to correct the residual VSD, which is contributing to the left-to-right shunt and further RV dilation. Surgical intervention is expected to improve symptoms, prevent further RV dilation, reduce the risk of arrhythmias, and improve the overall prognosis. In summary, the patient's clinical presentation and imaging findings suggest that he would benefit from surgical intervention to address the residual defects from his previous Tetralogy of Fallot repair. Surgical pulmonary valve replacement and VSD closure [[C]] are indicated to improve his symptoms and prevent further deterioration of his cardiac function.

House AV et al. Impact of clinical follow-up and diagnostic testing on intervention for tetralogy of Fallot. Open Heart. 2015 Apr 30;2(1):e000185. PMID: 25973212

Case Note

After the age of 45, atrial fibrillation, reentrant atrial arrhythmias, and ventricular ectopy are common. It seems that arrhythmias are more common with left heart disease compared to right heart disease.

Case 76B

A 38-year-old man with a history of repaired tetralogy of Fallot in childhood presents for a routine follow-up. He has been doing well with no cardiovascular symptoms. His physical examination is unremarkable, with no murmurs, cyanosis, or clubbing, and his oxygen saturation is 98% on room air. A recent transthoracic echocardiogram showed mild pulmonary valve regurgitation and a mildly dilated right ventricle. Cardiac MRI revealed an RV end-diastolic volume index (RVEDVI) of 165 mm/m^2 and an RV end-systolic volume index (RVESVI) of 82 mm/m^2. There is no evidence of residual infundibular stenosis or branch pulmonary artery stenosis. His exercise tolerance is excellent, and he has no arrhythmias on recent Holter monitoring.
Which of the following is the most appropriate next step in the management of this patient?

- A. Schedule for surgical pulmonary valve replacement.
- B. Initiate medical therapy for pulmonary hypertension.
- C. Continue with routine follow-up and reassess in 6 months.
- D. Refer for percutaneous pulmonary valve replacement.

The correct answer is A. Schedule for surgical pulmonary valve replacement. The patient has a history of repaired tetralogy of Fallot and now presents with cardiac MRI findings of an RVEDVI greater than 160 mm/m2 and an RVESVI greater than 80 mm/m^2, which are above the recommended cutoffs for intervention despite being asymptomatic. Early surgical intervention for pulmonary valve replacement is increasingly favored to prevent further RV dilation and potential dysfunction, even in asymptomatic patients. The absence of significant pulmonary hypertension, arrhythmias, and symptoms, along with good exercise tolerance, suggests that the patient is at a good point in time for elective surgery with a likely favorable outcome. Option B is incorrect because there is no evidence of significant pulmonary hypertension that requires medical therapy, and the primary issue is the volume load on the RV due to pulmonary regurgitation. Option C is incorrect because, despite the absence of symptoms, the MRI findings indicate that the RV is at risk of progressive dilation and dysfunction, which warrants intervention rather than watchful waiting. Option D is incorrect because the patient's pulmonary root size may be too large for the currently available percutaneous valve diameters, and surgical replacement is the preferred option when the RV volumes exceed the recommended thresholds. Some patients with a moderate level of subpulmonic stenosis reach adulthood without undergoing surgery. In the management of adult patients, the standard surgical repair typically involves closure of the ventricular septal defect (VSD), excision of infundibular muscle, and placement of an outflow tract patch to alleviate subpulmonic obstruction. Patients with pulmonary valve regurgitation require vigilant monitoring to prevent progressive enlargement of the right ventricle. For individuals with tetralogy of Fallot, it is recommended to undergo transthoracic echocardiogram assessments for pulmonary valve regurgitation every 12–24 months, adjusted based on the severity of regurgitation. Detecting low-pressure pulmonary valve regurgitation can be challenging due to the disparity between right ventricular diastolic pressures and pulmonary arterial diastolic pressure, resulting in minimal gradient between the pulmonary artery and right ventricle during diastole, leading to limited murmur or turbulence visible on color flow Doppler. Any right ventricular enlargement should raise suspicion of pulmonary valve regurgitation until confirmed otherwise. Early surgical pulmonary valve replacement is increasingly favored, with cardiac MRI right ventricular volumes playing a pivotal role in determining the optimal timing for intervention in less symptomatic patients. Guidelines suggest considering intervention if the right ventricular end-diastolic volume index exceeds 160 mm/m2 or the end-systolic volume index surpasses 80 mm/m2. Various factors outlined in the American Heart Association/American College of Cardiology (AHA/ACC) and European Society of Cardiology (ESC) guidelines may prompt intervention. Limitations exist in using a percutaneous approach for pulmonary valve regurgitation due to constraints in available valve diameters compared to the size of the pulmonary annulus. The Melody valve is designed for placement in the superior vena cava, with the largest size measuring 22 mm in diameter. Percutaneous stented valves, like the Edwards SAPIEN XT, have shown efficacy in patients with larger pulmonary root sizes. Typically, a standard stent is first inserted into the pulmonary artery (PA), followed by positioning the stented valve within this initial stent. It is critical to ensure that PA expansion does not impede coronary artery flow, verified by inflating a trial balloon while simultaneously imaging the coronary artery (a class I requirement). An uptick in stented valve endocarditis has been noted post-Melody valve placement, prompting close monitoring. In cases of an anomalous coronary artery, an extracardiac conduit from the right ventricle to the PA may be necessary during tetralogy repair. Long-term follow-up reveals that approximately 10-15% of patients may necessitate reoperation for issues such as severe pulmonary valve regurgitation and residual infundibular stenosis. Typically, the pulmonary valve is substituted with a pulmonary homograft, although a porcine bioprosthetic valve is also suitable. Stented bioprosthetic valves have been effectively employed for percutaneous valve-in-valve procedures in instances of surgical bioprosthetic valve malfunction. Cryoablation of arrhythmogenic tissue may be performed during reoperation. Branch pulmonary stenosis can be addressed percutaneously through stenting. For individuals with prior RV outflow obstruction repair using a conduit, a percutaneous approach with a stented pulmonary valve may be considered. Endocarditis prophylaxis is imperative for all patients. Adults with stable hemodynamics can lead an active lifestyle, and women can successfully carry a pregnancy if RV function remains optimal. Beyond age 45, atrial fibrillation, reentrant atrial arrhythmias, and ventricular ectopy are prevalent. Arrhythmias appear more frequent in left heart disease than in right heart disease. Biventricular dysfunction often manifests as patients age. Left ventricular dysfunction can stem from various causes and may not always be clearly elucidated. Similarly, aortic enlargement can occur with aortic regurgitation, potentially necessitating surgical intervention for severe cases. Individuals with right ventricular (RV) or left ventricular (LV) dysfunction or dysfunction in both ventricles may require a preventive defibrillator.

Dłużniewska N et al.Long-term follow-up in adults after tetralogy of Fallot repair. Cardiovasc Ultrasound. 2018 Oct 29;16(1):28. PMID: 30373624

5 VALVULAR HEART DISEASE

5.1 Exertional Dyspnea in a Patient with CKD and Severe MS

Case 77

A 68-year-old woman with a history of end-stage renal disease on hemodialysis presents with exertional dyspnea and orthopnea. She denies any history of rheumatic fever. On physical examination, she has a diastolic rumbling murmur best heard at the apex with the patient in the left lateral decubitus position. Her blood pressure is 130/80 mm Hg, and her heart rate is 88 beats per minute. An electrocardiogram shows left atrial enlargement. Transthoracic echocardiography reveals severe mitral stenosis with a mitral valve area of 1.0 cm^2, thickened mitral leaflets, and extensive calcification of the mitral annulus extending into the leaflets. The left atrium is significantly enlarged, and there is no evidence of mitral regurgitation. Pulmonary pressures are estimated to be mildly elevated.
Which of the following is the most appropriate next step in the management of this patient?

- A. Initiate medical management with diuretics and beta-blockers.
- B. Refer for percutaneous mitral balloon valvotomy.
- C. Schedule for mitral valve replacement surgery.
- D. Perform a transesophageal echocardiogram to further evaluate the mitral valve.

The correct answer is C. Schedule for mitral valve replacement surgery. This patient presents with symptomatic severe mitral stenosis likely due to calcific degeneration, a condition common in older patients and those undergoing dialysis. Given the extensive calcification extending into the leaflets and the severe restriction of the mitral valve area, percutaneous mitral balloon valvotomy (PMBV) is less likely to be successful and carries a higher risk of complications such as embolization of the calcific material. Mitral valve replacement surgery is the most appropriate intervention for symptomatic relief and to improve her quality of life. Option A is incorrect because while medical management with diuretics and beta-blockers may help reduce symptoms, they do not address the underlying mechanical obstruction caused by the calcified mitral valve. Option B is incorrect because PMBV is typically reserved for patients with pliable, non-calcified mitral valves, particularly in the context of rheumatic mitral stenosis. In this case, the extensive calcification makes PMBV less suitable and more hazardous. Option D is incorrect because the transthoracic echocardiogram has already provided sufficient information to diagnose severe mitral stenosis with extensive calcification. A transesophageal echocardiogram (TEE) is unlikely to offer additional information that would change the management in this case. Intervention for mitral stenosis is warranted if symptoms such as pulmonary edema, reduced exercise capacity, or signs of pulmonary hypertension (peak systolic pulmonary pressure over 50 mm Hg) are present. Some physicians suggest that the presence of atrial fibrillation should also be considered when determining the need for intervention. Most therapies are not initiated until the patient reaches the symptomatic stage (stage D). Symptoms may arise in certain patients when the mitral valve area ranges from 1.5 cm2 to 1.0 cm2. The decision to intervene in these patients should be based on symptoms or evidence of pulmonary hypertension, not solely on the estimated valve area. Open mitral commissurotomy is currently uncommon and has been largely replaced by percutaneous balloon valvuloplasty. Long-term statistics comparing surgery and balloon valvuloplasty over ten years indicate no significant difference in outcomes. Valve replacement is necessary when there is a combination of stenosis and regurgitation, or when the mitral valve echocardiographic score exceeds 8-10. The valve score is determined by assigning numbers 1 to 4 to four valve characteristics: mobility, calcification, thickness, and submitral scar, with a highest possible score of 16. Percutaneous balloon valvuloplasty has a mortality rate of less than 0.5% and a morbidity rate of 3–5%. Operative mortality rates are typically between 1% and 3% in most facilities. If the valve's morphology remains suitable, a repeat balloon valvuloplasty can be performed. A Maze procedure may be performed during surgery to reduce the likelihood of recurrent atrial arrhythmias. The procedure involves creating multiple incisions in the endocardium of both the right and left atria to interrupt the electrical activity responsible for sustaining atrial arrhythmias. In many institutions, the left atrial appendage is surgically closed to prevent future blood clot formation.

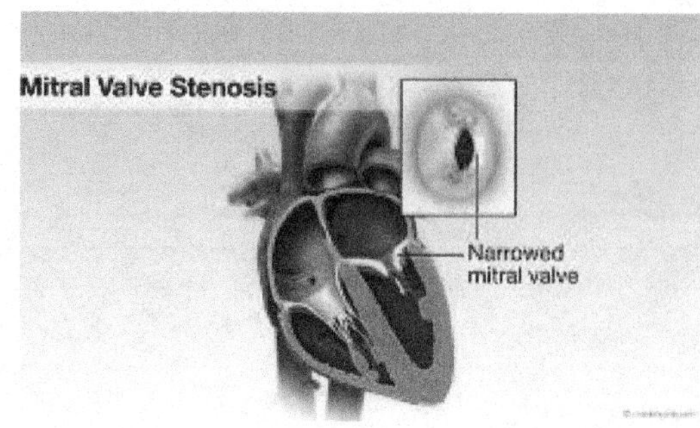

Figure 5.1: MS

Mechanical mitral prosthetic valves have a higher susceptibility to thrombosis compared to mechanical aortic prosthetic valves. The recommended INR range is higher, specifically between 2.5 and 3.5, with an average of 3.0. Low-dose aspirin should be taken with warfarin when the risk of bleeding is minimal. Direct oral anticoagulants (DOACs) are not recommended for use as an anticoagulant in this setting. It is strongly recommended to utilize warfarin for up to 6 months following the implantation of a bioprosthetic mitral valve. Bioprosthetic valves typically deteriorate after around 10 to 15 years. Percutaneous balloon valvuloplasty is ineffective for bioprosthetic valve stenosis, while transcatheter valve-in-valve procedures have shown efficacy. Transcatheter valve-in-valve procedures are increasingly being performed on patients with a high risk of requiring another cardiac surgical valve replacement. Initial results have shown favorable outcomes in patients with bioprosthetic valves, ring annuloplasty, and even in some individuals with calcific mitral stenosis. Younger patients and individuals with end-stage kidney disease are typically thought to have worse outcomes with bioprosthetic heart valves, although there is research challenging the significance of chronic kidney disease as a major risk factor.

Harb SC et al. Mitral Valve Disease: a Comprehensive Review. Curr Cardiol Rep. 2017 Aug;19(8):73. PMID: 28688022

Case Note

Endocarditis prevention is recommended for patients with prosthetic heart valves but not for those with native valve disease.

Table 5.1: Heart Murmur Types

Type	Description	Conditions linked
Systolic murmur	Heard during contraction phase of cardiac cycle	Aortic valve stenosis, hypertrophic obstructive cardiomyopathy, aortic flow murmurs
Holosystolic murmur	Heard throughout contraction phase of cardiac cycle	Mitral regurgitation, tricuspid regurgitation
Early diastolic murmur	Heard during relaxation stage of cardiac cycle after second heart sound	Aortic valve regurgitation, pulmonic valve regurgitation
Continuous murmur	Heard for most of the cardiac cycle	Coronary AV fistula, patent ductus arteriosus, ruptured sinus of Valsalva aneurysm
Mid-to-late diastolic murmur	Heard in mid-to-late phase of relaxation stage of cardiac cycle	Mitral or tricuspid stenosis, flow murmur across mitral or tricuspid valves

5.2 Progressive Dyspnea and Palpitations in a Patient with History of RF

Case 78

A 55-year-old woman presents to the clinic with complaints of progressive dyspnea on exertion and intermittent palpitations over the past 6 months. She has a past medical history significant for rheumatic fever during childhood. On physical examination, her blood pressure is 120/70 mm Hg, heart rate is 78 beats per minute and regular, and she has no lower extremity edema. Cardiac auscultation reveals a loud S1 and an opening snap that is closely followed by S2. There is a low-pitched diastolic rumble heard best at the apex with the patient in the left lateral decubitus position. There are no additional murmurs.
Which of the following is the most appropriate next step in the management of this patient?

- A. Initiate anticoagulation with warfarin.
- B. Perform transthoracic echocardiography.
- C. Refer for percutaneous mitral balloon valvotomy.
- D. Schedule for mitral valve replacement surgery.

The correct answer is B. Perform transthoracic echocardiography. The patient's history of rheumatic fever and the presence of a loud S1 and an opening snap following S2, along with a diastolic rumble, are classic findings for mitral stenosis. Transthoracic echocardiography is the diagnostic test of choice to confirm the diagnosis, assess the severity of the stenosis, evaluate the valve anatomy, and measure the pressure gradients across the mitral valve and the size of the left atrium. This information is crucial for determining the appropriate management strategy. Option A is incorrect because while anticoagulation may be indicated in patients with mitral stenosis, especially if they have atrial fibrillation or a history of thromboembolism, the decision to initiate anticoagulation should be based on a comprehensive assessment including echocardiographic findings. Option C is incorrect because although percutaneous mitral balloon valvotomy is a potential treatment for mitral stenosis, it is indicated after confirming the diagnosis and assessing the suitability of the valve anatomy for this procedure via echocardiography. Option D is incorrect because mitral valve replacement surgery is a treatment option for severe mitral stenosis, particularly when the valve is not amenable to repair or valvotomy. However, this decision should be made after detailed imaging and assessment of the valve anatomy and severity of stenosis. Chronic rheumatic heart disease arises from one or multiple episodes of rheumatic fever, resulting in the stiffening and distortion of valve cusps, fusion of commissures, or shortening and fusion of chordae tendineae. Valvular stenosis or regurgitation commonly coexist within this condition. In chronic rheumatic heart disease, the mitral valve is the primary anomaly in 50-60% of cases, while 20% exhibit combined aortic and mitral valve issues; pure aortic valve abnormalities are less frequent. Tricuspid involvement occurs in around 10% of cases, usually alongside mitral or aortic disease, with a higher prevalence in cases with recurrent infections. Long-term effects on the pulmonary valve are rare. Notably, only 60% of individuals with rheumatic heart disease have a confirmed history of rheumatic fever. Despite advancements in treatment, chronic rheumatic heart disease remains a significant cardiovascular challenge in impoverished regions worldwide. Patients with mitral stenosis typically manifest two clinical symptoms. In mild to moderate cases, left atrial pressure and cardiac output are usually normal, with symptoms appearing post-exertion or remaining asymptomatic. Severe mitral stenosis, characterized by a valve area below 1.0 cm2, can lead to severe pulmonary hypertension due to secondary stenosis in the pulmonary vascular bed. Distinctive features of rheumatic mitral stenosis include an opening snap following A2 due to the rigid mitral valve. The time interval between the opening snap and aortic closure sound varies with left atrial pressure levels. As mitral stenosis progresses, a low-pitched diastolic murmur becomes more pronounced and prolonged, correlating with the degree of stenosis. Mitral regurgitation may also be present, with 50-80% of patients eventually developing atrial fibrillation. Regulating heart rate is crucial in optimizing diastolic filling of the left ventricle; slower heart rates facilitate this process by extending diastole duration and reducing pressure gradients across the mitral valve. An abrupt increase in heart rate can precipitate pulmonary edema, emphasizing the importance of heart rate control in managing chronic rheumatic heart disease effectively.

Table 5.2: Effects of Respiration on Heart Murmurs and Sounds

Respiration	Effect on Murmurs and Sounds
Inspiration	Systolic murmurs caused by tricuspid regurgitation or pulmonic blood flow through a normal or stenotic valve, as well as right sided S3 and S4 murmurs, typically increase
Expiration	Murmurs and sounds on the left side are typically louder

Case 78B

A 62-year-old woman with a history of rheumatic heart disease and moderate mitral stenosis presents with new-onset palpitations. She reports that these symptoms started about 2 months ago. Her physical examination reveals an irregularly irregular pulse, and an echocardiogram confirms the presence of atrial fibrillation with a left atrial diameter of 4.2 cm. Her CHA2DS2-VASc score is 4, indicating a high risk for thromboembolic events. She has no history of bleeding disorders or contraindications to anticoagulation.
Which of the following is the most appropriate management for this patient's atrial fibrillation?

- A. Initiate anticoagulation with a direct oral anticoagulant (DOAC).
- B. Initiate anticoagulation with warfarin.
- C. Perform electrical cardioversion without anticoagulation.
- D. Prescribe an antiarrhythmic drug for rhythm control without anticoagulation.

The correct answer is B. Initiate anticoagulation with warfarin. In patients with rheumatic mitral stenosis and atrial fibrillation, warfarin is the preferred anticoagulant due to the increased risk of thromboembolic events associated with this condition. The INVICTUS trial showed that patients with rheumatic mitral valve disease and atrial fibrillation had a higher rate of adverse vascular events when treated with a DOAC (rivaroxaban) compared to those treated with a vitamin K antagonist (warfarin). Given the patient's CHA2DS2-VASc score of 4 and the recent onset of atrial fibrillation, anticoagulation is indicated to reduce the risk of stroke and systemic embolism. Option A is incorrect because DOACs are not recommended for patients with rheumatic mitral stenosis and atrial fibrillation, as evidenced by the results of the INVICTUS trial, which showed a higher rate of adverse events with rivaroxaban compared to warfarin. Option C is incorrect because electrical cardioversion without prior or concurrent anticoagulation increases the risk of thromboembolic events, especially in patients with mitral stenosis and atrial fibrillation. Anticoagulation should be initiated before considering cardioversion. Option D is incorrect because while rhythm control may be a component of managing atrial fibrillation, it does not obviate the need for anticoagulation in a patient with a high risk of thromboembolism. Antiarrhythmic drugs alone without anticoagulation would not adequately protect against the risk of stroke in this patient. The onset of atrial fibrillation typically presents symptoms that can be managed by controlling the ventricular rate or restoring sinus rhythm. Successfully transitioning to and sustaining sinus rhythm is more achievable when atrial fibrillation is of short duration (less than 6-12 months) and the left atrium is not significantly enlarged (diameter less than 4.5 cm). Following an episode of atrial fibrillation, patients are advised to be prescribed warfarin regardless of whether sinus rhythm is restored. This precaution is necessary as atrial fibrillation often recurs despite antiarrhythmic therapy, and untreated individuals face a 20-30% risk of systemic embolization. In cases of systemic embolization in mild to severe conditions, surgical intervention is not typically warranted; instead, management with warfarin is recommended. Current guidelines do not endorse the use of DOACs (dabigatran, apixaban, rivaroxaban, edoxaban) for individuals with atrial fibrillation due to their exclusion from approval studies. A randomized clinical trial published in 2022 supports this stance. The INVICTUS trial assigned patients with rheumatic mitral valve disease and atrial fibrillation to receive either rivaroxaban or a vitamin K antagonist for treatment. Over a 3.1-year period, those administered rivaroxaban exhibited a notably higher incidence of the primary outcome, encompassing death from vascular or unexplained causes, stroke, systemic embolism, or myocardial infarction. Vascular mortality and ischemic stroke as secondary endpoints were more prevalent in the rivaroxaban group.

Connolly SJ et al; INVICTUS Investigators. Rivaroxaban in rheumatic heart disease-associated atrial fibrillation. N Engl J Med. 2022;387:978. PMID: 36036525

Table 5.3: Effects of Valsalva Maneuver on Heart Murmurs

Maneuver	Effect on Murmurs
Majority of murmurs	Get shorter and less intense over time.
Exceptions	Hypertrophic cardiomyopathy (HCM) murmurs typically get much louder, and mitral valve prolapse (MVP) murmurs typically get longer and louder.
Right-sided murmurs	Typically return to control intensity earlier than left-sided murmurs after release of Valsalva maneuver.
HCM murmur	Gets louder when standing up.
MVP murmur	Lengthens and frequently gets stronger when standing up. Most murmurs get louder when squatting, but HCM and MVP murmurs usually get softer and might even go away.
Isotonic and submaximal isometric (handgrip) exercise	Causes murmurs caused by blood flow across healthy or obstructed valves to become louder.
Exercise involving the handgrip	Causes an increase in murmurs of mitral regurgitation, ventricular septal defect, and aortic regurgitation.
HCM murmur	Frequently lessens when exercising the handgrip to its near maximum.

5.3 Anticoagulation in a Patient with Mechanical Mitral Valve Replacement

Case 79

A 58-year-old man with a history of mechanical mitral valve replacement 5 years ago presents for a routine follow-up. He has been on warfarin therapy with a target INR of 2.5-3.5. He reports compliance with his medication and denies any bleeding symptoms. His other medications include low-dose aspirin, a statin, and an ACE inhibitor. On examination, his vitals are stable, and his cardiac exam is notable for a mechanical valve click without any additional murmurs. His most recent INR, checked 1 week ago, was 3.2. He has no history of thromboembolism or atrial fibrillation.
Which of the following is the most appropriate management for this patient's anticoagulation therapy?

- A. Continue current warfarin and aspirin therapy with routine INR monitoring.
- B. Increase warfarin dose to achieve an INR of 3.5-4.5.
- C. Switch anticoagulation therapy to a direct oral anticoagulant (DOAC).
- D. Discontinue aspirin and continue warfarin therapy with the same target INR.

The correct answer is A. Continue current warfarin and aspirin therapy with routine INR monitoring. Patients with mechanical mitral valves are at a higher risk of thromboembolic events compared to those with mechanical aortic valves. The recommended INR range for mechanical mitral valves is 2.5-3.5 to reduce the risk of thrombosis. Low-dose aspirin is often added to warfarin therapy if the patient has a low bleeding risk, as it can provide additional protection against thromboembolism. Since the patient's INR is within the target range and he is not experiencing any complications, it is appropriate to continue his current regimen with routine INR monitoring to ensure it remains within the therapeutic range. Option B is incorrect because increasing the warfarin dose to achieve an INR of 3.5-4.5 would put the patient at an unnecessarily high risk of bleeding without additional benefit, as his current INR is already within the recommended therapeutic range. Option C is incorrect because DOACs are not recommended for patients with mechanical heart valves due to an increased risk of thromboembolic events and valve thrombosis when compared to warfarin. Option D is incorrect because there is no indication to discontinue aspirin in this patient. Aspirin provides an additional antithrombotic effect, and since the patient is not experiencing any bleeding, it is beneficial to continue it along with warfarin. Dabigatran, a direct oral anticoagulant (DOAC), has been found to be associated with increased rates of thromboembolic and bleeding complications in patients with mechanical heart valves compared to warfarin. This was revealed in research studies like the RE-ALIGN trial, which aimed to validate a new dabigatran dosing regimen for the prevention of thromboembolic complications in these patients. However, the trial was halted early due to an excess of thromboembolic and bleeding events in the dabigatran group. The study found that most thromboembolic events among patients in the dabigatran group occurred in those who had started the drug within 7 days after valve surgery, with fewer occurring in patients who had undergone valve implantation more than 3 months before randomization . This suggests that the timing of initiation of dabigatran in mechanical valve patients may be a critical factor to consider. The use of dabigatran in patients with mechanical heart valves showed no benefit and an excess risk, leading to the conclusion that dabigatran was not effective in preventing thromboembolic complications in these patients and was linked to an increased risk of bleeding. Due to these safety concerns, regulatory bodies like the FDA and the European Medicines Agency have recommended against using dabigatran in patients with mechanical heart valves pradaxa-dabigatran-etexilate-mesylate-should-not-be-used-patients). This highlights the importance of appropriate anticoagulant selection in this patient population and suggests that warfarin remains the preferred choice for anticoagulation in patients with mechanical heart valves.

Eikelboom JW et al. Dabigatran versus warfarin in patients with mechanical heart valves. N Engl J Med. 2013 Sep 26;369(13):1206-14. PMID: 23991661

5.4 Managing Acute Dyspnea and AF in a Patient with Hypertension

Case 80

A 68-year-old man with a history of hypertension presents to the emergency department with acute onset of shortness of breath and palpitations that started suddenly while he was mowing the lawn. He denies any chest pain. His past medical history is unremarkable except for hypertension, which is controlled with hydrochlorothiazide. On examination, his blood pressure is 150/90 mm Hg, heart rate is 110 beats per minute and irregularly irregular, respiratory rate is 22 breaths per minute, and oxygen saturation is 88% on room air. Lung auscultation reveals bilateral rales halfway up both lung fields. Cardiac examination shows a hyperdynamic precordium, a brisk carotid upstroke, and a pansystolic murmur at the apex radiating to the axilla. There is no murmur change post-premature ventricular contraction. An electrocardiogram shows atrial fibrillation with no ST changes, and a chest X-ray demonstrates pulmonary edema.
Which of the following is the most appropriate next step in the management of this patient?

- A. Immediate electrical cardioversion.
- B. Initiation of intravenous diuretics and afterload reduction.
- C. Urgent transthoracic echocardiography.
- D. Immediate mitral valve surgery.

The correct answer is C. Urgent transthoracic echocardiography. This patient presents with signs and symptoms suggestive of acute mitral regurgitation (MR) given the new onset of shortness of breath, palpitations (which may indicate atrial fibrillation), a pansystolic murmur radiating to the axilla, and evidence of pulmonary edema on physical examination and chest X-ray. In the setting of acute MR, the left atrium (LA) has not had time to dilate and accommodate the regurgitant volume, leading to a sudden increase in LA and pulmonary pressures, which can precipitate pulmonary edema. Urgent transthoracic echocardiography is indicated to confirm the diagnosis, assess the severity of MR, identify the mechanism of regurgitation, and guide further management, including potential surgical intervention. Option A is incorrect because immediate electrical cardioversion is not the first-line treatment for acute MR. While it may be considered to restore sinus rhythm in patients with atrial fibrillation, the priority is to stabilize the hemodynamics and confirm the diagnosis and severity of MR. Option B is incorrect because, although intravenous diuretics and afterload reduction can help reduce symptoms of pulmonary edema and improve hemodynamics, it is essential to first confirm the diagnosis and severity of MR with echocardiography to guide the management. Option D is incorrect because immediate mitral valve surgery may eventually be necessary for acute severe MR, but it is not the first step before confirming the diagnosis and assessing the valve anatomy and function with echocardiography. Mitral regurgitation can develop suddenly due to various factors such as papillary muscle failure following a myocardial infarction, valve perforation in infective endocarditis, hypertrophic cardiomyopathy (HCM), or ruptured chordae tendineae in patients with mitral valve prolapse, potentially necessitating emergency surgical intervention. In instances of hemodynamic instability, the use of vasodilators or intra-aortic balloon counterpulsation may be necessary to reduce retrograde regurgitant flow by lowering systemic vascular resistance and enhancing forward stroke volume. The effectiveness of reducing afterload in chronic mitral regurgitation is a subject of debate due to the inherent decrease in afterload resulting from the condition itself, with limited evidence supporting chronic afterload reduction for preventing left ventricular failure or the need for surgery. While some experts propose considering beta-blockade routinely to address heightened sympathetic activity, this remains a theoretical concept. Notably, patients with tachycardia-induced cardiomyopathy may experience an improvement in mitral regurgitation upon normalization of heart rate. Individuals with severe mitral regurgitation are at an increased risk of in-hospital mortality. For those with functional mitral regurgitation, timely percutaneous coronary intervention (PCI) directed at the culprit artery may provide benefits, while urgent surgery can be life-saving for individuals with primary mitral regurgitation. These points emphasize the crucial role of timely and appropriate interventions in managing mitral regurgitation and its associated complications.

Leitman M et al. Assessment and Management of Acute Severe Mitral Regurgitation in the Intensive Care Unit. J Heart Valve Dis. 2017 Mar;26(2):161-168. PMID: 28820545

5.5 Asymptomatic Patient with Mild MR and Rising BNP

Case 81

A 55-year-old woman with a history of mild mitral regurgitation diagnosed two years ago presents for a routine follow-up. She is asymptomatic and has been participating in her regular activities without limitation. Her blood pressure is 130/80 mm Hg, heart rate is 72 beats per minute, and she is in sinus rhythm. On examination, she has a grade 2/6 pansystolic murmur at the apex radiating to the axilla. She has no signs of heart failure on examination, and her lung fields are clear. An echocardiogram six months ago showed mild mitral regurgitation with normal left ventricular size and function. Her current NT-proBNP level is 450 pg/mL, which has increased from 150 pg/mL over the past six months.
Which of the following is the most appropriate next step in the management of this patient?

- A. Repeat echocardiography now.
- B. Initiate treatment with an ACE inhibitor.
- C. Schedule for mitral valve surgery.
- D. Continue routine follow-up with no additional testing.

The correct answer is A. Repeat echocardiography now. In patients with mitral regurgitation, BNP or NT-proBNP levels can be useful for the early identification of left ventricular (LV) dysfunction, even in asymptomatic patients. An upward trend in NT-proBNP levels over time, as seen in this patient, may indicate worsening mitral regurgitation or the development of LV dysfunction and has prognostic importance. Given the significant increase in NT-proBNP levels in this patient, it is appropriate to perform repeat echocardiography to reassess the severity of mitral regurgitation, LV size, and function, and to determine if there has been a change that would warrant a modification in management. Option B is incorrect because there is no current indication to initiate treatment with an ACE inhibitor in this patient, who is asymptomatic with previously documented mild mitral regurgitation and normal LV function. ACE inhibitors are typically used in the management of heart failure or significant LV dysfunction, neither of which has been established in this patient without updated echocardiographic data. Option C is incorrect because mitral valve surgery is generally reserved for patients with symptomatic severe mitral regurgitation, evidence of LV dysfunction, or other specific indications such as new-onset atrial fibrillation or pulmonary hypertension. This patient is asymptomatic with only a previous diagnosis of mild mitral regurgitation, and there is no current evidence from an updated echocardiogram to suggest that surgery is indicated. Option D is incorrect because the significant rise in NT-proBNP levels suggests that there may be a change in the patient's cardiac status that warrants further investigation. Continuing routine follow-up without additional testing may miss the opportunity to detect and manage potential progression of mitral regurgitation or LV dysfunction. The degree of left ventricular enlargement serves as an indicator of the severity and duration of blood backflow. Left ventricular volume overload can lead to left ventricular failure and reduced cardiac output. In cases of chronic mitral regurgitation, significant expansion of the left atrium may occur, and the heart can endure a considerable volume of regurgitation without immediate symptoms. Individuals with chronic conditions may remain asymptomatic for an extended period. Surgery becomes necessary upon symptom onset or evidence of left ventricular dysfunction, as progressive and irreversible deterioration of left ventricular function can occur before symptoms manifest. Early surgical intervention is advised for asymptomatic individuals with a reduced ejection fraction (EF less than 60%) or notable left ventricle dilation with decreased contractility (end-systolic size larger than 4.0 cm). Mitral valve surgery is recommended when the left ventricular ejection fraction is above 60% and the left ventricular end-systolic dimension is less than 4.0 cm, but subsequent imaging reveals a continuous increase in end-systolic dimension or a consistent decline in ejection fraction. The presence of pulmonary hypertension signifies significant mitral regurgitation and warrants intervention. If mitral regurgitation stems from cardiac dysfunction, improvement may occur as the infarction heals or left ventricular dilation diminishes. Regurgitation is often attributed to papillary muscle displacement and an enlarged mitral annulus rather than papillary muscle ischemia. Improper leaflet alignment during systole, due to leaflet prolapse or retraction, is a primary concern. Papillary muscle rupture can result from acute myocardial infarction with severe repercussions. Intermittent yet occasionally severe mitral regurgitation may arise during myocardial ischemia, leading to sudden pulmonary edema. Patients with dilated cardiomyopathies may develop secondary mitral regurgitation due to papillary muscle displacement, annular dilation, or both. Preserving chordae during mitral valve replacement surgery can help prevent further ventricular dilation. Historically, positive outcomes have been achieved by various organizations performing mitral valve replacement on patients with a left ventricular ejection fraction below 30% and subsequent mitral regurgitation. Guidelines recommend considering mitral valve repair or replacement for individuals with severe mitral regurgitation and an ejection fraction below 30% or a left ventricular end-systolic size exceeding 5.5 cm, or both, provided repair and chordae maintenance are feasible.

Otto CM et al. 2020 ACC/AHA guideline for the management of patients with valvular heart disease. J Am Coll Cardiol. 2021;77:450. PMID: 33342587

5.6 Chronic Mitral Regurgitation with Declining LV Function

Case 82

A 63-year-old woman with a known history of chronic mitral regurgitation presents for an annual follow-up. She reports no symptoms of heart failure and is able to perform her daily activities without limitation. Her medical history is significant for hyperlipidemia, which is well-controlled with atorvastatin. On physical examination, her blood pressure is 135/85 mm Hg, heart rate is 78 beats per minute, and she is in sinus rhythm. Cardiac auscultation reveals a grade 3/6 holosystolic murmur best heard at the apex and radiating to the axilla. There is no jugular venous distension, lung examination is clear, and there are no peripheral edema. A transthoracic echocardiogram performed one year ago showed mild to moderate mitral regurgitation with a left ventricular ejection fraction (LVEF) of 65% and left ventricular end-systolic dimension (LVESD) of 3.5 cm. Current echocardiogram shows a LVEF of 58% and LVESD of 4.2 cm. Pulmonary artery systolic pressure is estimated at 35 mm Hg.
Which of the following is the most appropriate next step in the management of this patient?

- A. Continue annual follow-up with echocardiography.
- B. Initiate treatment with an angiotensin-converting enzyme (ACE) inhibitor.
- C. Refer for mitral valve repair or replacement surgery.
- D. Perform cardiac magnetic resonance imaging (MRI) to further assess LV size and function.

The correct answer is C. Refer for mitral valve repair or replacement surgery. This patient has chronic mitral regurgitation and is currently asymptomatic. However, the echocardiogram shows a decrease in LVEF from 65% to 58% and an increase in LVESD from 3.5 cm to 4.2 cm over the past year. These changes indicate a progressive decline in LV function and an increase in LV size, which are markers of worsening mitral regurgitation and predictors of poor outcome if left untreated. Early surgical intervention is indicated in asymptomatic patients with chronic mitral regurgitation who have a reduced LVEF (less than 60%) or marked LV dilation with reduced contractility (LVESD greater than 4.0 cm). Additionally, the development of pulmonary hypertension (pulmonary artery systolic pressure of 35 mm Hg) further supports the need for surgical intervention. Option A is incorrect because, despite the absence of symptoms, the patient has echocardiographic evidence of progressive LV dysfunction and enlargement, which warrants surgical intervention rather than continued observation. Option B is incorrect because, while ACE inhibitors may be used in the management of heart failure or LV dysfunction, this patient's echocardiographic findings indicate the need for surgical intervention, which should not be delayed by medical therapy. Option D is incorrect because the current echocardiographic findings are sufficient to make a decision regarding surgery. Cardiac MRI may provide additional details about LV size and function but is not necessary in this case as the echocardiogram has already provided the necessary information to guide management. Mitral valve replacement with chordal preservation is the preferred approach for patients with persistent ischemic cardiomyopathy over mitral valve repair. In cases of cardiomyopathy associated with mitral regurgitation, cardiac resynchronization therapy with biventricular pacemaker insertion may help alleviate the regurgitation. Guidelines recommend considering biventricular pacing prior to surgical intervention for symptomatic individuals with functional mitral regurgitation who meet specific criteria, such as a QRS duration exceeding 150 msec, presence of left bundle branch block, or both. Ongoing trials are exploring percutaneous techniques to reduce mitral regurgitation. These methods include using a MitraClip device to create a double-orifice mitral valve, various coronary catheter devices to reduce the mitral annular area, and devices to decrease septal-lateral ventricular dimensions and subsequently the mitral orifice size. Among these devices, the edge-to-edge MitraClip has demonstrated the most favorable outcomes. The guidelines endorse the use of the MitraClip in patients with secondary mitral regurgitation at high surgical risk. Vascular plugging and occluder devices are employed in select cases to seal perivalvular leaks around prosthetic mitral valves. Additionally, a transcatheter stented valve, commonly used for transcatheter aortic valve replacement (TAVR), can be utilized to address a dysfunctional mitral bioprosthetic valve in various positions like aortic, mitral, tricuspid, or pulmonary Transcatheter valve replacement has been explored in limited studies to correct mitral regurgitation post-mitral valve repair, yielding diverse outcomes

Overtchouk P et al. Comparison of Mitral Valve Replacement and Repair for Degenerative Mitral Regurgitation: a Meta-analysis and Implications for Transcatheter Mitral Procedures. Curr Cardiol Rep. 2020 Jul 9;22(9):79. PMID: 32648008

5.7 Worsening Functional MR in a Patient with Ischemic Cardiomyopathy

Case 83

A 72-year-old man with a history of ischemic cardiomyopathy and a left ventricular ejection fraction (LVEF) of 25% presents with worsening dyspnea on exertion and orthopnea over the past 2 months. He has a history of a myocardial infarction 3 years ago and has been on optimal medical therapy for heart failure, including an ACE inhibitor, beta-blocker, and spironolactone. His blood pressure is 110/70 mm Hg, heart rate is 70 beats per minute, and he is in sinus rhythm with a QRS duration of 160 msec and left bundle branch block on the electrocardiogram. On examination, he has a displaced apical impulse, a grade 3/6 holosystolic murmur at the apex radiating to the axilla, and bibasilar crackles on lung auscultation. A recent echocardiogram shows severe mitral regurgitation with an LV end-systolic dimension of 6.0 cm. There is no evidence of mitral valve prolapse or intrinsic mitral valve disease, suggesting functional mitral regurgitation.
Which of the following is the most appropriate next step in the management of this patient?

- A. Refer for mitral valve replacement with chordal preservation.
- B. Initiate cardiac resynchronization therapy (CRT) with biventricular pacemaker insertion.
- C. Refer for percutaneous mitral valve repair with a MitraClip device.
- D. Continue optimal medical therapy without further intervention.

The correct answer is B. Initiate cardiac resynchronization therapy (CRT) with biventricular pacemaker insertion. This patient has symptomatic heart failure with reduced ejection fraction (HFrEF) and functional mitral regurgitation, which is often related to the dilatation of the left ventricle and displacement of the papillary muscles. He also has a wide QRS complex and left bundle branch block, which are criteria for CRT according to current guidelines. CRT has been shown to improve LV function, reduce mitral regurgitation, and improve symptoms in many patients with functional mitral regurgitation and a conduction delay. Therefore, before considering valve surgery or percutaneous interventions, CRT should be attempted in this patient. Option A is incorrect because mitral valve replacement with chordal preservation is generally considered after CRT in patients with persistent severe mitral regurgitation despite optimal medical therapy and resynchronization therapy. Option C is incorrect because percutaneous mitral valve repair with a MitraClip device is typically considered for patients with significant symptomatic mitral regurgitation who are at high surgical risk. This patient should first receive CRT, which could potentially reduce the severity of mitral regurgitation and improve his symptoms. Option D is incorrect because the patient's symptoms have worsened despite optimal medical therapy, and he has a QRS duration greater than 150 msec with left bundle branch block, which are indications for CRT. Continuing medical therapy alone is unlikely to address the functional mitral regurgitation or improve his heart failure symptoms adequately. Cardiac Resynchronization Therapy (CRT) is a vital intervention for patients with heart failure, particularly those in sinus rhythm with specific criteria. It is primarily recommended for symptomatic individuals with heart failure and a left ventricular ejection fraction (LVEF) of 35% or less, a QRS duration of 150 ms or more, and left bundle branch block (LBBB) QRS morphology. Furthermore, CRT can be considered for symptomatic patients with heart failure in sinus rhythm who meet the criteria of an LVEF of 35% or less, a QRS duration between 130-149 ms, and LBBB QRS morphology. Additionally, it may be an option for individuals with heart failure in sinus rhythm, an LVEF of 35% or less, a QRS duration of 150 ms or more, and non-LBBB QRS morphology. Patients in New York Heart Association (NYHA) class III or IV with heart failure and an LVEF of 35% or less who are in atrial fibrillation (AF) may also be candidates for CRT. In cases where high-degree atrioventricular block (AVB) and cardiac pacing are indicated for heart failure with reduced EF (LVEF under 40%), CRT is preferred over right ventricular (RV) pacing. It is crucial to highlight that CRT should not be utilized in patients with heart failure and a QRS duration less than 130 ms unless ventricular pacing is necessary. In instances of non-LBBB QRS morphology, the evidence supporting the benefits of CRT is less compelling, especially when PR and QRS durations are normal and below 150 ms. The indications for CRT have evolved over time, with recent data expanding its use to include patients with mild-to-moderate heart failure and atrial fibrillation, as well as those requiring antibradycardia pacing with reduced left ventricular function. However, patients with a wide QRS above 150 ms and LBBB morphology derive the most benefit from CRT. Conversely, in individuals with a narrower QRS complex under 130 ms, CRT may not be beneficial despite evidence of ventricular dyssynchrony on echocardiography. Additionally, it is important to note that there is currently no prospective randomized study demonstrating a mortality benefit from a combined CRT defibrillating device compared to a CRT pacer alone.

Schiavone M, Cardiac resynchronization therapy: present and future. Eur Heart J Suppl. 2023 Apr 26;25(Suppl C):C227-C233. PMID: 37125274

5.8 Managing Progressive Exertional Symptoms in a Patient with Severe AS

Case 84

A 78-year-old man with a history of hypertension and hyperlipidemia presents with exertional chest pain and dyspnea. He reports that his symptoms have been progressively worsening over the past 6 months. He denies any episodes of syncope. His blood pressure is 145/85 mm Hg, heart rate is 68 beats per minute, and he is in sinus rhythm. On examination, there is a late peaking systolic murmur heard best at the right upper sternal border that radiates to the carotids. An echocardiogram reveals calcific aortic stenosis with an aortic valve area of 0.8 cm^2, a mean gradient of 30 mm Hg, and a peak aortic velocity of 4.0 m/sec. The left ventricular ejection fraction (LVEF) is 55%, and the stroke volume index is calculated to be 32 mL/m2/min.
Which of the following is the most appropriate next step in the management of this patient?

- A. Initiate medical management with a beta-blocker and follow up in 6 months.
- B. Perform a dobutamine stress echocardiogram to further assess the aortic valve gradient.
- C. Refer for aortic valve replacement (AVR) given the presence of symptoms and severe aortic stenosis.
- D. Continue observation until symptoms worsen or mean gradient exceeds 40 mm Hg.

The correct answer is C. Refer for aortic valve replacement (AVR) given the presence of symptoms and severe aortic stenosis. This patient has symptomatic severe aortic stenosis, as evidenced by exertional chest pain and dyspnea, with an aortic valve area of less than 1.0 cm^2. Despite the mean gradient being less than 40 mm Hg, the presence of symptoms in the setting of severe aortic stenosis is an indication for AVR. The patient's stroke volume index is low, indicating that he has a low-flow state despite a preserved LVEF, which is consistent with paradoxical low-flow severe aortic stenosis. In such patients, the presence of symptoms is a clear indication for intervention, and further stress testing is not required to make this decision. Option A is incorrect because medical management with a beta-blocker is not the primary treatment for symptomatic severe aortic stenosis and may actually worsen the outflow obstruction by reducing the heart rate and increasing the time the LV is in systole, thereby exacerbating the gradient across the stenotic aortic valve. Option B is incorrect because a dobutamine stress echocardiogram is used to differentiate true severe aortic stenosis from pseudo-severe aortic stenosis in patients with low-flow, low-gradient aortic stenosis with reduced LVEF. In this patient with normal LVEF and symptoms, the indication for surgery is already clear, and further stress testing is not necessary. Option D is incorrect because waiting for the mean gradient to exceed 40 mm Hg in the presence of symptoms and severe aortic stenosis could lead to unnecessary delays in treatment and increased risk for the patient. Symptomatic severe aortic stenosis is an indication for valve replacement regardless of the gradient measurements. Severe aortic stenosis is typically characterized by an aortic valve area less than 1.0 cm2 and echocardiographic confirmation of a fixed aortic valve. In individuals with normal left ventricular ejection fraction and cardiac output, intervention is recommended when the peak aortic gradient exceeds 64 mm Hg and the mean aortic gradient exceeds 40 mm Hg. Super-severe aortic stenosis is identified by a mean gradient exceeding 55 mm Hg or peak aortic velocity surpassing 5 m/sec as assessed by Doppler. Some patients with an aortic valve area smaller than 1.0 cm2, limited cardiac output, and stroke volume may exhibit a mean gradient below 40 mm Hg. This scenario can occur in cases where the left ventricle's contractile function is compromised (low-gradient severe aortic stenosis with reduced left ventricular ejection fraction) or when the left ventricle functions normally (paradoxical low-flow severe aortic stenosis with normal left ventricular ejection fraction). Low flow in these instances is characterized by an echocardiographic stroke volume index below 35 mL/min/m2. Patients with low gradient, reduced valve area, diminished output, and normal LVEF in aortic stenosis may have a poorer prognosis compared to those with high gradient, restricted valve area, normal output, and normal LVEF. In situations where low-flow severe aortic stenosis coincides with reduced left ventricular ejection fraction, provocative testing using dobutamine or nitroprusside may be necessary to enhance stroke volume and ascertain if a mean aortic valve gradient of at least 40 mm Hg can be achieved without altering the aortic valve area. If the aortic valve area remains unchanged despite an increase in stroke volume from inotropic stimulation failing to show a mean gradient above 40 mm Hg, it suggests that the low gradient is due to cardiomyopathy rather than aortic valve stenosis, obviating the need for intervention. Intervention is advised for cases of super-severe aortic stenosis, even in the absence of symptoms (grade C), as well as when symptoms are present in any other scenarios. Classification includes D1 for patients with symptomatic high-gradient features, D2 for those with low-flow, low-gradient symptoms and poor LVEF, and D3 for individuals exhibiting low-flow, low-gradient symptoms alongside normal LVEF.

Banovic M et al. Aortic Valve Replacement Versus Conservative Treatment in Asymptomatic Severe Aortic Stenosis: The AVATAR Trial. Circulation. 2022 Mar;145(9):648-658. doi: 10.1161/CIRCULATIONAHA.121.057639. PMID: 34779220

5.9 Hypertension Management in an Asymptomatic Patient with Severe AS

Case 85

A 65-year-old woman with a history of severe aortic stenosis and hypertension presents for a routine follow-up. She is asymptomatic from a cardiac perspective and reports compliance with her antihypertensive medications. She has no history of coronary artery disease (CAD) and her lipid profile is within normal limits. Her current medications include amlodipine 10 mg daily and lisinopril 20 mg daily. Her blood pressure today is 148/92 mm Hg. Physical examination reveals a systolic ejection murmur that is loudest at the right upper sternal border and radiates to the neck. Recent echocardiography showed an aortic valve area of 0.9 cm^2, a mean gradient of 35 mm Hg, and a peak velocity of 4.2 m/sec. Her left ventricular ejection fraction is 60%.
Which of the following is the most appropriate next step in the management of this patient's hypertension?

- A. Discontinue lisinopril due to concerns about afterload reduction in aortic stenosis.
- B. Add a beta-blocker to further control blood pressure.
- C. Increase the dose of lisinopril to achieve better blood pressure control.
- D. Initiate a statin for presumed atherosclerotic benefit in aortic stenosis.

The correct answer is C. Increase the dose of lisinopril to achieve better blood pressure control. In patients with aortic stenosis, controlling systemic hypertension is important because the left ventricle is subjected to the total afterload, which includes both the systemic blood pressure and the aortic valve gradient. Adequate control of systemic blood pressure can help to reduce the myocardial workload and potentially slow the progression of left ventricular hypertrophy. Lisinopril, an angiotensin-converting enzyme (ACE) inhibitor, is effective for blood pressure control and is not contraindicated in aortic stenosis, especially in the absence of symptoms. The patient's blood pressure is above the target range, so increasing the dose of lisinopril is a reasonable step to improve blood pressure control. Option A is incorrect because there is no need to discontinue lisinopril solely due to concerns about afterload reduction in aortic stenosis. While it is important to avoid hypotension, ACE inhibitors can be used safely in patients with aortic stenosis for the treatment of hypertension. Option B is incorrect because while beta-blockers can be used to control hypertension, there is no specific indication to add a beta-blocker in this scenario, especially when the dose of the current medication (lisinopril) has not been maximized. Option D is incorrect because statins have not been shown to slow the progression of aortic stenosis. While statins should be used in patients with aortic stenosis who have concomitant CAD or hyperlipidemia according to the guidelines for CAD, this patient has a normal lipid profile and no history of CAD, so there is no indication to start a statin for the aortic stenosis itself.

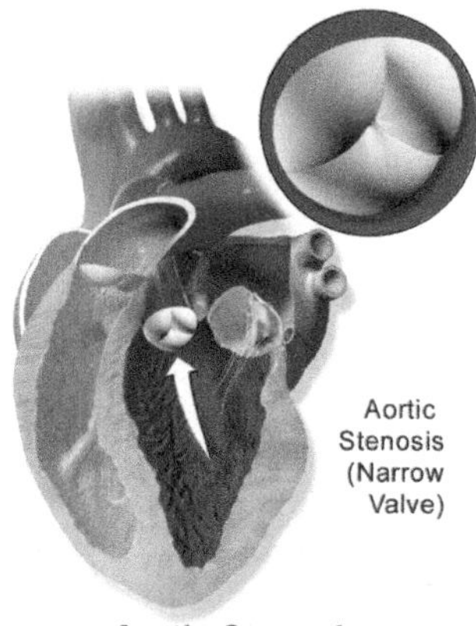

stenosis.png

Figure 5.2: AS

In asymptomatic patients with severe aortic stenosis, the recommended frequency for serial Doppler echocardiography is crucial for monitoring disease progression. According to the guidelines, follow-up assessments should focus on the progression of stenosis severity, changes in left ventricular ejection fraction (LVEF), secondary mitral regurgitation (MR) and tricuspid regurgitation (TR), as well as alterations in pulmonary artery pressure and ascending aorta size. It is emphasized that methodological precision and careful interpretation are essential during follow-up assessments to avoid artificial changes in measurements The key points to consider during follow-up assessments include monitoring peak aortic jet velocity, severe valve calcification with a rapid increase in peak transvalvular velocity, and an increase of mean pressure gradient with exercise. These markers play a significant role in determining the need for surgery in asymptomatic severe aortic stenosis patients.

The following prognostic markers have been considered to impact decision for surgery in asymptomatic severe aortic stenosis patients:

- Peak aortic jet velocity $> 5.5\,\text{m/s}$
- Combination of severe valve calcification with a rapid increase in peak transvalvular velocity of $\geq 0.3\,\text{m/s/year}$
- Increase of mean pressure gradient with exercise by $> 20\,\text{mmHg}$

During follow-up assessments, ensure that aortic jet velocity is recorded from the same window with the same quality. When effective AVA changes, look for changes in the different components incorporated in the assessment. Attempts to slow down the progression of aortic stenosis by inhibiting the renin-angiotensin system have not been successful. However, these inhibitors are advised for patients who have undergone TAVR. Managing systemic hypertension is crucial, as unwarranted concerns about reducing afterload too much in aortic stenosis patients can lead to insufficient control of systemic blood pressure. Maintaining normal systemic blood pressure is essential due to its impact on the left ventricle from the combined afterload of systemic blood pressure and the aortic valve gradient. Valve intervention is necessary for all individuals with symptomatic severe aortic stenosis, while asymptomatic cases may require intervention based on specific criteria. Treatment is often recommended for asymptomatic patients with severe aortic stenosis if they meet certain standards, such as undergoing coronary artery bypass grafting (CABG), having an LVEF less than 50%, experiencing exercise intolerance or a drop in blood pressure during exercise, among other factors outlined in the guidelines.

Case Note

After the development of heart failure, angina, or syncope, the outlook without surgery is grim, with a 50% mortality rate within three years. Medical treatment can stabilize individuals with heart failure, but intervention is necessary for all symptomatic patients with severe aortic stenosis. Patients who show no symptoms but have severe aortic stenosis (aortic valve area less than 1.0 cm2) should often receive treatment based on specific standards.

- undergoing coronary artery bypass grafting (CABG)
- LVEF is less than 50%
- mean gradient exceeds 55 mm Hg (peak velocity over 5 m/sec)
- exercise intolerance or a drop in blood pressure over 10 mm Hg during exercise
- severe valvular calcification
- rapid increase in peak aortic gradient (over 0.3 m/sec/year)
- progressive decrease in LVEF
- NT-proBNP levels are three times higher than normal

5.10 Anticoagulation In Pregnant Woman with Mechanical Valve

Case 86

A 42-year-old woman with a history of rheumatic heart disease presents with exertional dyspnea and chest tightness. She has no significant past medical history other than a mechanical mitral valve replacement 10 years ago. She is currently on warfarin with a target INR of 2.5-3.5. She has no history of bleeding or thromboembolic events and her INR values have been consistently within the therapeutic range. She is now considering pregnancy and is concerned about the risks associated with her anticoagulation therapy. She does not have atrial fibrillation.
Which of the following is the most appropriate management of her anticoagulation during pregnancy?

- A. Continue warfarin throughout the entire pregnancy.
- B. Switch to low molecular weight heparin (LMWH) before conception and throughout the pregnancy.
- C. Switch to a direct oral anticoagulant (DOAC) before conception and throughout the pregnancy.
- D. Switch to unfractionated heparin (UFH) during the first trimester, LMWH during the second trimester, and warfarin in the third trimester until close to delivery.

The correct answer is B. Switch to low molecular weight heparin (LMWH) before conception and throughout the pregnancy. Warfarin is teratogenic and is associated with a risk of fetal bleeding, especially in the first trimester and close to delivery. LMWH does not cross the placenta and is the preferred anticoagulant in pregnant women with mechanical heart valves who cannot be on warfarin. It is important to monitor anti-Xa levels to ensure therapeutic anticoagulation due to the increased risk of valve thrombosis during pregnancy. Option A is incorrect because warfarin is teratogenic and can cause fetal warfarin syndrome, especially when used during the first trimester and near delivery. It is generally avoided in pregnant women with mechanical heart valves unless they are at very high risk for thromboembolism and other options are not viable. Option C is incorrect because DOACs are not recommended for use with mechanical heart valves due to an increased risk of thromboembolic events and valve thrombosis, as shown in clinical trials Option D is incorrect because the use of UFH in the first trimester is associated with a higher risk of valve thrombosis compared to LMWH. Warfarin is typically avoided throughout pregnancy in women with mechanical heart valves due to its teratogenic effects. The strategy of switching anticoagulants during pregnancy is complex and should be individualized, but warfarin is generally avoided due to the risks to the fetus. Patients with mechanical heart valves (MHVs) face a heightened risk of thromboembolic events compared to those with atrial fibrillation (AF). This disparity is evident in the necessity for a higher maintenance international normalized ratio (INR) range in MHV patients and the consideration of anticoagulation bridge therapy when warfarin is temporarily discontinued perioperatively. Enoxaparin has emerged as a viable option for bridge therapy in MHV patients requiring temporary cessation of warfarin therapy for various reasons, such as prior to invasive procedures with bleeding risks. A prospective cohort study has demonstrated the efficacy and safety of enoxaparin as a bridging anticoagulant in patients with mechanical prosthetic heart valves necessitating brief interruptions in warfarin therapy due to elective surgeries or other invasive procedures.

Lee YS et al. Enoxaparin as an Anticoagulant in a Multipara with a Mechanical Mitral Valve: A Case Report. J Chest Surg. 2023 Nov 5;56(6):452-455. PMID: 37518948

Wang X et al. Successful Long-term Anticoagulation with Enoxaparin in a Patient with a Mechanical Heart Valve. Pharmacotherapy. 2020 Feb;40(2):174-177. PMID: 31885093

Dixon D et al Safety of enoxaparin bridge therapy in patients with mechanical heart valves. Ann Pharmacother. 2008 Jan;42(1):143-4. PMID: 18042810.

5.11 Managing Severe Aortic Regurgitation

Case 87

A 52-year-old man with no significant past medical history presents to the clinic with exertional dyspnea and a sensation of heart pounding for the past 6 months. He denies chest pain, syncope, or symptoms of heart failure. On examination, his blood pressure is 155/55 mm Hg, and his pulse is 90 bpm and bounding. You note a high-pitched, blowing, decrescendo diastolic murmur best heard along the left sternal border. Additionally, you observe a bobbing motion of the head with each heartbeat. There is no peripheral edema. An echocardiogram reveals severe aortic regurgitation with a normal left ventricular ejection fraction and no evidence of left ventricular hypertrophy.
Which of the following is the most appropriate next step in the management of this patient?

- A. Initiate treatment with an ACE inhibitor and schedule a follow-up in 6 months.
- B. Refer for immediate surgical aortic valve replacement.
- C. Perform a cardiac MRI to assess the degree of aortic root dilation.
- D. Prescribe a beta-blocker to reduce the heart rate and improve diastolic filling time.

The correct answer is C. Perform a cardiac MRI to assess the degree of aortic root dilation. In a patient with severe aortic regurgitation and a normal left ventricular ejection fraction (LVEF) without symptoms of heart failure, the next step is often to assess the aortic root and ascending aorta for dilation, which can accompany aortic valve disease and may influence the timing and type of surgery. Cardiac MRI is an excellent modality for assessing aortic root size, aortic regurgitation severity, and LV volumes and function. This information is crucial for surgical planning and can help determine if valve repair or replacement is necessary and whether any aortic root surgery is indicated. Option A is incorrect because while ACE inhibitors can be used in the management of chronic aortic regurgitation to reduce afterload, this patient has no symptoms of heart failure, and the primary issue at this point is to assess for indications for surgery, not to initiate medical therapy. Option B is incorrect because immediate surgical intervention is not indicated in asymptomatic patients with severe aortic regurgitation unless there is evidence of left ventricular dysfunction (LVEF under 50%), symptoms of heart failure, or significant dilation of the aorta. This patient is asymptomatic with a normal LVEF. Option D is incorrect because beta-blockers are not the first-line treatment for aortic regurgitation. They may be used in certain cases to control heart rate and improve diastolic filling time, but this patient's heart rate is not significantly elevated, and there is no mention of symptoms that would be relieved by slowing the heart rate. The clinical presentation of aortic regurgitation is influenced by the rate at which the regurgitation develops. Initially, a faint aortic diastolic murmur may be the sole indicator of chronic aortic regurgitation over an extended period. As the condition progresses, diastolic blood pressure decreases, and the left ventricle gradually enlarges. Many individuals may remain asymptomatic for prolonged periods, even as the left ventricle failure develops and can manifest suddenly. Common symptoms include exertional dyspnea, fatigue, paroxysmal nocturnal dyspnea, and pulmonary edema, with angina pectoris or atypical chest discomfort occasionally present. Unlike aortic stenosis, coronary artery disease (CAD), presyncope, or syncope are less commonly associated with aortic regurgitation. Compensatory left ventricular dilation allows patients to maintain adequate forward cardiac output by ejecting a large stroke volume until the disease progresses to later stages. Surgical intervention is indicated in cases of abnormal left ventricular systolic function characterized by a reduced ejection fraction (under 50%) and an increasing end-systolic left ventricle volume (above 5.0 cm). In chronic aortic regurgitation, physical findings are related to the rapid pumping of a large volume of blood into the body's vascular system due to the regurgitation. This results in a wide arterial pulse pressure and distinctive observations such as a water-hammer pulse or Corrigan pulse (rapid rise and fall in intensity), Quincke pulses (capillary pulsations in the nailbed), Duroziez sign (to-and-fro murmur with femoral artery compression), and Musset sign (head nodding with each heartbeat). Younger patients may exhibit higher systolic pressure in the lower extremities due to elevated stroke volume combined with reflected pressure waves from the periphery, known as Hill sign. Severe aortic regurgitation may present with a pronounced apical impulse, laterally displaced and hyperdynamic, along with murmurs like Austin Flint murmur during mid to late diastole due to mitral valve closure interference from rising left ventricular diastolic pressure caused by aortic regurgitation. In chronic aortic regurgitation, the indications for surgical intervention, according to ESC and US guidelines, include the presence of symptoms, which is considered a class I indication for surgery. Additionally, surgical intervention may be warranted in cases where there is worsening aortic regurgitation, increasing left ventricular size, or aortic root dilatation. Regular echocardiograms are recommended every 12 months for asymptomatic patients with severe aortic regurgitation and more frequently (every six months) for patients with specific left ventricular dimensions. Serial echocardiograms are crucial for monitoring disease progression and guiding the timing of surgical intervention. Magnetic resonance imaging (CMR) can also be used as an alternative for longitudinal follow-up in certain cases.

Galusko V et al. Aortic regurgitation management: a systematic review of clinical practice guidelines and recommendations. Eur Heart J Qual Care Clin Outcomes. 2022 Mar 2;8(2):113-126. PMID: 35026012

Case 87B

A 60-year-old man with a history of chronic aortic regurgitation presents to the clinic for a routine follow-up. He is asymptomatic with no history of chest pain, syncope, or heart failure symptoms. His blood pressure is 130/80 mm Hg, and his heart rate is 78 bpm. Physical examination reveals a high-pitched, blowing, decrescendo diastolic murmur along the left sternal border and a bounding pulse. An echocardiogram shows severe aortic regurgitation with a left ventricular ejection fraction of 55% and no significant aortic root dilation. His current medications include a multivitamin and low-dose aspirin.
Which of the following is the most appropriate management of this patient's aortic regurgitation?

- A. Initiate an angiotensin receptor blocker (ARB) for afterload reduction.
- B. Start a beta-blocker to reduce the rate of aortic dilation.
- C. Schedule for surgical aortic valve replacement given the severity of regurgitation.
- D. Continue current management and arrange for annual follow-up with echocardiography.

The correct answer is D. Continue current management and arrange for annual follow-up with echocardiography. In asymptomatic patients with chronic severe aortic regurgitation and preserved left ventricular function (LVEF above 50%) without significant aortic root dilation, the current guidelines recommend regular follow-up with echocardiography to monitor for signs of left ventricular dysfunction or other changes that would prompt surgical intervention. Since the patient is asymptomatic, has normal blood pressure, and there is no evidence of left ventricular dysfunction or significant aortic root dilation, there is no indication for afterload reduction or surgery at this time. Option A is incorrect because afterload reduction with an ARB is recommended in patients with chronic aortic regurgitation only when there is associated systolic hypertension (systolic BP greater than 140 mm Hg), which this patient does not have. Option B is incorrect because beta-blockers are not indicated solely for the reduction of aortic dilation in the absence of other indications such as hypertension, aortic aneurysm, or Marfan syndrome with aortic involvement. This patient does not have an enlarged aorta or hypertension. Option C is incorrect because surgical aortic valve replacement is not indicated in asymptomatic patients with preserved LV function and no significant aortic root dilation. Surgery is considered when there is evidence of LV dysfunction, symptoms, or significant aortic root dilation. Chronic aortic regurgitation can be managed conservatively for an extended period, but the prognosis significantly deteriorates once symptoms manifest if surgical intervention is delayed. Aortic regurgitation imposes increased preload (volume) and afterload on the left ventricle. While medications targeting afterload reduction may alleviate regurgitation severity, there is limited evidence supporting their impact on mortality. Current recommendations advise reducing afterload in aortic regurgitation only in the presence of concurrent systolic hypertension (systolic BP above 140 mm Hg), deeming it unnecessary in normotensive patients. In cases where aortic dilation is present, particularly in conditions like Marfan syndrome, angiotensin II receptor blockers (ARBs) are preferred over beta-blockers as an adjunct to medical therapy due to their potential to reduce aortic stiffness by inhibiting TGF-beta and potentially slowing aortic dilation progression. However, clinical trials assessing the efficacy of ARBs in reducing aortic stiffness and delaying aortic dilatation have not yielded conclusive results to support their routine use. Surgical intervention is recommended upon symptom onset or any signs of left ventricular dysfunction, such as a decrease in left ventricular ejection fraction below 55% or an increase in left ventricular end-systolic diameter exceeding 50 mm on echocardiography. Surgery should also be considered if the left ventricle becomes severely enlarged, with a left ventricular end-diastolic diameter surpassing 65 mm. Guidelines suggest contemplating surgery as a class IIb indication if serial imaging reveals progressive left ventricular enlargement. Early surgical consideration based on these criteria can help prevent adverse outcomes associated with advanced stages of chronic aortic regurgitation.

Galusko V et al. Aortic regurgitation management: a systematic review of clinical practice guidelines and recommendations. Eur Heart J Qual Care Clin Outcomes. 2022 Mar 2;8(2):113-126. PMID: 35026012

5.12 Navigating Management Options for Severe AR

Case 88

A 58-year-old man with a bicuspid aortic valve presents with exertional dyspnea and occasional palpitations. He has no family history of aortic dissection. His blood pressure is 135/85 mm Hg, and his heart rate is 72 bpm. Physical examination reveals a diastolic murmur heard best at the right second intercostal space. An echocardiogram shows severe aortic regurgitation, a left ventricular ejection fraction of 60%, and an end-diastolic diameter of 68 mm. The aortic root diameter measures 5.2 cm with no evidence of increase in size over the past year.
Which of the following is the most appropriate next step in the management of this patient?

- A. Medical management with an ACE inhibitor and serial echocardiography every 6 months.
- B. Surgical aortic valve replacement and consideration of aortic root replacement.
- C. Transcatheter aortic valve replacement (TAVR) with a new-generation device.
- D. Continue current management and reassess in 1 year with repeat echocardiography.

The correct answer is B. Surgical aortic valve replacement and consideration of aortic root replacement. This patient has severe aortic regurgitation with a bicuspid aortic valve, symptoms of heart failure (exertional dyspnea), and an enlarged left ventricle (end-diastolic diameter of 68 mm), which are indications for surgical intervention. Additionally, the aortic root diameter is greater than 5.0 cm, which is a Class IIa indication for aortic root replacement, especially in the setting of valve surgery. Given the absence of risk factors for dissection and no increase in aortic root size over the past year, immediate surgery is not mandated by a Class I indication but is strongly suggested by Class IIa indications. Option A is incorrect because the patient has symptoms and LV enlargement, which are indications for surgery rather than medical management alone. Option C is incorrect because TAVR is generally not the first-line treatment for patients with bicuspid aortic valves and aortic regurgitation, especially when there is a need for aortic root intervention. TAVR has been associated with higher rates of procedural complications in bicuspid valves compared to tricuspid valves, and the patient's aortic root diameter also needs to be addressed. Option D is incorrect because the patient already has symptoms and LV enlargement, which are indications for surgery rather than watchful waiting. Initial TAVR trials showed a significant occurrence of postprocedural persistent aortic regurgitation, reaching 19% in one experiment. Recent TAVR valves significantly decrease residual aortic regurgitation in individuals with pure natural aortic regurgitation to 4%. Postprocedural at least moderate 1-year all-cause mortality in multivariable analysis. When using new-generation devices, Transcatheter Aortic Valve Replacement (TAVR) showed better procedural outcomes than early-generation devices for treating patients with pure native aortic regurgitation. In individuals with native aortic regurgitation, a significant post-procedural occurrence of aortic regurgitation has been associated with higher mortality rates. Paravalvular prosthetic valve defects leading to aortic regurgitation can sometimes be managed using percutaneous occluder devices. The choice of prosthetic valve for aortic valve replacement (AVR) is influenced by the patient's age and suitability for warfarin anticoagulation, similar to considerations in aortic stenosis AVR procedures. The mortality rate following aortic valve replacement (AVR) typically ranges from 3% to 5%. Aortic regurgitation stemming from aortic root pathology often requires concomitant root repair or replacement alongside aortic valve surgery. While there have been advancements in valve-sparing techniques, most patients necessitating root intervention also undergo simultaneous valve replacement. When performing root replacement alongside valve replacement, coronary artery anastomosis may be required, adding complexity compared to standalone valve replacement procedures. The Wheat procedure involves replacing the aortic root while preserving the coronary artery attachment sites to obviate the need for reimplantation. Following aortic valve surgery, left ventricular size often decreases, and function typically improves, even if the ejection fraction is initially low. In patients with a bicuspid valve, it is recommended to repair the aortic root when its diameter exceeds 5.5 cm, regardless of the severity of aortic valve disease. Studies indicate that aortic dissection is more prevalent when the aortic root diameter surpasses 6.0 cm, emphasizing the importance of intervention before reaching this threshold. Patients with risk factors like familial dissection history or rapid root diameter increase should undergo aorta repair when the maximum dimension reaches 5.0 cm. The guidelines outline specific criteria for surgical intervention on the aortic root in individuals with a bicuspid aortic valve:

1. Class I indication (Level of Evidence C): Aortic root diameter at sinuses or ascending aorta exceeding 5.5 cm, irrespective of the need for aortic valve replacement.
2. Class IIa indication (Level of Evidence C): Aortic root diameter at sinuses or ascending aorta exceeding 5.0 cm in the presence of additional risk factors like familial dissection history or rapid size increase.
3. Class IIa indication (Level of Evidence C): Aortic root width exceeding 4.5 cm in patients undergoing aortic valve replacement for valvular causes.

Amano M et al. Optimal Management of Chronic Severe Aortic Regurgitation- How to Determine Cutoff Values for Surgical Intervention? Circ J. 2022 Oct 25;86(11):1691-1698. doi: 10.1253/circj.CJ-21-0652. PMID: 34456205

5.13 Managing Severe TR in a Post-Mitral Valve Repair

Case 89

A 67-year-old woman with a history of severe mitral regurgitation status post mitral valve repair 5 years ago presents with worsening fatigue and shortness of breath on exertion. She reports increasing abdominal girth and lower extremity edema. Her medications include furosemide, lisinopril, and spironolactone. On physical examination, her jugular venous pressure is elevated at 10 cm H2O, and there is notable hepatomegaly and 2+ pitting edema in the lower extremities. Auscultation of the heart reveals a holosystolic murmur at the left lower sternal border that increases with inspiration. A transthoracic echocardiogram shows normal left ventricular function, severe tricuspid regurgitation with a tricuspid annular dilation of 4.5 cm, and no mitral valve stenosis or regurgitation.
Which of the following is the most appropriate next step in the management of this patient?

- A. Increase the dose of furosemide and add a thiazide diuretic.
- B. Initiate intravenous diuretic therapy to manage volume overload.
- C. Refer for surgical tricuspid valve annuloplasty.
- D. Perform a right heart catheterization to measure pulmonary artery pressures.

The correct answer is C. Refer for surgical tricuspid valve annuloplasty. This patient has severe tricuspid regurgitation with symptoms of right heart failure (fatigue, shortness of breath, abdominal girth increase, lower extremity edema) and evidence of tricuspid annular dilation (4.5 cm). Given that she has had a previous mitral valve repair and now presents with severe tricuspid regurgitation and annular dilation, surgical intervention is indicated. According to the guidelines, tricuspid valve surgery is recommended for patients with symptomatic severe tricuspid regurgitation and annular dilation when undergoing left-sided valve surgery. Although she is not currently undergoing left-sided valve surgery, her symptoms and the degree of annular dilation warrant consideration of surgical repair. Option A is incorrect because while increasing diuretic therapy may help manage symptoms temporarily, it does not address the underlying mechanical issue of severe tricuspid regurgitation and annular dilation. Option B is incorrect because, although intravenous diuretics can be used to manage acute volume overload, this patient's chronic symptoms and echocardiographic findings suggest that a more definitive treatment is needed. Option D is incorrect because right heart catheterization to measure pulmonary artery pressures may be part of the preoperative evaluation but is not the next step in management. The echocardiogram has already provided sufficient information to indicate the need for surgical intervention. Mild tricuspid regurgitation is common and can be effectively managed with diuretics. In cases of severe tricuspid regurgitation, the efficacy of oral diuretics like furosemide may be compromised due to intestinal edema, necessitating the initiation of intravenous diuretics. Torsemide or bumetanide are preferred in this context as they demonstrate improved absorption when co-administered orally with diuretics. The use of aldosterone antagonists is beneficial, particularly in the presence of ascites. Combining loop diuretics with thiazide diuretics can enhance their effectiveness (refer to Treatment, Heart Failure). Given that most instances of tricuspid regurgitation are secondary, the optimal approach typically involves addressing the root cause of right ventricle dysfunction. Surgical valve replacement for secondary tricuspid regurgitation is not advised until the underlying issue of right ventricular failure is resolved. Managing left heart disease can lead to decreased pulmonary pressures, reduced right ventricle size, and resolution of tricuspid regurgitation. Addressing both primary and secondary causes of pulmonary hypertension often results in a reduction in tricuspid regurgitation. Guidelines suggest considering tricuspid valve surgery if the tricuspid annular dilatation at end-diastole exceeds 4.0 cm and the patient is symptomatic. Tricuspid annuloplasty should be contemplated in cases of severe tricuspid regurgitation concurrent with mitral valve replacement or repair for mitral regurgitation. De-Vega annuloplasty, which omits the use of a prosthetic ring, can effectively reduce tricuspid annular dilatation in certain instances.Bioprosthetic valves are preferred over mechanical valves due to the higher risk of mechanical valve thrombosis when INR levels are unstable. Anticoagulation is unnecessary for bioprosthetic valves unless there is concurrent atrial fibrillation or flutter. Transcatheter valve replacement has been proven effective in treating tricuspid regurgitation caused by bioprosthetic degeneration. Initial findings indicate that percutaneous tricuspid valve replacement for native valve tricuspid regurgitation has been successful.

Meijerink F et al. Tricuspid regurgitation after transcatheter mitral valve repair: Clinical course and impact on outcome. Catheter Cardiovasc Interv. 2021 Sep;98(3):E427-E435. PMID: 33458911

5.14 Long-Term Prophylaxis for Recurrent Rheumatic Fever

Case 90

A 26-year-old woman with a history of acute rheumatic fever (ARF) at the age of 12 presents for a routine follow-up. She had carditis during her initial episode but has no evidence of residual valvular disease on her most recent echocardiogram. She works as a kindergarten teacher and has not had any episodes of streptococcal pharyngitis since her initial diagnosis. Her only medication is benzathine penicillin G, which she receives every 4 weeks as secondary prophylaxis.

Which of the following is the most appropriate management for prevention of recurrent rheumatic fever in this patient?

- A. Continue benzathine penicillin G every 4 weeks indefinitely.
- B. Discontinue benzathine penicillin G now that she is over 21 years of age.
- C. Switch to oral penicillin twice daily until the age of 40.
- D. Continue benzathine penicillin G every 4 weeks until 10 years after her acute rheumatic fever episode.

The correct answer is D. Continue benzathine penicillin G every 4 weeks until 10 years after her acute rheumatic fever episode. According to the guidelines for secondary prevention of rheumatic fever, patients who have had carditis without residual valvular disease should continue prophylaxis for 10 years after the last episode of ARF or until they reach 21 years of age, whichever is longer. Since this patient had her episode of ARF at age 12, she should continue prophylaxis until she is at least 22 years old. However, because she is in a high-risk occupation as a kindergarten teacher, where exposure to streptococcal infections is more likely, it would be prudent to continue prophylaxis until 10 years after her ARF episode, which would be until she is 22 years old. Option A is incorrect because indefinite continuation of prophylaxis is not necessary unless the patient has residual valvular disease or is at high risk of recurrent exposure beyond the recommended prophylaxis duration. Option B is incorrect because, although prophylaxis can be stopped at age 21 for patients without carditis, this patient had carditis and is in a high-risk occupation, warranting a longer duration of prophylaxis. Option C is incorrect because oral penicillin is considered less reliable than intramuscular benzathine penicillin G, and the guidelines do not recommend switching to oral penicillin in this scenario. The duration of prophylaxis for rheumatic fever is determined by several factors, which are crucial for preventing the recurrence of the disease and the development of rheumatic heart disease (RHD). These factors include:

1. Patient's Age: The age of the patient at the time of treatment plays a significant role in determining how long prophylaxis should be continued.
2. Date of Last Attack: The time elapsed since the last episode of acute rheumatic fever (ARF) influences the duration of prophylaxis.
3. Presence and Severity of Rheumatic Heart Disease: The existence and severity of rheumatic heart disease following ARF are perhaps the most critical factors. Patients with more severe valvular disease may require lifelong prophylaxis.
4. History of Carditis: Patients with a history of rheumatic fever with carditis and residual heart disease (persistent valvular disease) are recommended to continue prophylaxis for more than 10 years since the last episode and at least until age 40 years, sometimes requiring lifelong prophylaxis. In contrast, those with carditis but no residual heart disease are advised to continue for 10 years after the last attack or at least until 21 years of age, whichever is longer. Patients without carditis may need prophylaxis for 5 years or until 21 years, whichever is longer.
5. After Valve Surgery: Patients who have undergone valve surgery are recommended to continue prophylaxis lifelong due to the persistent risk of recurrence of RHD.
6. Occupational and Environmental Exposure: For individuals in high-risk settings, such as those frequently exposed to group A streptococcal infections, the duration of prophylaxis might be adjusted to account for the increased risk of reinfection.
7. Patient or Family Preference: In some cases, the decision to cease prophylaxis may also consider the patient or family's preference, especially in the context of advancing age or end-of-life care, provided that the patient has stable valvular disease/cardiac function on serial echocardiography for 3 years.

These guidelines are designed to reduce the acquisition of new group A streptococcal strains that might induce rheumatic fever and are a major determinant of cardiac outcomes. The choice of antibiotic and the route of administration are based on the clinical assessment of the patient's condition, with benzathine benzylpenicillin G via intramuscular injection every 4 weeks being a common choice for secondary prophylaxis.

McDonald M et al. Preventing recurrent rheumatic fever: the role of register based programmes. Heart. 2005 Sep;91(9):1131-3. PMID: 16103536

Valve Type	Target INR	Anticoagulation Regimen
Mechanical Mitral Valve	2.5 - 3.5	Warfarin (Vitamin K antagonist)
Mechanical Aortic Valve (no risk factors)	2.0 - 2.5	Warfarin
Mechanical Aortic Valve (with risk factors*)	2.5 - 3.5	Warfarin
On-X Mechanical Aortic Valve	1.5 - 2.0	Warfarin (Class IIb recommendation)
Bioprosthetic Valve (first 3-6 months)	2.5	Warfarin (Class IIa recommendation)
Bioprosthetic Valve (after 3-6 months)	-	Aspirin 75-100mg daily (Class IIb)
TAVR Valve (first 3-6 months)	-	Dual antiplatelet therapy (aspirin + clopidogrel)
TAVR Valve (after 3-6 months)	-	Aspirin monotherapy
TAVR Valve (alternative for 3 months)	2.5	Warfarin (Class IIa recommendation)

**Risk factors: Atrial fibrillation, previous thromboembolism, LV dysfunction, hypercoagulable state, older valve models*

Key Points:

- Mechanical valves require lifelong anticoagulation with warfarin.
- Bioprosthetic valves have lower thromboembolism risk than mechanical valves.
- Mechanical mitral valves have higher thrombosis risk than aortic valves.
- Guidelines recommend expanded use of warfarin after bioprosthetic valve replacement.
- Dual antiplatelet therapy recommended for 3-6 months after TAVR, then aspirin monotherapy.
- Pregnant women with mechanical valves have higher risk of adverse events than bioprosthetic valves.

6 SPECIAL TOPICS

6.1 Pulmonary Hypertension

Case 91

A 58-year-old woman with a history of systemic sclerosis presents to the clinic with progressive dyspnea on exertion and fatigue over the past 6 months. She denies any chest pain, palpitations, or syncope. On physical examination, she has a loud P2 heart sound, and a 2/6 systolic murmur is heard over the left sternal border. There is no peripheral edema. A transthoracic echocardiogram shows right ventricular hypertrophy with an estimated right ventricular systolic pressure of 45 mm Hg. Pulmonary function tests reveal a mild restrictive pattern without significant impairment of diffusion capacity. High-resolution CT of the chest shows no evidence of significant interstitial lung disease.
What is the most appropriate next step in the evaluation of this patient's pulmonary hypertension?

- A. Right heart catheterization
- B. Initiate treatment with an endothelin receptor antagonist
- C. Perform a V/Q scan
- D. Initiate treatment with a phosphodiesterase-5 inhibitor
- E. Refer for lung transplantation evaluation

The correct answer is A. Right heart catheterization. This patient has systemic sclerosis, a connective tissue disease that is associated with pulmonary arterial hypertension (PAH), classified as Group I pulmonary hypertension according to the Sixth World Symposium on Pulmonary Hypertension. The presence of a loud P2 and echocardiographic findings suggestive of right ventricular hypertrophy and elevated systolic pressure are consistent with PAH. However, the definitive diagnosis of PAH requires hemodynamic confirmation by right heart catheterization, which can accurately measure mean pulmonary artery pressure (PA pressure), pulmonary vascular resistance (PVR), and pulmonary capillary wedge pressure (PCWP).

Initiating treatment with an endothelin receptor antagonist (Option B) or a phosphodiesterase-5 inhibitor (Option D) is premature without a definitive diagnosis and classification of pulmonary hypertension, which can only be accurately determined by right heart catheterization.

A V/Q scan (Option C) is typically performed to evaluate for chronic thromboembolic pulmonary hypertension

(CTEPH), which is classified as Group IV pulmonary hypertension. Although this is an important consideration, the patient's history of systemic sclerosis and the absence of suggestive findings for CTEPH on imaging make PAH a more likely diagnosis.

Referral for lung transplantation evaluation (Option E) is not the appropriate next step at this stage of the patient's disease without a complete evaluation and attempt at medical management of her condition.

Therefore, right heart catheterization is the most appropriate next step to confirm the diagnosis of PAH, assess the severity of the disease, and guide subsequent therapy.

The categorization of pulmonary hypertension, as defined by the Sixth World Symposium on Pulmonary Hypertension, is structured into distinct groups based on underlying causes and associated conditions.

1. Group I: This category encompasses pulmonary arterial hypertension (PAH) linked to a pulmonary vasculopathy. Formerly known as "primary pulmonary hypertension," it is now termed "idiopathic pulmonary hypertension." This condition is characterized by elevated pulmonary vascular resistance and pulmonary hypertension without concurrent lung or cardiac diseases. Approximately 6-10% of cases are attributed to inherited PAH. Drug-induced and toxic forms of pulmonary hypertension are associated with anorexigenic drugs that modulate serotonin release, such as aminorex fumarate, fenfluramine, and dexfenfluramine. Rare instances of pulmonary hypertension are also linked to the consumption of rapeseed oil, L-tryptophan, and recreational drugs like amphetamines and cocaine. Additionally, connective tissue diseases like systemic sclerosis contribute to around 8-12% of cases in this group.
2. Group II: This group includes cases related to left heart disease.
3. Group III: Cases in this category are attributed to parenchymal lung diseases, compromised respiratory control, or residing in high-altitude regions. Examples include idiopathic pulmonary fibrosis and chronic obstructive pulmonary disease (COPD).
4. Group IV: Patients in this group have persistent thromboembolic disease or other obstructions in the pulmonary arteries.
5. Group V: This category encompasses cases with multiple etiologies, including hematologic, systemic, and metabolic disorders.

By classifying pulmonary hypertension into these distinct groups, healthcare professionals can better understand the underlying causes and tailor treatment strategies accordingly for improved patient outcomes.

Mandras SA et al. Pulmonary Hypertension: A Brief Guide for Clinicians. Mayo Clin Proc. 2020 Sep;95(9):1978-1988. PMID: 32861339

Case 91B

A 45-year-old woman with a history of systemic sclerosis presents with a 6-month history of progressive dyspnea on exertion and fatigue. She denies any chest pain, syncope, or hemoptysis. Her physical examination reveals a loud P2 on auscultation, and 2+ pitting edema in her ankles. A transthoracic echocardiogram estimates a right ventricular systolic pressure of 45 mm Hg and shows evidence of right ventricular hypertrophy with normal left ventricular function. Pulmonary function tests show a mild restrictive pattern without significant reduction in diffusion capacity. An overnight oximetry is normal, and she lives at sea level. Which of the following is the most appropriate next step in the evaluation of this patient?

- A. Initiate treatment with an endothelin receptor antagonist.
- B. Perform right heart catheterization to confirm the diagnosis and assess hemodynamics.
- C. Prescribe long-term oxygen therapy.
- D. Refer for lung transplantation evaluation.

The correct answer is B. Perform right heart catheterization to confirm the diagnosis and assess hemodynamics. This patient has systemic sclerosis, a connective tissue disease that is associated with pulmonary arterial hypertension (PAH), which falls under Group I of the clinical classification of pulmonary hypertension. The echocardiogram suggests pulmonary hypertension with an estimated right ventricular systolic pressure of 45 mm Hg and right ventricular hypertrophy. However, a definitive diagnosis of pulmonary hypertension requires confirmation by right heart catheterization, which is the gold standard for measuring mean pulmonary artery pressure (PA pressure), pulmonary vascular resistance (PVR), and pulmonary capillary wedge pressure (PCWP). This will help to differentiate between pre-capillary and post-capillary pulmonary hypertension and guide appropriate therapy. Option A is incorrect because treatment should not be initiated before a definitive diagnosis is made with right heart catheterization. Specific therapies for PAH, such as endothelin receptor antagonists, are indicated only after confirming the diagnosis and the type of pulmonary hypertension. Option C is incorrect because there is no evidence of hypoxemia on overnight oximetry, and the patient does not have a parenchymal lung disease or live at high altitude, which would suggest Group III pulmonary hypertension requiring oxygen therapy. Option D is incorrect because lung transplantation is considered a last resort for patients with advanced lung disease who do not respond to medical therapy. This patient first requires a definitive diagnosis and an attempt at medical management before considering transplantation. In 2019, the European Society of Cardiology (ESC) and the European Respiratory Society updated guidelines concerning the diagnosis and management of pulmonary hypertension. Patients deemed high-risk for pulmonary arterial hypertension (PAH) should undergo confirmatory right heart catheterization. When investigating idiopathic pulmonary hypertension in a clinical setting, it is imperative to exclude secondary causes. Screening for a hypercoagulable state involves assessing protein C and S levels, lupus anticoagulant presence, factor V Leiden, prothrombin gene mutations, and D-dimer levels. To rule out chronic pulmonary emboli, a ventilation-perfusion lung scan or contrast spiral CT scan is necessary. While the ventilation-perfusion scan is more sensitive, it lacks specificity. If persistent thromboembolic pulmonary hypertension is absent, the likelihood is low. A chest X-ray can help eliminate primary lung causes, with patchy pulmonary edema suggesting pulmonary veno-occlusive disease due to a blockage in pulmonary venous drainage. In cases of suspected sleep apnea, a sleep study may be warranted. Findings on an electrocardiogram may reveal right ventricular hypertrophy and right atrial enlargement. Echocardiography with Doppler can exclude an intracardiac shunt and typically shows an enlarged right ventricle (RV) and right atrium (RA), sometimes significantly enlarged with reduced contractility. Severe regurgitation of the pulmonic or tricuspid valve may be observed. Interventricular septal flattening on echocardiogram indicates pulmonary hypertension. Doppler assessment of tricuspid regurgitation jet provides an estimate of right ventricular systolic pressure. Pulmonary function tests are valuable for excluding other conditions. Indicators of primary pulmonary hypertension may include low carbon monoxide DLCO or significant desaturation, particularly if a stretched patent foramen ovale (PFO) leads to a right-to-left shunt. A decrease in DLCO can precede the onset of pulmonary hypertension in systemic sclerosis patients. Chest CT scans reveal enlarged pulmonary arteries and rule out alternative explanations like emphysema or interstitial lung disease.

Imaging modalities such as pulmonary angiography, magnetic resonance angiography, or CT angiography demonstrate the absence of minor acinar pulmonary arteries and narrowing of larger ones. Catheterization allows for monitoring of pulmonary pressures and assessment of vasoreactivity using various agents; nitric oxide is preferred due to its simplicity and short duration of action. A positive response is characterized by a reduction in mean pulmonary pressure by over 10 mm Hg, resulting in a final mean pulmonary artery pressure below 40 mm Hg. An abdominal ultrasound is recommended to exclude portal hypertension, while lung biopsy is considered unnecessary for diagnosis purposes. The diagnostic criteria for pulmonary hypertension according to the ESC and European Respiratory Society guidelines are as follows:

1. Pulmonary hypertension (PH) is defined by a mean pulmonary arterial pressure above 20 mm Hg at rest. For pulmonary arterial hypertension (PAH), additional criteria include a pulmonary vascular resistance (PVR) above 2 Wood Units.
2. The diagnostic algorithm for PH involves a three-step approach: suspicion by first-line physicians, detection by echocardiography, and confirmation with right heart catheterization in specialized PH centers.
3. To address underdiagnosis of chronic thromboembolic pulmonary hypertension (CTEPH), improved recognition of computed tomography (CT) and echocardiographic signs of chronic thromboembolic pulmonary hypertension is emphasized, along with systematic follow-up of patients with acute pulmonary embolism.
4. The treatment algorithm for PAH has been simplified, focusing on risk assessment, cardiopulmonary comorbidities, and treatment goals. Initial combination therapy and treatment escalation at follow-up are standard practices.
5. Recommendations aim to bridge the gap between pediatric and adult PAH care, with strategies based on risk stratification and treatment response adapted for different age groups
6. Updated recommendations address sex-related issues in PAH patients, including pregnancy. Women

with PH who are pregnant or develop newly diagnosed PAH during pregnancy should ideally receive treatment in centers with experienced multidisciplinary teams. Certain medications like endothelin receptor antagonists, riociguat, and selexipag should be discontinued due to potential teratogenic effects.

These guidelines provide a comprehensive framework for diagnosing and managing pulmonary hypertension, emphasizing the importance of accurate diagnosis, risk assessment, tailored treatment strategies, and specialized care for specific patient populations.

Maron BA et al. Pulmonary Arterial Hypertension: Diagnosis, Treatment, and Novel Advances. Am J Respir Crit Care Med. 2021 Jun 15;203(12):1472-1487. PMID: 33861689

Case 91C

A 34-year-old woman presents with a 6-month history of progressive dyspnea on exertion and fatigue. She has no significant past medical history and takes no medications. She denies any history of drug use, and her family history is non-contributory. On physical examination, she has a loud P2 heart sound, jugular venous distension, and a 2/6 systolic murmur over the left sternal border. There is no peripheral edema. A transthoracic echocardiogram shows right ventricular hypertrophy with an estimated right ventricular systolic pressure of 60 mm Hg. Pulmonary function tests reveal a reduced diffusion capacity for carbon monoxide (DLCO). A ventilation-perfusion (V/Q) scan shows no evidence of pulmonary embolism. Laboratory tests, including antinuclear antibodies and anti-centromere antibodies, are negative. An abdominal ultrasound shows no evidence of portal hypertension.
What is the most appropriate next step in the evaluation of this patient's suspected pulmonary arterial hypertension (PAH)?

- A. Initiate empiric anticoagulation therapy
- B. Perform a right heart catheterization
- C. Start treatment with an oral endothelin receptor antagonist
- D. Refer for genetic counseling and testing for heritable PAH
- E. Conduct a six-minute walk test to assess functional capacity

The correct answer is B. Perform right heart catheterization to confirm the diagnosis and assess hemodynamics. This patient has systemic sclerosis, a connective tissue disease that is associated with pulmonary arterial hypertension (PAH), which falls under Group I of the clinical classification of pulmonary hypertension. The echocardiogram suggests pulmonary hypertension with an estimated right ventricular systolic pressure of 45 mm Hg and right ventricular hypertrophy. However, a definitive diagnosis of pulmonary hypertension requires confirmation by right heart catheterization, which is the gold standard for measuring mean pulmonary artery pressure (PA pressure), pulmonary vascular resistance (PVR), and pulmonary capillary wedge pressure (PCWP). This will help to differentiate between pre-capillary and post-capillary pulmonary hypertension and guide appropriate therapy. Option A is incorrect because treatment should not be initiated before a definitive diagnosis is made with right heart catheterization. Specific therapies for PAH, such as endothelin receptor antagonists, are indicated only after confirming the diagnosis and the type of pulmonary hypertension. Option C is incorrect because there is no evidence of hypoxemia on overnight oximetry, and the patient does not have a parenchymal lung disease or live at high altitude, which would suggest Group III pulmonary hypertension requiring oxygen therapy. Option D is incorrect because lung transplantation is considered a last resort for patients with advanced lung disease who do not respond to medical therapy. This patient first requires a definitive diagnosis and an attempt at medical management before considering transplantation.

Maron BA et al. Pulmonary Arterial Hypertension: Diagnosis, Treatment, and Novel Advances. Am J Respir Crit Care Med. 2021 Jun 15;203(12):1472-1487. PMID: 33861689

6.2 Management of Pulmonary Arterial Hypertension

Case 92

A 35-year-old woman presents to the clinic with a 6-month history of progressive dyspnea on exertion and occasional syncope. She has no significant past medical history. Her physical examination shows a loud pulmonic component of the second heart sound and a 3/6 systolic ejection murmur best heard over the left upper sternal border. Her electrocardiogram shows right ventricular hypertrophy and her echocardiogram reveals right ventricular dilatation with an estimated right ventricular systolic pressure of 70 mm Hg. Her pulmonary function tests are normal, and her V/Q scan shows no evidence of pulmonary embolism. She has been diagnosed with pulmonary arterial hypertension (PAH).
Given her clinical presentation, which of the following will be the most appropriate next step in her management?

- A. Start her on calcium channel blockers.
- B. Start her on bosentan.
- C. Recommend balloon pulmonary angioplasty.
- D. Advise her to start an aerobic exercise regimen.

Correct Answer: B. Start her on bosentan. The patient's presentation is consistent with pulmonary arterial hypertension (PAH), and the most appropriate next step in management is to start her on bosentan, an endothelin-receptor blocker. Bosentan is a dual endothelin receptor antagonist that has been shown to improve symptoms and exercise capacity in patients with PAH. Option A is incorrect because calcium channel blockers are reserved for patients who have a positive response to a vasoreactivity test (a decrease in mean pulmonary artery pressure by at least 10 mm Hg to a total mean pressure of less than 40 mm Hg without a decrease in cardiac output), and we don't have information about this in the given scenario. Option C is not the best choice because balloon pulmonary angioplasty is typically reserved for patients with inoperable chronic thromboembolic pulmonary hypertension, which this patient does not have. Option D is not the most appropriate initial step in management, although aerobic exercise is recommended for patients with PAH, it is not a substitute for medical therapy. In Group I patients with a normal pulmonary capillary wedge pressure (PCWP), treatment is guided by their response to a nitric oxide challenge. Those showing a positive initial response may be considered for calcium channel blockers, although the majority do not exhibit acute vasoreactivity. In such cases, pulmonary arterial hypertension (PAH) therapy is recommended, typically starting with monotherapy and progressing to sequential drug regimens if pulmonary pressures do not improve. Critically ill hypotensive patients may require inotropic support and could be candidates for lung transplantation. Balloon atrial septostomy, although classified as a IIb guideline, is infrequently performed due to the belief that increasing right-to-left shunting could potentially enhance cardiac output.

The efficacy of medication monotherapy varies based on the underlying etiology. Only individuals in functional class I who demonstrate responsiveness to nitric oxide should be considered for calcium channel blockers.

Treatment options include endothelin receptor blockers (such as ambrisentan, bosentan, and macitentan), phosphodiesterase type-5 inhibitors (like sildenafil, tadalafil, and vardenafil), a guanylate cyclase stimulator (riociguat), prostanoids (including epoprostenol, iloprost, treprostinil, and beraprost), and an IP-receptor agonist (selexipag). Various approved combination therapies exist, with sequential drug regimens being an option if initial treatments prove ineffective. It is essential to assess potential drug interactions with HIV medications when necessary. Specific medications for PAH associated with underlying lung disease or left heart dysfunction are currently lacking. Bosentan, an endothelin receptor antagonist, is recommended as first-line therapy for individuals with Eisenmenger syndrome. Anticoagulation is often recommended and should be continued indefinitely in cases of persistent thromboembolic pulmonary hypertension.

The utilization of balloon pulmonary angioplasty has significantly increased in patients with inoperable chronic thromboembolic pulmonary hypertension due to positive outcomes observed. Riociguat stands as the sole approved pharmacological treatment for individuals with chronic thromboembolic pulmonary hypertension within this specific population.

Mayeux JD et al. Management of Pulmonary Arterial Hypertension. Curr Cardiovasc Risk Rep. 2021;15(1):2. PMID: 33224405

Case 92B

A 32-year-old man with a recent diagnosis of idiopathic pulmonary arterial hypertension (IPAH) presents to the clinic for management. He has a WHO functional class III symptoms and has no significant past medical history. His baseline 6-minute walk distance is 380 meters. He has undergone acute vasodilator testing with inhaled nitric oxide, which did not demonstrate a significant response. His current medications include furosemide and supplemental oxygen to maintain oxygen saturation above 90%. His echocardiogram shows right ventricular enlargement and hypokinesis with an estimated right ventricular systolic pressure of 85 mm Hg. Right heart catheterization confirms a mean pulmonary artery pressure of 55 mm Hg, pulmonary vascular resistance of 8 Wood units, and a normal pulmonary capillary wedge pressure.
Which of the following is the most appropriate next step in the management of this patient?

- A. Initiate monotherapy with an oral calcium channel blocker.
- B. Start combination therapy with an endothelin receptor antagonist and a phosphodiesterase type-5 inhibitor.
- C. Refer for immediate lung transplantation.
- D. Perform a balloon atrial septostomy.

The correct answer is B. Start combination therapy with an endothelin receptor antagonist and a phosphodiesterase type-5 inhibitor. This patient with IPAH is symptomatic with WHO functional class III symptoms and has not responded to acute vasodilator testing with nitric oxide, which rules out the use of calcium channel blockers as a treatment option. Current guidelines recommend the initiation of combination therapy in patients with IPAH who have WHO functional class II or III symptoms and who are non-responders to acute vasodilator testing. Combination therapy with an endothelin receptor antagonist and a phosphodiesterase type-5 inhibitor has been shown to improve exercise capacity, WHO functional class, and hemodynamics in patients with PAH. Option A is incorrect because the patient did not demonstrate a significant response to acute vasodilator testing, which is a prerequisite for the use of calcium channel blockers in the treatment of IPAH. Option C is incorrect because lung transplantation is considered a treatment option for patients with PAH who have progressive disease despite optimal medical therapy. This patient has not yet been given a trial of medical therapy. Option D is incorrect because balloon atrial septostomy is a palliative procedure reserved for patients with advanced PAH who are refractory to medical therapy and either awaiting lung transplantation or not candidates for it. It is not a first-line treatment and carries significant risks. Current guidelines recommend initiating combination therapy in patients with idiopathic pulmonary arterial hypertension (IPAH) who exhibit World Health Organization (WHO) functional class II or III symptoms and do not respond to acute vasodilator testing. The suggested combination therapy involves an endothelin receptor antagonist and a phosphodiesterase type-5 inhibitor. Endothelin receptor antagonists (ERAs) serve as oral alternatives to parenteral prostacyclin agents. By competitively binding to endothelin 1 (ET-1) receptors endothelin-A and endothelin-B, they lead to reductions in pulmonary artery pressure (PAP), pulmonary vascular resistance (PVR), and mean right atrial pressure (RAP). These agents are indicated for treating PAH in patients with WHO class III or IV symptoms to enhance exercise capacity and reduce clinical deterioration. Bosentan, a mixed endothelin-A and endothelin-B receptor antagonist, is approved for PAH, including IPAH. Clinical trials have demonstrated that bosentan enhances exercise capacity, reduces clinical deterioration rates, improves functional class, and enhances hemodynamics.

Tadalafil, a phosphodiesterase type-5 inhibitor, is prescribed to enhance exercise capacity. Combination therapy involving multiple drug classes concurrently has been utilized in systemic hypertension and heart failure treatment. The use of combination therapy in PAH is growing, with applications either sequentially or as initial therapy (upfront). This approach has proven effective in enhancing exercise capacity, cardiac hemodynamics, WHO functional class, and quality of life in PAH patients.

In summary, the combination therapy of an endothelin receptor antagonist and a phosphodiesterase type-5 inhibitor has demonstrated improvements in exercise capacity, WHO functional class, and hemodynamics in patients with PAH. This regimen presents a viable treatment option for individuals with IPAH experiencing symptomatic WHO functional class III symptoms who have not responded to acute vasodilator testing with nitric oxide.

Mayeux JD et al. Management of Pulmonary Arterial Hypertension. Curr Cardiovasc Risk Rep. 2021;15(1):2. PMID: 33224405

6.3 Right Heart Failure in Pulmonary Hypertension

Case 93

A 60-year-old male with a past medical history of hypertension presents to the emergency department with a 3-month history of progressive shortness of breath and bilateral leg swelling. He denies any chest pain, palpitations, or syncope. His medications include hydrochlorothiazide and lisinopril. On examination, his heart rate is 69 bpm, blood pressure is 196/92 mm Hg, respiratory rate is 24/min, and oxygen saturation is 91% on 10 liters of oxygen via a non-rebreather mask. Physical examination reveals jugular venous pressure of 5 cm at 45 degrees, a regular cardiac rhythm with an S4 gallop, bilateral crackles in the lungs, and 2+ pitting edema around his ankles. Laboratory tests show hemoglobin of 12.7 g/dL, white cell count of 9.5, normal liver function tests, BUN/Creatinine of 29/1.4 mg/dL, troponin ¡0.01 ng/mL, and NT-proBNP of 90 pg/mL. Given this clinical scenario, what is the most appropriate next step in the management of this patient?

- A. Initiate warfarin anticoagulation therapy.
- B. Start loop diuretics and spironolactone.
- C. Perform acute vasodilator testing with nitric oxide.
- D. Administer supplemental oxygen to maintain saturation greater than 90

Correct Answer: B. Start loop diuretics and spironolactone. The patient presents with signs and symptoms suggestive of right-sided heart failure (HF), likely secondary to pulmonary hypertension given the elevated systolic blood pressure in the pulmonary artery (as indicated by the high right ventricular systolic pressure on echocardiogram). The presence of an S4 gallop, jugular venous distension, and bilateral leg edema further supports this diagnosis. Option B is correct because diuretics are useful in the management of right-sided HF, which is likely contributing to the patient's symptoms of shortness of breath and leg swelling. Loop diuretics, such as torsemide or bumetanide, are preferred in the presence of bowel edema as they are better absorbed, and spironolactone is added for its potassium-sparing effects and potential benefits in heart failure management. Option A is incorrect because warfarin anticoagulation is recommended in all patients with idiopathic PAH and no contraindication, but there is no evidence of idiopathic PAH or thromboembolic disease in this patient's presentation. Option C is not the best choice at this time because acute vasodilator testing is typically performed in patients with idiopathic PAH who may be candidates for calcium channel blocker therapy. This patient's PAH is likely secondary to left heart disease due to longstanding hypertension, and he would not be expected to respond well to calcium channel blockers . Option D, while important for symptomatic relief, is not the most appropriate next step in management. Supplemental oxygen should be used to maintain oxygen saturation greater than 90%, but this alone does not address the underlying cause of the patient's right-sided HF. Given the clinical scenario, the patient's management should focus on addressing the volume overload with diuretics, which can provide symptomatic relief and improve his functional status. Right ventricular failure in pulmonary hypertension is characterized by changes in cellular metabolism, the onset of right ventricular ischemia, and activation of the renin–angiotensin–aldosterone system.

Right heart failure (RHF) stands as the leading cause of mortality in individuals with pulmonary arterial hypertension (PAH) and arises from a complex process initiated by persistent elevations in right ventricular (RV) afterload. Despite the availability of various PAH-specific treatments, mortality rates remain notably high in this patient population. Improving understanding of the intricate pathophysiological changes underlying PAH, encompassing metabolic dysregulation and the neurohormonal effects on the right heart, is crucial.

RV dysfunction significantly impacts the survival of individuals with pulmonary hypertension, presenting as modifications in both overall RV systolic function and abnormalities in contraction patterns and synchronization. Research has predominantly concentrated on the influence of pH levels on the right ventricle in individuals with pulmonary arterial hypertension (PAH). With a growing elderly population, heart failure with preserved ejection fraction (HFpEF) has emerged as a notable contributor to pulmonary hypertension (PH) in recent years.The renin-angiotensin-aldosterone system plays a significant role in the development of right heart failure in individuals with pulmonary hypertension. In pulmonary arterial hypertension (PAH), there is evidence of activation of this system, leading to increased levels of angiotensin

Table 6.1: Summary of the treatment for Pulmonary Arterial Hypertension (PAH)

Treatment Method	Description
Calcium Channel Blockers	Used for group I patients with a normal PCWP who respond to nitric oxide challenge.
Specific PAH Therapy	Recommended for patients who do not respond to the acute vasoreactivity testing. This begins with monotherapy but expands to sequential medication therapy when pulmonary pressures are not improved.
Inotropic Support	May be required for critically ill hypotensive patients.
Lung Transplantation	Considered when other treatments are ineffective.
Balloon Atrial Septostomy	Considered a IIb recommendation but is very rarely utilized.
Medication Therapies	Include endothelin-receptor blockers (ambrisentan, bosentan, macitentan), phosphodiesterase type-5 inhibitors (sildenafil, tadalafil, and vardenafil), a guanylate cyclase stimulator (riociquat), prostanoids (epoprostenol, iloprost, teprostinil, and beraprost), and an IP-receptor agonist (selexipag).
Sequential Medication Therapies	Used when medication combinations are ineffective.
Anticoagulation	Often recommended and is required lifelong in chronic thromboembolic pulmonary hypertension.
Balloon Pulmonary Angioplasty	Used for inoperable chronic thromboembolic pulmonary hypertension patients.
Counseling and Patient Education	Important part of the treatment process.
Aerobic Exercise	Recommended but no heavy physical exertion or isometric exercise.
Routine Immunizations	Advised for patients.
Pregnancy Prevention	Strongly discouraged due to high maternal mortality in severe PAH.
Warfarin Anticoagulation	Recommended in all patients with idiopathic PAH and no contraindication.
Diuretics	Useful for the management of right-sided HF.
Oxygen	Should be used to maintain oxygen saturation greater than 90%.
Acute Vasodilator Testing	Should be performed in all patients with idiopathic PAH who may be potential candidates for long-term therapy with calcium channel blockers.

and aldosterone in both plasma and lung tissue. These elevated levels contribute to various detrimental effects, including oxidative stress signaling pathways activation, reduced nitric oxide availability, increased inflammation, cell proliferation, migration, extracellular matrix remodeling, and fibrosis. Clinically, heightened renin-angiotensin activity and elevated aldosterone levels have been observed in PAH patients, indicating a potential role for angiotensin and mineralocorticoid receptor antagonists in PAH treatment. The pathophysiological impact of the renin-angiotensin-aldosterone system on PAH involves promoting vascular remodeling, increasing pulmonary vascular resistance, and impairing right ventricular function. This system's activation contributes to the progression of right heart failure by inducing maladaptive remodeling processes in the right ventricle. Despite the complexity of managing right heart failure in the context of pulmonary hypertension, understanding and targeting the renin-angiotensin-aldosterone system may offer therapeutic opportunities to mitigate the adverse effects on the cardiovascular system.

Cassady SJ et al. Right Heart Failure in Pulmonary Hypertension. Cardiol Clin. 2020 May;38(2):243-255. doi: PMID: 32284101

6.4 Cardiac Mass In Echo

Case 94

A 57-year-old woman presents to the emergency department with acute onset shortness of breath and orthopnea. She has a history of hypertension and hyperlipidemia but no known cardiac history. On physical examination, her blood pressure is 150/90 mm Hg, heart rate is 110 beats per minute, and oxygen saturation is 92% on room air. She has jugular venous distension, bilateral rales halfway up both lung fields, and a low-pitched diastolic murmur best heard at the apex. She also has a mid-diastolic sound that is not clearly a murmur. Laboratory studies show normal white blood cell count, elevated brain natriuretic peptide (BNP), and a normal troponin. A chest X-ray reveals pulmonary venous congestion. An urgent transthoracic echocardiogram demonstrates a 4 cm x 3 cm mass in the left atrium attached to the interatrial septum, swinging back and forth across the mitral valve during diastole.
Which of the following is the most appropriate next step in the management of this patient?

- A. Initiate broad-spectrum antibiotics and order blood cultures.
- B. Perform a transesophageal echocardiogram to further characterize the mass.
- C. Refer the patient for urgent surgical excision of the cardiac mass.
- D. Start anticoagulation therapy and schedule an outpatient cardiac MRI.

The correct answer is C. Refer the patient for urgent surgical excision of the cardiac mass. The patient's presentation is consistent with a cardiac myxoma causing obstruction of mitral inflow, as evidenced by symptoms of heart failure (shortness of breath, orthopnea, and pulmonary edema) and the echocardiographic findings of a mass in the left atrium swinging across the mitral valve. The presence of a diastolic murmur and a mid-diastolic sound ("tumor plop") further supports the diagnosis. Surgical excision is the treatment of choice for atrial myxomas, especially when they are causing hemodynamic compromise, as in this case. Urgent surgical intervention is indicated to relieve the obstruction and to prevent further complications such as systemic embolization. Option A is incorrect because the clinical scenario and echocardiographic findings are more suggestive of a cardiac tumor than infective endocarditis. While infective endocarditis can present with similar constitutional symptoms, the echocardiographic findings of a large mass are not typical for vegetations seen in endocarditis. Option B is incorrect because the transthoracic echocardiogram has already provided sufficient information to make a diagnosis and to indicate the need for surgery. While transesophageal echocardiography (TEE) can provide more detailed imaging, it is not necessary in this urgent situation where the diagnosis is clear and the patient requires prompt surgical intervention. Option D is incorrect because anticoagulation therapy is not the primary treatment for a cardiac myxoma, and while cardiac MRI can provide detailed imaging of cardiac masses, it is not the appropriate next step in the setting of acute hemodynamic compromise. Primary cardiac tumors are rare and represent a small fraction of all malignancies affecting the heart or pericardium. Atrial myxoma stands out as the most common primary tumor, constituting approximately 50% of cases in adult series. Typically attached to the atrial septum, these tumors tend to occur more frequently on the left atrial side rather than the right. Patients with myxomas may manifest symptoms resembling a systemic illness, encounter obstruction of blood flow at the mitral valve, or present with signs of peripheral embolization. The clinical picture may include fever, malaise, weight loss, leukocytosis, elevated erythrocyte sedimentation rate (ESR), and emboli, which can be peripheral or pulmonary depending on the tumor's location. This condition can sometimes be misdiagnosed as infective endocarditis, lymphoma, other cancers, or autoimmune disorders.

As the tumor grows in size, it can lead to symptoms by impeding mitral inflow. Episodes of pulmonary edema may occur upon assuming an upright position, resulting in manifestations of reduced cardiac output. During a physical examination, a diastolic sound associated with tumor movement ("tumor plop") or a diastolic murmur resembling mitral stenosis may be detected. Right-sided myxomas can present with signs of right-sided heart failure.The primary treatment option for atrial myxoma is surgical resection, which is considered the most appropriate and effective approach. Surgery should be performed promptly after diagnosis to prevent complications associated with the tumor. The surgical prognosis for cardiac myxomas is excellent, with a mortality rate of less than 3%. The surgical technique should aim to minimize manipulation of the tumor, provide adequate exposure for complete mass resection, allow inspection of all heart chambers, and ensure safety and efficacy. A bi-atrial approach through a median sternotomy has been reported to yield excellent results. In cases of low-risk, small masses, a minimally invasive approach can be considered as a feasible treatment option. Recurrence of atrial myxomas can occur in about 3% of patients and is usually due to incomplete excision of the tumor or growth from a second focus. Extensive resection of the myxoma attached to the atrial septum or wall can reduce the likelihood of recurrence. Long-term clinical and echocardiographic follow-up is essential to monitor for any signs of recurrence

Familial myxomas are a hallmark of the Carney complex, a condition characterized by myxomas, pigmented skin lesions, and endocrine neoplasia. Diagnosis of atrial myxoma is typically confirmed through echocardiography or pathological examination of embolic material. Cardiac MRI serves as a valuable adjunctive diagnostic tool, while angiography, although often unnecessary, can reveal a characteristic "tumor blush" in vascular masses. Surgical excision is the primary treatment modality, with regular echocardiographic monitoring recommended due to the potential for recurrences. Valvular papillary fibroelastomas and atrial septal lipomas are among the second most commonly encountered primary cardiac tumors. These lesions are generally benign and often do not require active intervention. Papillary fibroelastomas, commonly found on the pulmonary or aortic valves, have the potential to cause embolisms or valvular dysfunction and should be surgically removed if they are large and mobile. Other primary cardiac tumors include rhabdomyomas (frequently located in both ventricles), fibrous histiocytomas, hemangiomas, and various rare sarcomas. Some sarcomas can grow significantly before being detected. Primary pericardial tumors, such as mesotheliomas associated with asbestos exposure, can also arise. An abnormal cardiac silhouette on radiography can aid in diagnosis. While echocardiography is generally useful, it may not always detect malignancies infiltrating the ventricular wall. Cardiac MRI is the preferred diagnostic modality for all cardiac malignancies, complemented by gated CT imaging. Metastases from malignant tumors can also affect the heart. Common sites of metastasis include malignant melanoma, bronchogenic carcinoma, breast carcinoma, lymphoma, renal cell carcinoma, sarcomas, and Kaposi sarcoma in individuals with AIDS. Early detection and appropriate management are crucial in addressing cardiac involvement in metastatic disease.

Griborio-Guzman AG et al. Cardiac myxomas: clinical presentation, diagnosis and management. Heart. 2022 May 12;108(11):827-833. PMID: 34493547

6.5 Cardiac Tamponade Post Road Accident

Case 95

A 35-year-old man is brought to the emergency department after being involved in a high-speed motor vehicle collision. He was the restrained driver, and airbags were deployed. On arrival, he is alert but appears anxious and is complaining of chest pain. His blood pressure is 90/60 mm Hg, heart rate is 120 beats per minute, and respiratory rate is 22 breaths per minute. Physical examination reveals distended neck veins, muffled heart sounds, and clear lungs. The electrocardiogram (ECG) shows low voltage QRS complexes and electrical alternans. Focused Assessment with Sonography for Trauma (FAST) exam shows a large pericardial effusion. Which of the following is the most appropriate next step in the management of this patient?

- A. Immediate pericardiocentesis.
- B. Urgent coronary angiography.
- C. Administration of intravenous fluids and inotropic agents.
- D. Observation and serial echocardiography.

The correct answer is A. Immediate pericardiocentesis. The patient's presentation is suggestive of cardiac tamponade, which is a life-threatening condition characterized by the accumulation of fluid in the pericardial space leading to impaired ventricular filling. The clinical triad of hypotension, distended neck veins, and muffled heart sounds, along with the ECG findings of low voltage QRS complexes and electrical alternans, are classic for tamponade. The FAST exam confirms the presence of a large pericardial effusion. Immediate pericardiocentesis is indicated to relieve the pressure on the heart and to prevent cardiovascular collapse. Option B is incorrect because, although coronary artery injury could be a concern in blunt chest trauma, the immediate life-threatening issue is the cardiac tamponade, which needs to be addressed before any other investigations or interventions. Option C is incorrect because, while intravenous fluids and inotropic agents may temporarily support the blood pressure, they do not address the underlying problem of impaired ventricular filling due to the pericardial effusion. The definitive treatment is removal of the effusion. Option D is incorrect because observation and serial echocardiography are not appropriate in the setting of hemodynamic instability and evidence of cardiac tamponade. This condition requires immediate intervention. Blunt trauma is a common cause of cardiac injury, often observed in motor vehicle accidents and various forms of chest trauma, including during CPR procedures. Myocardial contusions or hematomas are typical injuries, with the right ventricle (RV) being particularly vulnerable due to its proximity to the sternum.

Nonischemic cardiac damage can also result from metabolic factors like burns, electrical injuries, or infections. These injuries may present asymptomatically, especially in severe cases, or manifest as vague chest discomfort with a pericardial component. While cardiac enzyme elevations are frequent and can be substantial, they do not always correlate with prognosis. Specific cardiac biomarkers such as NT-proBNP may offer a stronger association with significant myocardial injury. Echocardiography can reveal motionless myocardial segments or pericardial effusion, while cardiac MRI can indicate acute damage.

Coronary CT angiography is valuable for detecting coronary dissection or acute occlusion when indicated. Pericardiocentesis is essential in cases of cardiac tamponade, and stress-induced Tako-tsubo transient myocardial dysfunction can occur.

Severe trauma may lead to myocardial or heart valve rupture, with survival rates highest when injuries affect the atria or right ventricle. Hemopericardium or pericardial tamponade typically necessitate surgical intervention. Mitral and aortic valve ruptures can occur in cases of significant blunt trauma, with the mitral valve more likely affected during systole and the aortic valve during diastole. Urgent surgical management is crucial for patients presenting in shock or severe heart failure.

Transthoracic and transesophageal echocardiography are valuable diagnostic tools, while CT and MRI may provide additional insights before surgical intervention. Blunt trauma can also impact coronary arteries, leading to acute or subacute coronary thrombosis presenting as acute myocardial infarction. Emergent revascularization through percutaneous intervention or coronary artery bypass surgery may be necessary. Left ventricular aneurysms can result from traumatic coronary blockages without collateral vascular support.

Coronary artery dissection or rupture can occur due to blunt cardiac trauma, highlighting the diverse range of potential cardiac injuries following blunt trauma incidents.

Qamar SR et al. State of the art imaging review of blunt and penetrating cardiac trauma. Can Assoc Radiol J. 2020;71:301. PMID: 32066272

6.6 Pregnancy-Related Acute Aortic Dissection

Case 96

A 29-year-old woman with a known history of Marfan syndrome and a dilated aortic root measuring 4.5 cm is admitted to the obstetric service for labor induction at 38 weeks of gestation. Her pregnancy has been complicated by new-onset hypertension without proteinuria. On admission, her blood pressure is 145/95 mm Hg, heart rate is 88 beats per minute, and respiratory rate is 18 breaths per minute. She is asymptomatic with no signs of heart failure or aortic dissection. The obstetric team asks for a cardiology consult regarding the mode of delivery.

Which of the following is the most appropriate recommendation for the mode of delivery in this patient?

- A. Vaginal delivery with epidural anesthesia.
- B. Vaginal delivery with no epidural anesthesia.
- C. Scheduled cesarean section with spinal anesthesia.
- D. Scheduled cesarean section with general anesthesi

The correct answer is D. Scheduled cesarean section with general anesthesia. Patients with Marfan syndrome and a dilated aortic root are at increased risk of aortic dissection, which can be life-threatening. The hemodynamic changes associated with labor and delivery, particularly the rapid fluid shifts and the stress of labor, can increase this risk. In this patient, who has a significantly dilated aortic root and new-onset hypertension, the risk of aortic dissection is further elevated. A scheduled cesarean section is recommended to avoid the hemodynamic stress of labor. Spinal anesthesia is typically avoided in this setting because it can cause a sudden drop in systemic vascular resistance, which can worsen hemodynamic instability and increase the risk of aortic complications. General anesthesia allows for controlled induction and maintenance of blood pressure, which is crucial in patients at risk for aortic dissection. Option A is incorrect because epidural anesthesia can lead to hypotension and a compensatory increase in cardiac output, which may increase the stress on the aorta and the risk of dissection. Option B is incorrect because vaginal delivery, even without epidural anesthesia, involves significant hemodynamic stress and fluid shifts that can increase the risk of aortic dissection in a patient with Marfan syndrome and a dilated aortic root. Option C is incorrect because spinal anesthesia can cause a significant decrease in systemic vascular resistance, which can be dangerous in patients with a dilated aortic root due to Marfan syndrome. Pregnancy can elevate the risk of aortic and arterial dissections, potentially attributed to alterations in connective tissue. Individuals with Marfan syndrome, Ehlers-Danlos syndrome, or Loeys-Dietz syndrome face a notably heightened risk. The third trimester poses the greatest risk, with coronary dissection, thrombosis, and atherosclerosis exhibiting similar prevalence rates. Notably, coronary dissection emerges as a primary cause, often peaking in the early postpartum period. In select cases, paradoxical emboli traversing from a patent foramen ovale (PFO) to the coronary arteries have been implicated. Clinical management typically mirrors that of individuals experiencing acute infarction unless an underlying connective tissue disorder is present. Coronary intervention may carry risks if nonatherosclerotic dissection is already evident, potentially exacerbating the condition. Conservative management is generally favored, although significant aortic dissections may necessitate surgical intervention. Pregnant individuals with Marfan syndrome face an increased risk of aortic dilation when the aortic diameter exceeds 4.5 cm (or 27 mm/m2). In such cases, pregnancy avoidance is advised. Evidence suggests a heightened risk of dissection during pregnancy, even in scenarios where elective repair may be deemed appropriate (e.g., when the aortic root surpasses 4.0 cm in women with Marfan syndrome planning pregnancy). For pregnancies less than 28 weeks, treatment for aortic disease should begin after an abortion if necessary. In critical conditions, surgery may be required before deciding to continue or stop the pregnancy. Pregnancies beyond 28 weeks should aim to save the fetus. Treatment can start after caesarean section if the aortic condition is stable; otherwise, surgery and caesarean section may be performed simultaneously. During pregnancy, the treatment of aortic dissection depends on various factors such as the type of dissection, gestational age, and severity of the condition. Here are the treatment options :

- Stanford Type A Aortic Dissection:
- Surgical management involves excision of the inti-

mal tear, obliteration of entry into the proximal false lumen, and reconstitution of the aorta.

- For pregnant patients with acute Stanford type A aortic dissection, surgical intervention should be delayed as much as possible.
- Stanford Type B Aortic Dissection:
- Endovascular treatment (EVAR) is recommended for patients with Stanford type B aortic dissection who qualify for it
- Ascending Aortic Aneurysm:
- Critical ascending aortic aneurysm requires treatment similar to that for Stanford type A aortic dissection.

Braverman AC et al. Clinical Features and Outcomes of Pregnancy-Related Acute Aortic Dissection. JAMA Cardiol. 2021 Jan 1;6(1):58-66. PMID: 33052376

6.7 Catheter Ablation Complication Case

Case 97

A 52-year-old man with a history of ischemic cardiomyopathy and recurrent ventricular tachycardia (VT) is referred for catheter ablation. He has an implantable cardioverter-defibrillator (ICD) in place and has experienced multiple appropriate shocks for VT despite being on maximally tolerated doses of beta-blockers and amiodarone. His left ventricular ejection fraction is 25%. A recent cardiac MRI showed a large area of transmural scarring in the left ventricular anterolateral wall. During the ablation procedure, the VT is successfully induced and localized to the area of scarring. However, shortly after the ablation, the patient becomes hypotensive with a blood pressure of 80/50 mm Hg, and an echocardiogram reveals a new pericardial effusion with evidence of tamponade.
Which of the following is the most appropriate next step in the management of this patient?

- A. Immediate pericardiocentesis.
- B. Intravenous fluid bolus and observation.
- C. Urgent coronary angiography.
- D. Administration of intravenous corticosteroids.

The correct answer is A. Immediate pericardiocentesis. The patient's clinical presentation of hypotension and echocardiographic findings of a new pericardial effusion with evidence of tamponade following a catheter ablation procedure is highly suggestive of cardiac perforation leading to pericardial tamponade. This is a known complication of catheter ablation procedures and requires immediate intervention to prevent hemodynamic collapse. Pericardiocentesis is the procedure of choice to drain the pericardial effusion and relieve the pressure on the heart. Option B is incorrect because, while intravenous fluids may temporarily support the blood pressure, they do not address the underlying problem of cardiac tamponade. The definitive treatment is drainage of the effusion. Option C is incorrect because, although coronary artery injury could be a concern during catheter ablation, the immediate life-threatening issue is the cardiac tamponade, which needs to be addressed before any other investigations or interventions. Option D is incorrect because corticosteroids have no role in the acute management of cardiac tamponade. They do not address the mechanical compression of the heart due to the effusion. Cardiac tamponade following a catheter ablation is a rare but serious complication that can be life-threatening. It typically requires emergency intervention to prevent hemodynamic collapse. The incidence of cardiac tamponade during atrial fibrillation (AF) ablation procedures is relatively low, with studies reporting rates around 1.2% and in-hospital mortality about 0.04%. Factors such as older age, female sex, lower body mass index, and comorbidities like hypertension and diabetes are associated with a higher risk of complications. Cardiac tamponade can occur due to various procedural factors, including trans-septal puncture, extensive catheter manipulation, application of radiofrequency energy, or steam pops under intense anticoagulation. It can happen during or shortly after the procedure, and in some cases, even later, as demonstrated by a case where delayed cardiac tamponade occurred 19 days post-procedure. Management typically involves pericardiocentesis to drain the

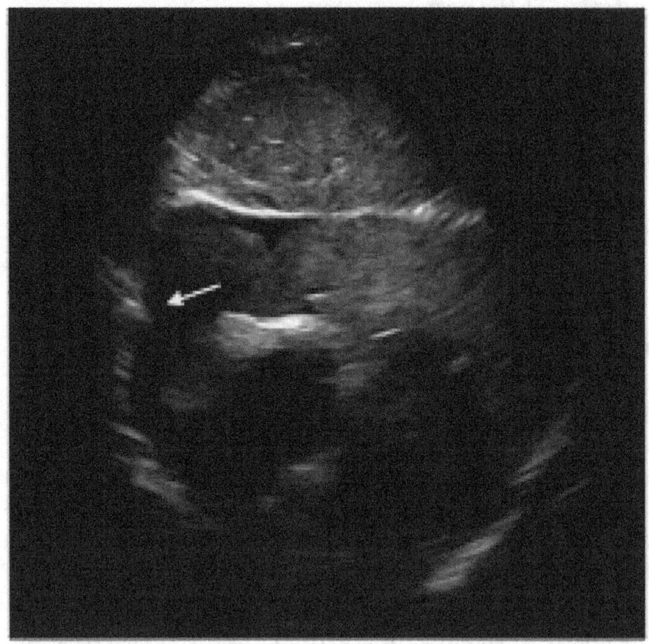

Figure 6.1: Pericardial Effusion

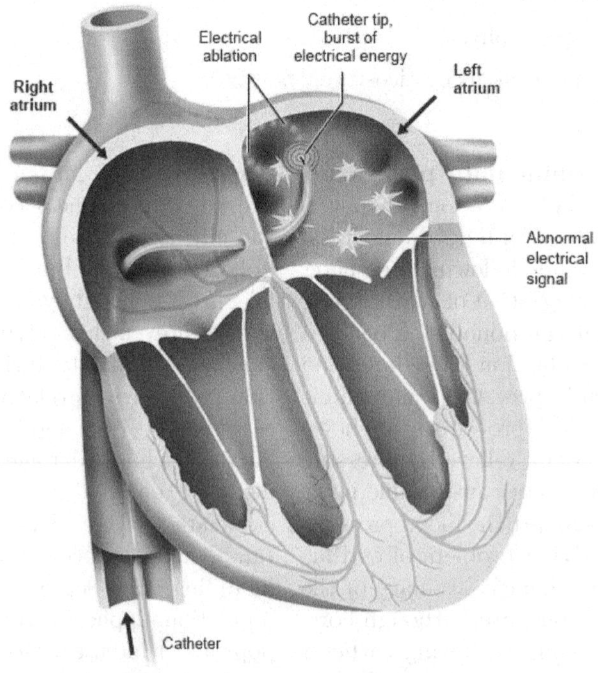

H

Figure 6.2: Catheter Ablation

pericardial effusion and relieve pressure on the heart. In some instances, surgical intervention may be required. The use of cryoballoon has been associated with a lower incidence of tamponade compared to other techniques. Women have been found to have an approximately two-fold higher risk of developing this complication. The diagnosis and management of cardiac tamponade following catheter ablation are critical, and clinicians must be vigilant for signs of this complication during and after the procedure. Regular post-procedural echocardiography is important for early detection, as a delayed diagnosis can be fatal

Hamaya R et al. Management of cardiac tamponade in catheter ablation of atrial fibrillation: single-centre 15year experience on 5222 procedures. Europace. 2018 Nov 1;20(11):1776-1782. PMID: 29161368

6.8 Peripartum Cardiomyopathy (PPCM)

Case 98

A 32-year-old African American woman presents to the clinic 2 weeks postpartum with progressive dyspnea, orthopnea, and lower extremity edema. She had a twin pregnancy and a history of preeclampsia. Her blood pressure is 130/85 mmHg, heart rate is 110 beats per minute, and respiratory rate is 22 breaths per minute. On examination, she has an S3 gallop, jugular venous distension, and bilateral rales halfway up her lung fields. Her echocardiogram shows a left ventricular ejection fraction (LVEF) of 35% with global hypokinesis and no valvular abnormalities. Serum B-type natriuretic peptide (BNP) level is markedly elevated. She is currently breastfeeding.

Which of the following is the most appropriate next step in the management of this patient?

- A. Initiate bromocriptine therapy to improve left ventricular function.
- B. Start anticoagulation with warfarin for thromboembolic prophylaxis.
- C. Begin treatment with diuretics, beta-blockers, and consider hydralazine with nitrates for heart failure management.
- D. Schedule for immediate delivery of the baby despite being postpartum.

The correct answer is C. Begin treatment with diuretics, beta-blockers, and consider hydralazine with nitrates for heart failure management. The patient is presenting with signs and symptoms of heart failure due to peripartum cardiomyopathy (PPCM), which is supported by her recent pregnancy, twin gestation, history of preeclampsia, and echocardiographic findings. Management of PPCM includes standard heart failure therapy, which involves the use of diuretics to relieve pulmonary congestion and peripheral edema, beta-blockers to improve myocardial function and survival, and hydralazine with nitrates, especially in African American patients, to reduce afterload. These medications are generally safe in breastfeeding mothers and can improve outcomes in patients with PPCM. Option A is incorrect because, while bromocriptine has shown some promise in the treatment of PPCM, it is not considered first-line therapy and is typically reserved for cases that are refractory to standard heart failure treatments or in specific clinical trials. Additionally, bromocriptine can suppress lactation, which may not be desirable for a breastfeeding mother unless the benefits outweigh the risks. Option B is incorrect because anticoagulation may be considered in PPCM patients with severe LV dysfunction (LVEF ¡ 30%) or evidence of intracardiac thrombus, which is not mentioned in this scenario. The decision to anticoagulate should be individualized based on the patient's risk factors for thromboembolism. Option D is incorrect as the patient is already postpartum, and the delivery of the baby has already occurred. The management should now focus on treating the heart failure symptoms and improving cardiac function. Dilated cardiomyopathy affects approximately 1 in 3000 to 4000 live infants, typically manifesting in the final month of pregnancy or within six months post-delivery. Risk factors for this condition include preeclampsia, twin pregnancies, and being of Black race, potentially influenced by societal factors like racism and social marginalization. The disease's progression varies, with many cases showing improvement or complete resolution over several months, while others may progress to refractory heart failure. Approximately 60% of patients experience full recovery.

Although elevated serum BNP levels are common during pregnancy, monitoring serial readings can aid in identifying individuals at higher risk for adverse outcomes. Beta-blockers have been cautiously administered to these patients, showing some anecdotal efficacy. Diuretics, hydralazine, and nitrates are effective in managing heart failure with minimal fetal risk. Sotalol is a suitable option for treating ventricular or atrial arrhythmias when other beta-blockers are ineffective. Anticoagulation may be recommended due to an increased risk of thrombotic events. In severe cases, temporary extracorporeal membrane oxygenation (ECMO) may be beneficial in saving lives. Recurrence in subsequent pregnancies is probable if cardiac function has not fully recovered, and it is advisable to avoid further pregnancies if the ejection fraction (EF) remains below 55%. The risk of recurrent heart failure in subsequent pregnancies is estimated at 21%. Delivery plays a critical role, with most complications occurring within the first week post-delivery, although some cases may arise up to five weeks after delivery. Peripartum cardiomyopathy is believed to be linked to an antiangiogenic cleaved prolactin fragment. Bromocriptine, a prolactin release inhibitor, has shown efficacy in this condition. A multicenter European trial demonstrated that individuals with peripartum cardiomyopathy who received bromocriptine exhibited greater improvement in left ventricular ejection fraction (LVEF) compared to those who did not receive the treatment. Additionally, bromocriptine therapy was associated with a high likelihood of complete left ventricle recovery.

6.9 Syncope in Young Athlete

Case 99

A 22-year-old professional basketball player presents for evaluation before returning to competitive sports. He had a mild case of COVID-19 infection 2 months ago, with symptoms of mild cough and fever that resolved within a week. He denies any chest pain, palpitations, or dyspnea on exertion. His physical examination is unremarkable, and his resting ECG and high-sensitivity troponin levels are normal. However, he is anxious to return to play and requests further assessment to ensure his cardiac function is not compromised.
Which of the following is the most appropriate next step in the management of this patient?

- A. Perform a transthoracic echocardiogram to assess for any subtle cardiac abnormalities.
- B. Obtain a cardiac MRI to rule out myocardial inflammation or fibrosis.
- C. Schedule a cardiopulmonary exercise test to evaluate his functional capacity.
- D. Clear the patient for return to play without further testing.

The correct answer is A. Perform a transthoracic echocardiogram to assess for any subtle cardiac abnormalities. According to the expert consensus statement from the American College of Cardiology (ACC), in athletes who have had COVID-19, a normal ECG and high-sensitivity troponin are reassuring. However, if there are any clinical concerns, a transthoracic echocardiogram should be obtained to assess for right ventricular dysfunction, diastolic left ventricular abnormalities, and early signs of left ventricular dysfunction, including abnormal global longitudinal strain. These findings are considered "red flags" and could indicate a need for further testing. Since the patient is asymptomatic with normal initial screening tests but desires further evaluation, an echocardiogram is a reasonable next step to ensure there are no subtle cardiac abnormalities before returning to high-intensity sports.

Option B is incorrect because cardiac MRI is typically reserved for cases where "red flags" are identified on echocardiogram or when there is a high index of suspicion for myocardial involvement despite normal initial screening tests. It is not indicated as a routine screening tool in asymptomatic athletes with normal ECG and troponin levels. Option C is incorrect because cardiopulmonary exercise testing is generally avoided during the acute phase of COVID-19 and is more valuable at 3–6 months after the illness if symptoms persist. It is also used as part of return-to-play guidelines, but not as an initial screening tool in asymptomatic individuals. Option D is incorrect because, despite the normal ECG and troponin levels, the patient has requested further assessment. Given the potential risks associated with myocardial involvement post-COVID-19 and the high level of athletic performance required, it is prudent to perform an echocardiogram before clearing the patient for return to play. Stress-induced syncope or chest discomfort may signal an anomalous origin of a coronary artery. This anomaly often occurs when the left anterior descending artery or left main coronary artery arises from the right coronary cusp and traverses between the aorta and pulmonary trunks. The constriction of the arterial opening due to angulation at its origin is thought to result in ischemia when the aorta and pulmonary arteries dilate during vigorous physical exertion, placing stress on the coronary artery. Differentiating between a healthy athlete with left ventricular hypertrophy (LVH) and an athlete with hypertrophic cardiomyopathy can pose a challenge. Typically, a healthy athlete's heart is less likely to exhibit abnormal features such as asymmetric septal hypertrophy, left atrial enlargement, abnormal ECG findings, left ventricular cavity diameter less than 45 mm at end-diastole, abnormal diastolic filling pattern, or a family history of hypertrophic cardiomyopathy. Men are more commonly athletes than individuals with hypertrophic cardiomyopathy, while women face an equal risk. Cardiac MRI is increasingly valuable in distinguishing between an athlete's heart and hypertrophic obstructive cardiomyopathy. Patients with Wolff-Parkinson-White (WPW) syndrome, prolonged QTc interval, or abnormal ST shifts in leads V1 and V2 suggestive of Brugada syndrome are at higher risk. Selective use of routine ECG and stress testing is recommended for men over 40 and women over 50 engaging in intense exercise, and at younger ages if there is a family history of premature coronary artery disease (CAD), hypertrophic cardiomyopathy, or multiple risk factors. Several risk factors like prolonged QT interval, LVH, Brugada syndrome, and WPW syndrome can be identified through regular ECG screenings, prompting various cost-effectiveness evaluations. While many experts advocate for preparticipation ECGs as potentially beneficial, the optimal approach for slightly elevated QTc intervals remains uncertain. The prevalence of false-positive ECG results significantly diminishes its efficacy as a screening tool due to the rarity of cardiac abnormalities in the general population. A Canadian study examining 74 sudden cardiac arrests during sports revealed that most occurred during noncompetitive activities. The incidence rate in competitive athletics was 0.76 per 100,000 athlete-years, with no apparent association with structural heart disease in the majority of cases. Genetic testing for athletes displaying T wave inversions on their ECG has shown limited utility, yielding a new diagnosis beyond standard clinical methods in only 2.5% of cases. Routine screening remains a topic of debate. A 2018 study in the United Kingdom examined adolescent soccer players between 1996 and 2016, utilizing screening methods like ECG and echocardiography. Out of 118,351 person-years assessed, only 0.38% of athletes were found to have conditions associated with sudden death. Approximately 7 out of 100,000 athletes experienced unexpected fatalities, primarily attributed to undetected cardiomyopathies during screenings. In 2017, a joint position paper by several European societies deliberated on preparticipation screening options, with input from international sports bodies. The consensus supported obtaining clinical history, conducting physical examinations, and performing a 12-lead ECG on all individuals based on available data. Echocardiography was not recommended as a routine screening tool. The American Medical Society for Sports Medicine released a consensus statement in 2017 outlining screening recommendations for various clinical scenarios. Following identification of high-risk individuals, guidelines from the Bethesda Conference and the European Society of Cardiology (ESC) can aid in determining the athlete's eligibility to continue participating in sports. recommendations from the 36th Bethesda Conference and the European Society of Cardiology regarding participation in competitive sports for athletes with various cardiac conditions. Here are the key points:Hypertrophic Cardiomyopathy (HCM):

- Both guidelines exclude athletes with a clinical diagnosis of HCM from all competitive sports.
- The Bethesda Conference allows genotype-positive but phenotype-negative athletes to still compete.

Arrhythmogenic Right Ventricular Cardiomyopathy (ARVC): Both guidelines exclude athletes diagnosed with ARVC from competitive sports. Coronary Artery Anomalies (CCAA):

- The Bethesda Conference excludes athletes from competitive sports.
- It allows participation 3 months after successful surgery if no ischemia, arrhythmia, or LV dysfunction during exercise testing.
- The European guideline does not provide recommendations for CCAA.

Wolff-Parkinson-White Syndrome (WPW):

- Both allow asymptomatic athletes without structural heart disease to participate in all sports.
- For symptomatic athletes, electrophysiology study and ablation are recommended before return to sports after ECG normalization.

Long QT Syndrome (LQTS):

- Bethesda excludes athletes with previous cardiac arrest or syncope from competitive sports, but allows genotype-positive/phenotype-negative athletes.
- European guideline restricts asymptomatic patients

to low-intensity sports and excludes those with clinical or genotype diagnosis.

Brugada Syndrome (BrS):

- Bethesda excludes from all competitive sports except low-intensity.
- European guideline excludes from all competitive sports.

Catecholaminergic Polymorphic Ventricular Tachycardia (CPVT):

- Both exclude patients with a clinical diagnosis from competitive sports.
- Bethesda allows genotype-positive/phenotype-negative patients in low-intensity sports.

Phelan D et al. Screening of potential cardiac involvement in competitive athletes recovering from COVID-19: an expert consensus statement. JACC Cardiovasc Imaging. 2020;13: 2635. PMID: 33303102

7 DISORDERS OF RATE/RHYTHM

7.1 Recurrent Dizziness and Palpitations in a 78-Year-Old Woman

Case 100

A 78-year-old woman presents to the clinic with complaints of recurrent dizziness and palpitations for the past several months. She has a history of hypertension and type 2 diabetes mellitus. Her medications include metoprolol, lisinopril, and metformin. On examination, her blood pressure is 130/80 mm Hg, heart rate is 48 beats per minute, and she is not orthostatic. An electrocardiogram (ECG) reveals sinus bradycardia with occasional premature atrial contractions. A 24-hour Holter monitor shows periods of atrial fibrillation with rapid ventricular rates up to 150 beats per minute, followed by long sinus pauses of up to 4.5 seconds after the termination of atrial fibrillation episodes.
Which of the following is the most appropriate next step in the management of this patient?

- A. Increase the dose of metoprolol.
- B. Initiate anticoagulation therapy.
- C. Implantation of a dual-chamber pacemaker.
- D. Referral for catheter ablation of atrial fibrillation.

The correct answer is C. Implantation of a dual-chamber pacemaker. The patient's clinical presentation and Holter monitor findings are consistent with sick sinus syndrome, specifically the tachy-brady variant. The long pauses following the termination of atrial fibrillation episodes are likely contributing to her symptoms of dizziness. In this scenario, the bradycardia component needs to be addressed to prevent symptomatic pauses. Implantation of a dual-chamber pacemaker will provide pacing support during periods of bradycardia and allow for appropriate rate response during periods of tachycardia. Option A is incorrect because increasing the dose of metoprolol would likely exacerbate the bradycardia and the sinus pauses, potentially worsening her symptoms. Option B is incorrect because, while anticoagulation therapy is important in the management of atrial fibrillation to prevent thromboembolic events, it does not address the symptomatic bradycardia and pauses that are the primary issue in this patient. Option D is incorrect because, although catheter ablation of atrial fibrillation may reduce the burden of atrial fibrillation, it does not address the underlying sinus node dysfunction that is causing the symptomatic pauses. Moreover, the patient would still require a pacemaker to manage the bradycardia.

Sick sinus syndrome encompasses sinus arrest, sinoatrial exit block, or prolonged sinus bradycardia. In older adults, the condition often presents with recurrent supraventricular tachycardias, commonly atrial fibrillation, alongside bradyarrhythmias, referred to as "tachy-brady syndrome". The extended pauses following tachycardia cessation contribute to associated symptoms. Additionally, sick sinus syndrome may manifest as chronotropic incompetence, characterized by an inadequate heart rate response to physiological demands during activity or stress, sometimes overlooked as a cause of reduced exercise tolerance. For symptomatic individuals with bradycardia or sick sinus syndrome, implanting a permanent pacemaker is typically advised. A single-chamber atrial pacemaker is suitable for those without AV nodal or bundle branch conduction issues. Atrial-based pacing, whether single or dual chamber, has shown greater efficacy than ventricular-only pacing in individuals with sinus node dysfunction, supported by multiple randomized controlled trials. During dual-chamber pacemaker implantation for sinus node dysfunction with intact AV conduction, it is crucial to avoid excessive ventricular pacing to prevent worsening heart failure, especially in patients with underlying left ventricular dysfunction. Sinus tachycardia usually improves with treatment of the underlying cause. Symptomatic inappropriate sinus tachycardia may be managed with beta-blockers or calcium channel blockers, although treatment can be challenging.

De Ponti R et al. Sick Sinus Syndrome. Card Electrophysiol Clin. 2018 Jun;10(2):183-195. doi: 10.1016/j.ccep.2018.02.002. PMID: 29784479.

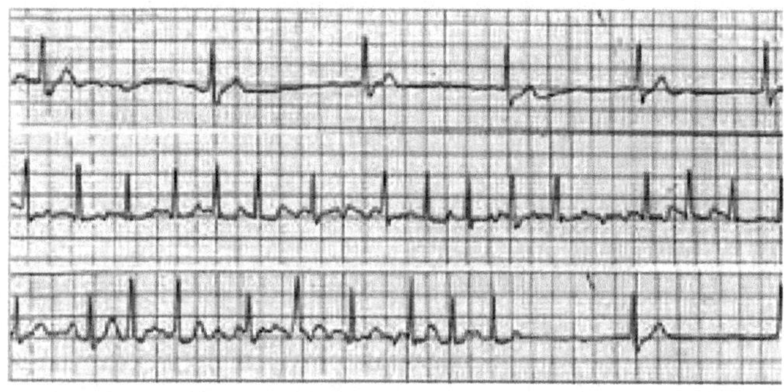

Figure 7.1: A 78-year-old woman

7.2 Syncope and Bradycardia in a 67-Year-Old

Case 101

A 67-year-old man with a history of hypertension and chronic obstructive pulmonary disease presents to the emergency department with syncope. He reports several episodes of lightheadedness over the past few months. His medications include amlodipine and tiotropium. On examination, his blood pressure is 130/85 mm Hg, heart rate is 45 beats per minute, and he is alert and oriented. His lung examination reveals mild expiratory wheezing, and the cardiac examination is notable for a regular bradycardic rhythm without murmurs. An ECG shows a normal sinus rhythm with a complete right bundle branch block and left anterior fascicular block. His echocardiogram shows normal left ventricular function with no valvular abnormalities.
Which of the following is the most appropriate next step in the management of this patient?

- A. Initiate beta-blocker therapy.
- B. Perform a head-up tilt table test.
- C. Implantation of a dual-chamber pacemaker.
- D. Observation and reassessment in 24 hours.

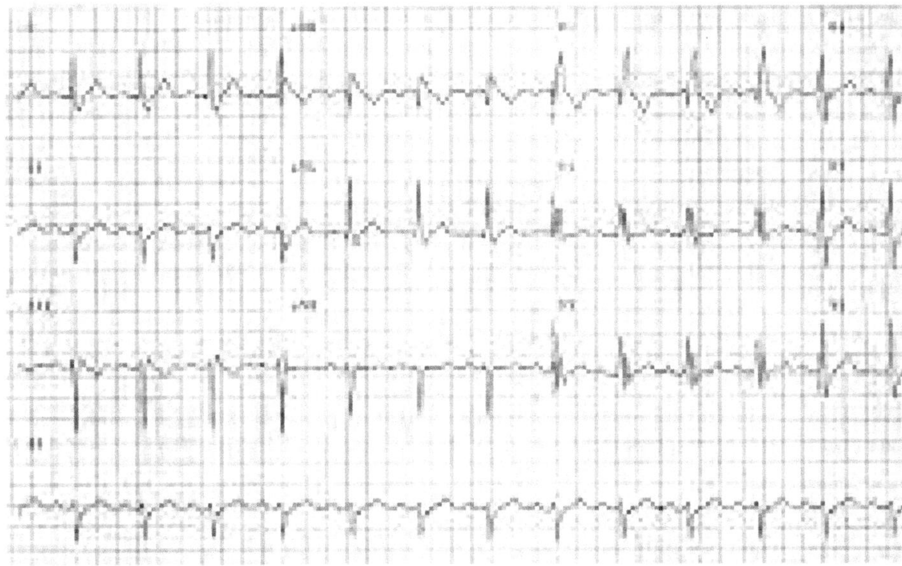

Figure 7.2: Right bundle branch block and left anterior fascicular block

The correct answer is C. Implantation of a dual-chamber pacemaker. The correct answer is C. Implantation of a dual-chamber pacemaker. The patient has experienced syncope, which can be attributed to bradycardia based on his heart rate of 45 beats per minute and the presence of bifascicular block (right bundle branch block and left anterior fascicular block) on the ECG. Given the syncope in the setting of bifascicular block, the patient is at risk for progression to complete heart block. A dual-chamber pacemaker is indicated in this scenario to prevent recurrent syncope and potential catastrophic bradyarrhythmic events. Option A is incorrect because beta-blockers would likely exacerbate the bradycardia and are not indicated in the setting of syncope with bifascicular block. Option B is incorrect because a head-up tilt table test is typically used to diagnose vasovagal syncope, which is less likely in this patient given the ECG findings suggestive of a high risk for bradyarrhythmias. Option D is incorrect because observation and reassessment do not address the immediate risk of progression to complete heart block and recurrent syncope or sudden cardiac arrest. Intraventricular conduction block is a frequently encountered phenomenon that may manifest as either transient (linked to heart rate elevation) or persistent. Right bundle branch block is commonly observed in individuals with structurally normal hearts. The left bundle comprises anterior and posterior fascicles, and the presence of left bundle branch block often indicates underlying cardiac conditions such as ischemic heart disease, inflammatory or infiltrative disorders, cardiomyopathy, and valvular heart disease. Asymptomatic individuals with bifascicular block have a low annual risk (1%) of progressing to concealed complete heart block. Bifascicular block involves impairment in two of the three infranodal components: the right bundle, left anterior, and left posterior fascicle.

A standardized naming convention for pacemaker devices typically utilizes four letters. The first letter denotes the paced chamber: A for atrium, V for ventricle, and D for dual (both). The second letter indicates the sensed chamber, which can be A, V, or D; an additional option (O) signifies absence of sensing. The third letter denotes the pacemaker's response to a detected event: I for inhibition, T for triggering, D for dual response modes, and O for no response. The fourth letter relates to programmability or rate response capability (R for rate modulation), a feature that adjusts the pacing rate based on activity or respiratory rate when the intrinsic heart rate is unacceptably low.

For patients in sinus rhythm, the most physiologically sound pacing approach involves a dual-chamber pacemaker capable of sensing and pacing in both chambers.The indication for a pacemaker in bradycardia is primarily based on symptomatic bradycardia, which refers to a documented bradyarrhythmia directly responsible for symptoms like dizziness, light-headedness, confusion, reduced exercise capacity, and even congestive heart failure due to cerebral hypoperfusion from low heart rates. The decision to implant a pacemaker is typically guided by the presence of these symptoms attributed to bradycardia. In patients with bradycardia and indications for pacemaker implantation, shared decision-making and patient-centered care are emphasized to ensure the best outcomes.

Specifically, the most common indications for permanent pacemaker implantation in cases of symptomatic bradycardia include sinus node dysfunction (SND) and advanced second- or third-degree atrioventricular (AV) block. For SND, permanent atrial or dual-chamber pacemaker implantation is recommended when symptoms correlate with age. Additionally, pacing may be considered for recurrent symptomatic neurocardiogenic syncope. associated with documented spontaneous events In summary, symptomatic bradycardia that leads to clinical manifestations such as dizziness, light-headedness, confusion, reduced exercise capacity, or congestive heart failure is a key indication for pacemaker implantation to address the underlying rhythm abnormalities and improve patient outcomes.

Ahmad M et al. Outcomes of dual-chamber implantable cardioverter defibrillator for left bundle branch area pacing: A systematic review of literature. Ann Noninvasive Electrocardiol. 2024 Jan;29(1):e13098. PMID: 37997513

7.3 Suspected Pacemaker Pocket Infection in a 73-Year-Old Woman

Case 102

A 73-year-old woman with a history of complete heart block underwent dual-chamber pacemaker implantation one week ago. She presents to the clinic with a 2-day history of increasing redness, warmth, and tenderness over the pacemaker pocket site. She denies fever or chills. Her other medical conditions include type 2 diabetes mellitus and chronic kidney disease. On examination, the temperature is 37.2C (99F), blood pressure is 145/86 mm Hg, heart rate is 70 beats per minute, and the respiratory rate is 16 breaths per minute. The pacemaker pocket site is erythematous, swollen, and tender to palpation. There is no fluctuance, and the overlying skin is intact without drainage. Laboratory studies show a white blood cell count of 12,000/L with 80% neutrophils. A chest X-ray is unremarkable, and the pacemaker leads appear to be in the appropriate position.
Which of the following is the most appropriate next step in the management of this patient?

- A. Oral antibiotics and close outpatient follow-up.
- B. Intravenous antibiotics and hospital admission for possible pacemaker pocket infection.
- C. Immediate pacemaker removal and intravenous antibiotics.
- D. Aspiration of the pacemaker pocket for culture and sensitivity.

The correct answer is B. Intravenous antibiotics and hospital admission for possible pacemaker pocket infection. The patient's presentation is suggestive of a pacemaker pocket infection, which is a serious complication of pacemaker implantation. The presence of localized signs of infection such as erythema, warmth, and tenderness, in the absence of systemic symptoms, may represent an early infection. Given her history of diabetes and chronic kidney disease, she is at higher risk for complications. Hospital admission for intravenous antibiotics after obtaining blood cultures is appropriate to provide adequate treatment and to monitor for any progression that might necessitate device removal. Option A is incorrect because oral antibiotics and outpatient follow-up are not adequate for a suspected pacemaker pocket infection, which can rapidly progress to a more serious infection involving the device and leads. Option C is incorrect because immediate pacemaker removal is generally reserved for confirmed device-related infections with systemic involvement or evidence of lead or valve endocarditis. There is no current evidence of systemic infection or device involvement that would necessitate immediate removal. Option D is incorrect because aspiration of the pacemaker pocket is not routinely performed due to the risk of introducing infection into the pocket or damaging the device and leads. It is typically reserved for cases where the diagnosis is uncertain and there is evidence of fluctuance suggesting an abscess. While pacemaker implantation is a common and generally safe procedure, it can give rise to various complications that can be broadly classified into those associated with the implantation process itself and those that manifest post-implantation. During the implantation procedure, complications may include pneumothorax, characterized by the presence of air in the pleural space leading to lung collapse, hemothorax, which involves the accumulation of blood in the pleural cavity, and cardiac perforation, a serious complication where inadvertent puncturing of the heart muscle occurs. Subsequent to the procedure, patients may encounter issues such as hematoma, a localized collection of blood outside blood vessels typically in liquid form within tissues or organs, often occurring at the pacemaker pocket site. Lead dislodgement is another common post-implantation complication where the leads connecting the pacemaker to the heart shift out of place, potentially disrupting the device's ability to effectively regulate the heart's rhythm. Infections are also a concern, typically within the first year post-implantation. Symptoms of a pacemaker infection may include fever, along with pain, swelling, and redness at the pacemaker site. Additionally, patients may experience pocket fibrosis, characterized by excessive formation of fibrous connective tissue in the pacemaker pocket leading to hardening or stiffening of the area. Other potential complications encompass lead infection, lead endocarditis (infection of the heart's inner lining), and venous thrombosis (blood clot in a vein). In rare instances, complications like right ventricular perforation and myocardial rupture can occur. To prevent lead dislodgement during pacemaker implantation, several strategies can be employed based on research findings:

1. **Creation of a Small Pocket:** By creating a small pocket during the implantation procedure, the risk of lead dislodgement can be reduced.
2. **Subpectoral Implantation:** Placing the device subpectorally, especially in aged obese patients with flabby subcutaneous tissue, can help prevent progressive displacement of the generator inside the pocket.
3. **Use of Non-absorbable Suture or Polyester Cases:** Fixating the leads with non-absorbable suture or polyester cases can enhance stability and reduce the likelihood of dislodgement.
4. **Active Fixation Leads:** Utilizing active fixation leads can provide better anchoring and stability, reducing the chances of lead movement.
5. **Immobilization of Upper Extremity:** Immobilizing the upper extremity in the first week post-implantation has been suggested as a preventive measure to minimize lead dislodgement.

While these techniques have been proposed to reduce lead dislodgement, it is important to note that recurrences have been reported despite these preventive measures. Additionally, using leadless pacemaker implantation may also be considered as a method to decrease lead dislodgement and prevent complications like Twiddler syndrome.

Haddadin F et al. Clinical outcomes and predictors of complications in patients undergoing leadless pacemaker implantation. Heart Rhythm. 2022 Aug;19(8):1289-1296. PMID: 35490710

7.4 Management of Bradycardia in a Patient with Palpitations

Case 103

A 68-year-old man with a history of hypertension and hyperlipidemia presents to the emergency department with lightheadedness and palpitations. He denies chest pain, shortness of breath, or syncope. His medications include atenolol and atorvastatin. On physical examination, his blood pressure is 130/80 mm Hg, heart rate is 45 beats per minute, and he is alert and oriented. Cardiac auscultation reveals an irregular rhythm without murmurs, rubs, or gallops. His lungs are clear to auscultation, and there is no peripheral edema. An electrocardiogram (ECG) shows a regular rhythm with narrow QRS complexes, a PR interval of 220 msec, and dropped beats occurring in a 3:2 pattern.
Diagnostic Test Results:

- ECG: Regular rhythm, narrow QRS complexes (¡120 msec), PR interval of 220 msec, 3:2 atrioventricular (AV) block pattern.

Question: What is the most appropriate next step in the management of this patient?

- A) Administer intravenous atropine
- B) Observe and monitor in a telemetry unit
- C) Implant a permanent pacemaker
- D) Perform an exercise stress test

The correct answer is B) Observe and monitor in a telemetry unit. The patient presents with a second-degree AV block, likely Mobitz type I (Wenckebach), given the narrow QRS complexes and prolonged PR interval. This type of block is often at the level of the AV node and can be physiologic, especially in well-conditioned athletes or during sleep. However, in this patient, it is more likely to be pathologic given his age and symptoms. The presence of lightheadedness suggests that the AV block is hemodynamically significant, but there is no evidence of acute instability requiring immediate intervention. Option A) Administer intravenous atropine is not the most appropriate next step as this patient is not bradycardic to the point of hemodynamic instability. Atropine is typically used in the acute management of symptomatic bradycardia, particularly if associated with hypotension or other signs of poor perfusion. Option C) Implant a permanent pacemaker may eventually be necessary if the patient's AV block is persistent and symptomatic, but it is not the immediate next step without further observation and assessment of the pattern and symptoms. Option D) Perform an exercise stress test is not appropriate at this time as the patient is currently symptomatic with a conduction abnormality that needs to be addressed before any stress testing. In conclusion, the most appropriate next step is to observe and monitor the patient in a telemetry unit to assess the stability of the AV block, the presence of symptoms, and to determine if there is progression to a higher degree of block that would necessitate pacemaker implantation. Atrioventricular (AV) block can present in two forms: physiologic, often due to heightened vagal tone, or pathologic, arising from factors like cardiac surgery, myocarditis, ischemia, or conduction system fibrosis. AV block is categorized into three degrees: complete (no atrial impulses reach the ventricles), second-degree (intermittent blocked rhythms), and first-degree (PR interval exceeding 200 msec with all atrial impulses conducting). Second-degree AV block is further divided into Mobitz type I (Wenckebach), characterized by a progressive PR interval elongation before a blocked beat, and Mobitz type II, featuring intermittently nonconducted atrial beats without preceding AV conduction changes. Differentiating between Mobitz types I and II with a 2:1 AV block on ECG can be challenging. Nodal (Mobitz type I) block is likely if the baseline PR interval is prolonged (>200 msec) or the QRS complex is narrow (<120 msec); infranodal (Mobitz type II) block is more probable with a wide QRS complex (≥120 msec). First-degree and Mobitz type I blocks typically present benignly with few symptoms.

Physiologic AV block can be triggered by increased parasympathetic activity, commonly observed during sleep, in athletes, or via carotid sinus massage. Pharmacological agents like calcium channel blockers, beta-blockers, digitalis, or antiarrhythmics can also induce this response. Pathologic considerations include myocardial ischemia or infarction, inflammatory conditions (e.g., Lyme disease), fibrosis, calcification, or infiltration (e.g., amyloidosis or sarcoidosis).

Manifestations of Mobitz type II block and complete (third-degree) heart block often present as fatigue, dyspnea, presyncope, or syncope, typically stemming from a pathological condition affecting the infranodal conduction system. In complete heart block, characterized by the absence of atrial impulses reaching the ventricle, the ventricular escape rate usually drops below 50 beats per minute. Symptom severity can vary based on the speed and stability of the escape rhythm. For milder forms of AV block, investigating the underlying pathological cause is crucial. Asymptomatic patients with Mobitz type I AV block of the first or second degree generally do not require specific therapy. Patients should seek treatment for reversible causes like myocardial ischemia or adverse drug reactions. Urgent intervention is necessary for symptomatic individuals with any degree of heart block, potentially involving atropine administration (initial intravenous dose of 0.5 mg) or temporary pacing (transcutaneous or transvenous). Permanent pacing is warranted for symptomatic bradyarrhythmias with any level of AV block or asymptomatic high-degree AV block (Mobitz type II or second-degree third-degree heart block) lacking a reversible or physiological explanation.

Kusumoto FM et al. 2018 ACC/AHA/HRS Guideline on the Evaluation and Management of Patients With Bradycardia and Cardiac Conduction Delay: Executive Summary: A Report of the American College of Cardiology/American Heart Association Task Force on Clinical Practice Guidelines, and the Heart Rhythm Society. J Am Coll Cardiol. 2019 Aug 20;74(7):932-987. PMID: 30412710

7.5 Palpitations and Lightheadedness in a Healthy Middle-Aged Man

Case 104

A 52-year-old man with no significant past medical history presents to the emergency department with palpitations and lightheadedness that began while he was jogging 30 minutes ago. He denies chest pain, shortness of breath, or syncope. His blood pressure is 110/70 mm Hg, heart rate is 170 beats per minute, and respiratory rate is 18 breaths per minute. Physical examination reveals a regular, tachycardic rhythm without murmurs, rubs, or gallops. Lung fields are clear. An ECG shows a narrow complex tachycardia without P waves before each QRS complex. Vagal maneuvers are attempted without success.
Which of the following is the most appropriate next step in the management of this patient?

- A. Administer intravenous adenosine 6 mg rapidly followed by a saline flush.
- B. Administer intravenous diltiazem.
- C. Administer intravenous esmolol.
- D. Perform immediate synchronized electrical cardioversion.

The correct answer is A. Administer intravenous adenosine 6 mg rapidly followed by a saline flush. The patient is presenting with paroxysmal supraventricular tachycardia (PSVT), which is a type of narrow complex tachycardia. The first-line treatment after unsuccessful vagal maneuvers is the administration of intravenous adenosine. Adenosine works by transiently blocking the AV node, which can terminate re-entrant tachycardias involving the AV node. The initial dose is 6 mg given rapidly over 1-2 seconds, followed by a rapid saline flush to ensure the drug reaches the central circulation before it is metabolized. Option B is incorrect because calcium channel blockers like diltiazem are typically considered after adenosine has failed to terminate the arrhythmia or if adenosine is contraindicated. They are also used with caution in patients with heart failure due to their negative inotropic effects. Option C is incorrect because beta-blockers are not the first-line treatment for acute PSVT. They are considered when adenosine is contraindicated or ineffective, and their role in terminating PSVT is less well established compared to adenosine and calcium channel blockers. Option D is incorrect because immediate synchronized electrical cardioversion is reserved for patients who are hemodynamically unstable. This patient is hemodynamically stable as evidenced by his blood pressure and absence of symptoms such as chest pain or syncope. As the initial-line treatment, intravenous adenosine is suggested owing to its short duration of action and negligible negative inotropic activity . Given that adenosine has a half-life of less than 10 seconds, the drug is administered swiftly (within 1–2 seconds) in the form of a 6 mg bolus followed by 20 mL of fluid. Should this treatment plan fail to induce cessation of the arrhythmia, an additional higher dose of 12 mg may be administered. Adenosine inhibits electrical conduction through the AV node, which in approximately 90% of instances terminates PSVT. Frequent minor adverse effects consist of temporary flushing, discomfort in the thorax, nausea, and headache. To mitigate the risk of atrial fibrillation (which can occur in up to 12% of patients) and ventricular arrhythmias (which are uncommon but possible), the administration of adenosine should be accompanied by continuous cardiac monitoring and the availability of an external defibrillator. Adenosine has the potential to induce bronchospasm in patients with reactive airway disease; therefore, it should be administered with caution in these individuals. In situations where adenosine is ineffective in terminating the arrhythmia or there are contraindications to its use, calcium channel blockers administered intravenously can be utilized. These include verapamil and diltiazem. Verapamil has demonstrated comparable efficacy to adenosine in terminating paroxysmal supraventricular tachycardia (PSVT) in the acute setting, with an approximate 90% success rate. Calcium channel blockers have negative inotropic effects, which necessitates their cautious administration in patients with heart failure. In contrast to adenosine, their extended half-life may lead to sustained hypotension even after the restoration of regular rhythm. Etripamil, a short-acting calcium channel blocker administered intranasally, has shown promising results in inducing rapid conversion of PSVT in preliminary studies, and phase 3 trials are currently underway. Intravenous beta-blockers, such as esmolol (a very short-acting agent), propranolol, and metoprolol, can also be considered. Although beta-blockers induce less myocardial depression than calcium channel blockers, there is limited evidence supporting their efficacy in terminating PSVT. In cases where adenosine, beta-blockers, and calcium channel blockers are contraindicated or ineffective, synchronized electrical cardioversion (starting at 100 J) should be implemented in patients who are hemodynamically unstable.

Kotadia ID et al. Supraventricular tachycardia: An overview of diagnosis and management. Clin Med (Lond). 2020 Jan;20(1):43-47. PMID: 31941731

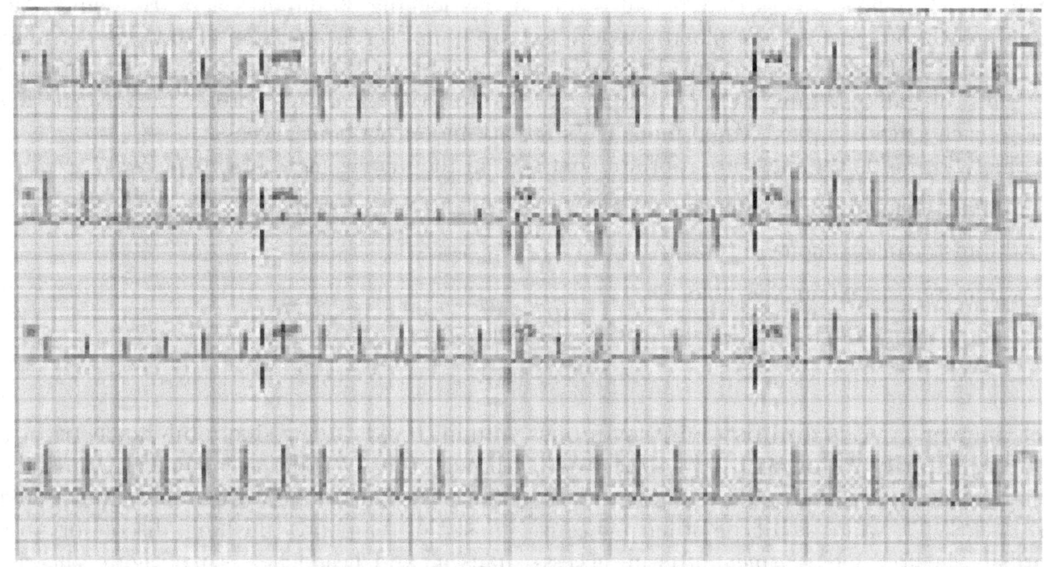

Figure 7.3: SVT

7.6 Acute Atrial Fibrillation with Rapid Ventricular Response

Case 105

A 68-year-old woman with a history of hypertension and diabetes presents to the emergency department with palpitations and dyspnea on exertion that started 12 hours ago. She has no history of atrial fibrillation. Her blood pressure is 90/60 mm Hg, heart rate is 150 beats per minute, and respiratory rate is 22 breaths per minute. She appears distressed and is unable to complete full sentences. Physical examination reveals an irregularly irregular rhythm, and lung auscultation suggests mild bibasilar crackles. An ECG confirms atrial fibrillation with a rapid ventricular response. The patient's renal function is normal, and there are no signs of active bleeding.
Which of the following is the most appropriate next step in the management of this patient?

- A. Administer intravenous diltiazem.
- B. Perform immediate synchronized electrical cardioversion.
- C. Administer intravenous ibutilide.
- D. Initiate oral anticoagulation therapy.

The correct answer is B. Perform immediate synchronized electrical cardioversion. This patient is hemodynamically unstable due to a rapid ventricular rate in the setting of new-onset atrial fibrillation, as evidenced by hypotension, tachycardia, and respiratory distress. Immediate rate control is necessary to stabilize the patient. In cases of hemodynamic instability, urgent electrical cardioversion is indicated to restore sinus rhythm and improve hemodynamics. The potential risk of thromboembolism is outweighed by the need for immediate rate control in this acutely unstable patient. Option A is incorrect because intravenous diltiazem, while useful for rate control in atrial fibrillation, is not appropriate in this scenario due to the patient's hypotension and acute hemodynamic instability. Diltiazem could potentially worsen the hypotension. Option C is incorrect because ibutilide is an option for chemical cardioversion but is not the first-line treatment in a hemodynamically unstable patient. Immediate electrical cardioversion is the preferred approach in this urgent situation. Option D is incorrect because while anticoagulation is an important consideration in the management of atrial fibrillation to prevent thromboembolic events, it is not the immediate priority in a hemodynamically unstable patient. The urgent need is to restore sinus rhythm and stabilize the patient's hemodynamics. Atrial fibrillation is the most prevalent chronic arrhythmia, affecting approximately 9% of individuals over 65 years old, with its incidence and prevalence increasing with age. It can occur in several cardiac conditions, such as rheumatic and valvular heart disease, dilated cardiomyopathy, hypertension, and coronary heart disease. It can also manifest in patients without any apparent heart disease and may be the first indicator of thyrotoxicosis, which should be ruled out during the initial episode. Atrial fibrillation typically presents in a paroxysmal manner before becoming the established rhythm. Pericarditis, chest trauma, thoracic or cardiac surgery, thyroid disorders, obstructive sleep apnea, or pulmonary disease (pneumonia, pulmonary embolism), as well as certain medications (beta-adrenergic agonists, inotropes, bisphosphonates, and some chemotherapeutic agents), can trigger episodes in individuals with otherwise healthy hearts. Excessive alcohol consumption and alcohol withdrawal, known as "holiday heart," can also precipitate atrial fibrillation. Abstaining from alcohol can reduce the likelihood of recurrent atrial fibrillation by approximately 50% in individuals who drink alcohol moderately and regularly. Atrial fibrillation, especially with an uncontrolled ventricular rate, can result in left ventricular dysfunction, heart failure, or myocardial ischemia in the presence of underlying coronary artery disease. Atrial fibrillation can lead to the formation of blood clots due to reduced blood flow in the atria, especially the left atrial appendage, which can result in the most severe consequence of embolization, particularly affecting the cerebral circulation.

The annual stroke risk is approximately 5% if left untreated. Patients with obstructive valvular disease, chronic heart failure, left ventricular dysfunction, diabetes mellitus, hypertension, age over 75 years, and a history of stroke or other embolic events are at a significantly increased risk, with rates of up to nearly 20% per year in individuals with multiple risk factors. Patients with cryptogenic stroke may have asymptomatic or "subclinical" atrial fibrillation identified using implantable loop recorders, which might lead to the initiation of oral anticoagulation if needed.

Lip GY et al. Atrial fibrillation. Nat Rev Dis Primers. 2016 Mar 31;2:16016. PMID: 27159789

7.7 New-Onset Atrial Fibrillation in a COPD Patient

Case 106

A 62-year-old man with a history of chronic obstructive pulmonary disease (COPD) presents to the emergency department with palpitations and mild dyspnea that began 10 hours ago. He has a history of hypertension but no prior episodes of atrial fibrillation. His blood pressure is 130/80 mm Hg, heart rate is 160 beats per minute, and respiratory rate is 20 breaths per minute. On examination, he is alert and oriented, with no signs of heart failure. Lung auscultation reveals diffuse wheezes. An ECG confirms atrial fibrillation with a rapid ventricular response. His renal function is normal, and there is no evidence of acute coronary syndrome or electrolyte imbalances.

Which of the following is the most appropriate next step in the management of this patient?

- A. Administer intravenous metoprolol.
- B. Administer intravenous diltiazem.
- C. Initiate oral anticoagulation therapy.
- D. Perform immediate synchronized electrical cardioversion.

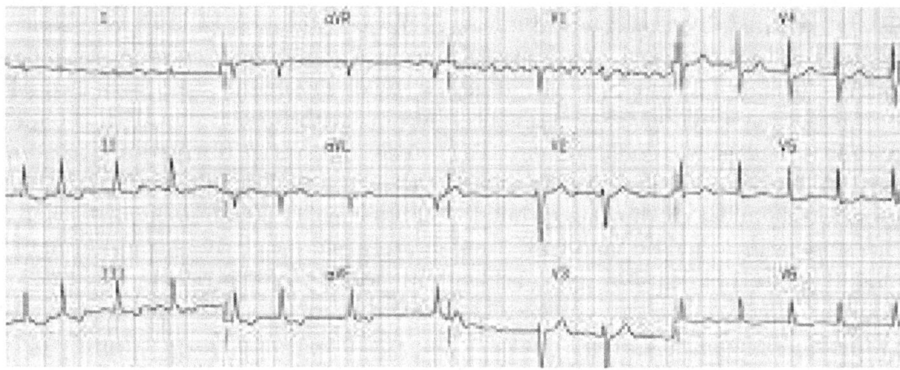

Figure 7.4: 62-year-old man

The correct answer is B. Administer intravenous diltiazem. This patient presents with new-onset atrial fibrillation with a rapid ventricular response and is hemodynamically stable. The first-line agent for ventricular rate control in a stable patient with atrial fibrillation is typically a beta-blocker or a calcium channel blocker. However, given the patient's history of COPD, a beta-blocker may exacerbate bronchospasm and should be avoided. Diltiazem is a calcium channel blocker that does not have significant negative effects on the respiratory system and is effective for rate control. It can be administered intravenously and titrated for effect, making it an appropriate choice in this scenario. Option A is incorrect because beta-blockers, such as metoprolol, can exacerbate underlying COPD by causing bronchoconstriction. Therefore, they should be used with caution or avoided in patients with reactive airway diseases. Option C is incorrect because while anticoagulation is an important consideration in atrial fibrillation to prevent thromboembolic events, the immediate priority is to achieve rate control. Anticoagulation can be considered once the patient is hemodynamically stable and the duration of atrial fibrillation is clarified. Option D is incorrect because immediate synchronized electrical cardioversion is reserved for patients who are hemodynamically unstable. This patient is hemodynamically stable and should be managed with pharmacologic rate control initially. While atrial fibrillation is generally not life-threatening in itself, it can lead to significant complications if the ventricular rate is fast enough to cause hypotension, myocardial ischemia, or tachycardia-induced myocardial dysfunction. In patients with risk factors, atrial fibrillation is a significant preventable cause of stroke. While some patients, especially those who are older or lead a sedentary lifestyle, may experience few symptoms if the ventricular rate is controlled, most patients will notice the irregular rhythm. Most patients will report fatigue, regardless of experiencing additional symptoms. The heart rate can vary from slow to fast, but it is consistently irregular unless there is complete heart block with a junctional escape rhythm or a permanent ventricular pacemaker. Atrial fibrillation is the only prevalent arrhythmia characterized by a rapid and highly irregular ventricular rate. While AF itself is not immediately life-threatening, it can have significant consequences if left unmanaged.

Hemodynamic Consequences:

- Rapid ventricular rates can lead to decreased cardiac output, hypotension, myocardial ischemia, and tachycardia-induced cardiomyopathy if sustained.
- Loss of atrial contraction (which accounts for about 20% of ventricular filling) can reduce cardiac output, especially in patients with diastolic dysfunction or hypertrophic cardiomyopathy.

Thromboembolic Risk:

- Stasis of blood in the atria, especially the left atrial appendage, can lead to thrombus formation and increase the risk of systemic embolization, primarily ischemic stroke.
- AF is a major risk factor for stroke, accounting for about 15% of all strokes annually.
- Risk factors that increase stroke risk in AF include advanced age, hypertension, diabetes, heart failure, prior stroke/TIA, and vascular disease.

Symptoms:

- Some patients, especially the elderly or sedentary, may be asymptomatic or have minimal symptoms if the ventricular rate is controlled.
- Common symptoms include palpitations, fatigue, dyspnea, chest discomfort, lightheadedness, and

reduced exercise tolerance.

- Symptoms are often related to the irregularity of the rhythm rather than the rate itself.

Types of AF:

- Paroxysmal AF: self-terminating episodes, usually lasting under 7 days
- Persistent AF: episodes lasting above 7 days and requiring cardioversion
- Longstanding persistent AF: continuous AF lasting above 1 year
- Permanent AF: continuous AF where cardioversion has failed or been foregone

Diagnosis:

- Electrocardiogram (ECG) is the primary diagnostic tool, showing irregular RR intervals and absence of distinct P waves.
- Additional tests may be required to assess underlying causes, such as echocardiography, thyroid function tests, and screening for sleep apnea.

Management:

- Rate control vs. rhythm control strategies are employed based on individual patient factors.
- Anticoagulation is often required to reduce stroke risk, especially in patients with additional risk factors.
- Treatment of underlying causes and lifestyle modifications are important adjuncts to pharmacological and interventional therapies.

Sagris M et al.Pathogenesis, Predisposing Factors, and Genetics. Int J Mol Sci. 2021 Dec 21;23(1):6. PMID: 35008432

7.8 Atrial Fibrillation : Deciding on Antithrombotic Therapy

Case 107

A 70-year-old female with a history of hypertension and hyperlipidemia presents to the clinic for a routine follow-up. She has no history of heart failure, diabetes mellitus, or prior thromboembolism. During the visit, she mentions experiencing occasional palpitations over the past few months, which prompted her to visit a local urgent care center last week. An ECG performed at that time showed atrial fibrillation, which she reports was asymptomatic. She has no current symptoms suggestive of stroke or TIA. Her blood pressure today is 145/85 mm Hg, and her heart rate is irregularly irregular at 78 beats per minute. Her CHADS2 score is 1, based on her age. Her echocardiogram shows normal left ventricular function with no valvular abnormalities.
Considering the CHA2DS2-VASc score, which of the following is the most appropriate next step in the management of this patient's atrial fibrillation?

- A. Initiate oral anticoagulation therapy.
- B. Prescribe aspirin therapy.
- C. Perform immediate cardioversion.
- D. Observe without antithrombotic therapy.

The correct answer is A. Initiate oral anticoagulation therapy. The patient's CHADS2 score is 1, based on her age, which is a risk factor for stroke in patients with atrial fibrillation. When considering the CHA2DS2-VASc score, additional risk factors include age 65–74 years, female sex, and presence of vascular disease. Since the patient is a 70-year-old female with hypertension, her CHA2DS2-VASc score is 3 (2 points for age 65–74 years, 1 point for female sex, and 1 point for hypertension). According to current guidelines, a CHA2DS2-VASc score of 2 or greater in females indicates that oral anticoagulation is recommended to reduce the risk of stroke. The patient should be started on an oral anticoagulant such as warfarin, dabigatran, rivaroxaban, apixaban, or edoxaban, taking into account her renal function, potential drug interactions, and patient preferences. Option B is incorrect because aspirin is no longer recommended for stroke prevention in atrial fibrillation due to lack of efficacy and potential harm, as indicated by the European guidelines. Option C is incorrect because immediate cardioversion is not indicated in this asymptomatic patient with atrial fibrillation of unknown duration without prior therapeutic anticoagulation or exclusion of left atrial appendage thrombus by transesophageal echocardiogram. Option D is incorrect because observation without antithrombotic therapy is not appropriate for this patient with a CHA2DS2-VASc score of 3, as she is at an increased risk for thromboembolic events. Patients with atrial fibrillation, including those with paroxysmal or infrequent episodes, should be evaluated for the need for oral anticoagulation therapy and treated if there are no significant contraindications. Patients under 65 years old with lone atrial fibrillation, meaning no evidence of associated cardiac conditions or risk factors such as hypertension, atherosclerosis, diabetes, or history of stroke, do not require antithrombotic therapy. Individuals experiencing temporary atrial fibrillation due to conditions like acute myocardial infarction or pneumonia, without any previous history of arrhythmia, are at an increased risk of developing atrial fibrillation in the future. Therefore, it is advisable to initiate anticoagulant treatment based on the identified risk factors. If the underlying cause can be reversed, such as after coronary artery bypass surgery or in cases of hyperthyroidism, then long-term anticoagulation may not be necessary.

In addition to the five conventional risk factors in the CHADS2 score (congestive heart failure, hypertension, age above or 75 years, diabetes mellitus, and history of stroke or transient ischemic attack), the European and American guidelines recommend considering three additional factors in the CHA2DS2-VASc score: age 65-74 years, female sex, and the presence of vascular disease.

The CHA2DS2-VASc score is particularly important for patients with a CHADS2 score of 0 or 1. If the CHA2DS2-VASc score is 2 or higher, oral anticoagulation is recommended. If the CHA2DS2-VASc score is 1, oral anticoagulation should be considered after evaluating the risk, benefit, and patient preferences. Female sex is considered a minor risk factor, although it has been excluded from the risk evaluation in the European guidelines. Research indicates that only 50% of individuals with atrial fibrillation who require oral anticoagulation actually receive it.Furthermore, even when these patients are prescribed warfarin, they spend almost half of the time outside the desired international normalized ratio (INR) range. Undertreatment may occur due to the misconception that aspirin is effective in preventing strokes caused by atrial fibrillation. According to European guidelines, aspirin is classified as a class III A recommendation, advising against its use due to potential harm and lack of clear evidence of benefit. Cardioversion should be performed after receiving 3-4 weeks of anticoagulation at a therapeutic level or after confirming the absence of a left atrial appendage thrombus using transesophageal echocardiography. Anticoagulation clinics that employ systematic management of warfarin dosing and adjustment have been proven to improve the maintenance of target anticoagulation levels.

Su CH et al. CHA2DS2-VASc score as an independent outcome predictor in patients hospitalized with acute ischemic stroke. PLoS One. 2022 Jul 13;17(7):e0270823. PMID: 35830440

Case 107B

A 78-year-old man with a history of non-valvular atrial fibrillation is currently managed on warfarin with a target INR of 2.5. He has a CHA2DS2-VASc score of 4, indicating a high risk of stroke. His other medical conditions include chronic kidney disease (CKD) stage III and a recent diagnosis of peptic ulcer disease. His current medications include warfarin, atorvastatin, and omeprazole. He presents to the clinic for a routine follow-up, and his laboratory tests show a creatinine clearance of 35 mL/min. He reports adherence to his medication regimen and has no new symptoms. His INR today is 2.4.
Given the patient's CKD and recent peptic ulcer disease, which of the following is the most appropriate management change?

- A. Continue warfarin with no change.
- B. Transition to a direct oral anticoagulant (DOAC).
- C. Add aspirin for gastroprotection.
- D. Discontinue anticoagulation therapy.

The correct answer is B. Transition to a direct oral anticoagulant (DOAC). This patient with non-valvular atrial fibrillation and a high risk of stroke (CHA2DS2-VASc score of 4) is currently managed on warfarin. However, he has developed CKD stage III and peptic ulcer disease, which may increase the risk of bleeding on warfarin. DOACs have been shown to have a lower risk of bleeding compared to warfarin, particularly in patients with CKD and gastrointestinal risk factors. Additionally, DOACs require less frequent monitoring and have fewer dietary and drug interactions. Given the patient's reduced renal function, a DOAC with a dosing regimen appropriate for his level of kidney function should be selected, and the patient should be monitored closely for any signs of bleeding or worsening renal function.

Option A is incorrect because, although the patient's INR is within the therapeutic range, his recent diagnosis of peptic ulcer disease and CKD stage III may increase the risk of bleeding on warfarin. Transitioning to a DOAC could be safer in terms of bleeding risk and requires less monitoring.

Option C is incorrect because aspirin is not indicated for gastroprotection and can increase the risk of bleeding, especially when combined with anticoagulants. Proton pump inhibitors (PPIs) like omeprazole are the preferred agents for gastroprotection in patients with a history of peptic ulcer disease. Option D is incorrect because discontinuing anticoagulation therapy would leave the patient at a high risk of stroke due to his atrial fibrillation and CHA2DS2-VASc score of 4. Anticoagulation is a critical component of stroke prevention in this patient population.

Drug	**Dose**	**Comparison to Warfarin**	**Trial**	**Notes**
Dabigatran	150 mg twice daily	Superior at preventing stroke	RE-LY	Results in less bleeding than warfarin. Not approved for treatment of atrial fibrillation in the US at 110 mg twice daily dose. Not recommended for patients with mechanical prosthetic heart valves.
Dabigatran	110 mg twice daily	Noninferior at preventing stroke	RE-LY	Results in less bleeding than warfarin. Not approved for treatment of atrial fibrillation in the US at this dose. Not recommended for patients with mechanical prosthetic heart valves.
Rivaroxaban	20 mg once daily (15 mg/day for patients with creatinine clearances between 15 and 50 mL/min)	Noninferior for stroke prevention	ROCKET-AF	Results in substantially less intracranial hemorrhage than warfarin. Should be administered with food for higher drug absorption.
Apixaban	5 mg twice daily (2.5 mg twice daily for patients with two of three high-risk criteria)	More effective at stroke prevention	ARISTOTLE	Lower risk of major bleeding and all-cause mortality than warfarin. Associated with less intracranial hemorrhage and well tolerated. Superior to aspirin in the AVERROES trial.
Edoxaban	60 mg once a day (30 mg/day for patients whose creatinine clearance is less than or equal to 50 mL/min)	Noninferior for stroke prevention	ENGAGE-AF	Lower rates of major bleeding and hemorrhagic stroke than warfarin. Not recommended for patients whose creatinine clearance is more than 95 mL/min.

Table 7.1: Summary of Anticoagulant Drugs

Table 7.2: Hemodynamically Unstable Patient

Condition	Treatment	Details
Hemodynamically unstable patient	Hospitalization and immediate treatment of atrial fibrillation	This is usually due to a rapid ventricular rate or associated cardiac or noncardiac conditions.
Use of Intravenous beta-blockers or calcium channel blockers	Esmolol, propranolol, metoprolol, diltiazem, and verapamil	These are usually effective at rate control in the acute setting.
Urgent electrical cardioversion	Indicated in patients with shock, severe hypotension, pulmonary edema, or ongoing MI or ischemia	An initial biphasic shock with 100–200 J is administered in synchrony with the R wave. If sinus rhythm is not restored, an additional attempt with 360 J is indicated.
Risk of thromboembolism	Present in patients undergoing cardioversion who have not received anticoagulation therapy	This is if atrial fibrillation has been present for more than 48 hours or is of unknown duration. However, in hemodynamically unstable patients the need for immediate rate control outweighs that risk.

1. DOACs (Direct Oral Anticoagulants) are recommended over Vitamin K antagonists (VKAs) like warfarin due to their advantages, including lower rates of intracerebral hemorrhage, making them particularly advantageous for older adults and frail patients.
2. DOACs should not be used in patients with mechanical prosthetic heart valves, advanced kidney disease, or moderate or severe mitral stenosis, and those who cannot afford the newer medications.
3. Apixaban may be considered for patients with creatinine clearance less than 25 mL/min.
4. Patients stable on warfarin with a high time in target INR range and lower risk for intracranial hemorrhage may have relatively less benefit from switching to a newer medication.
5. It's important to monitor kidney function at baseline and at least once a year, or more often for those with impaired kidney function.
6. Each of the medications interacts with other medications affecting the P-glycoprotein pathway, like oral ketoconazole, verapamil, dronederone, and phenytoin.
7. To transition patients from warfarin to a DOAC, wait until the INR decreases to about 2.0.
8. For elective procedures, stop the medications two to three half-lives (usually 24–48 hours) before procedures with low to moderate bleeding risk, and five half-lives before procedures like major surgery.
9. Aspirin should not be used with the DOACs unless there is a clear indication, such as coronary stents or ACS within the prior year.

Case 107C

A 68-year-old man with a history of atrial fibrillation is scheduled for elective cardioversion. He has been taking dabigatran for stroke prevention and has good renal function. On the day of the procedure, his creatinine clearance is calculated to be 90 mL/min. He took his last dose of dabigatran at 8 PM the night before the procedure, which is now 12 hours ago. His past medical history is significant for hypertension, which is well-controlled on lisinopril, and he has no history of bleeding disorders. His current vital signs are stable, and physical examination is unremarkable.
Which of the following is the most appropriate next step in the management of this patient's anticoagulation for the scheduled cardioversion?

- A. Proceed with cardioversion without additional anticoagulation measures.
- B. Administer idarucizumab prior to cardioversion.
- C. Delay cardioversion and administer four-factor prothrombin complex concentrate.
- D. Postpone cardioversion and resume dabigatran for at least 3–4 weeks.

The correct answer is A. Proceed with cardioversion without additional anticoagulation measures. In patients with atrial fibrillation who are undergoing elective cardioversion, it is important to ensure that they have been adequately anticoagulated for at least 3–4 weeks prior to the procedure to reduce the risk of thromboembolic events. This patient has been on dabigatran, which is a direct oral anticoagulant (DOAC) with a short half-life of about 12 hours in patients with normal renal function. Given that his creatinine clearance is 90 mL/min, indicating good renal function, and his last dose of dabigatran was 12 hours ago, he should have therapeutic levels of anticoagulation at the time of cardioversion. Therefore, it is safe to proceed with the cardioversion without additional anticoagulation measures. Option B is incorrect because idarucizumab is a reversal agent for dabigatran and is used in the event of severe bleeding or the need for an urgent procedure where rapid reversal of anticoagulation is necessary. This patient does not have active bleeding, nor is there an indication for immediate reversal of anticoagulation. Option C is incorrect because four-factor prothrombin complex concentrate may partially reverse the effects of DOACs and is not indicated in this scenario where the patient has been appropriately anticoagulated with dabigatran and is not experiencing bleeding. Option D is incorrect because there is no need to postpone cardioversion and resume dabigatran for at least 3–4 weeks if the patient has been on continuous anticoagulation with dabigatran and has adequate renal function. The patient is already anticoagulated, and cardioversion can be safely performed.

7.9 Acute Hematemesis in a 72-Year-Old Woman with Chronic AF

Case 108

A 72-year-old woman with a history of chronic atrial fibrillation is brought to the emergency department with acute onset of hematemesis. She has been on dabigatran for stroke prevention. Her past medical history is significant for hypertension and type 2 diabetes mellitus. On examination, she is pale and diaphoretic with a blood pressure of 90/60 mmHg and a heart rate of 110 beats per minute. Laboratory tests reveal a hemoglobin level of 7.2 g/dL, a creatinine clearance of 30 mL/min, and a normal aPTT. She has received two units of packed red blood cells and her blood pressure has improved to 110/70 mmHg. However, she continues to have active bleeding.
Which of the following is the most appropriate next step in the management of this patient's anticoagulation?

- A. Administer idarucizumab immediately.
- B. Give andexanet alfa as a reversal agent.
- C. Infuse four-factor prothrombin complex concentrate.
- D. Continue supportive measures and monitor hemoglobin.

The correct answer is A. Administer idarucizumab immediately. This patient is experiencing a life-threatening bleed while on dabigatran, a direct thrombin inhibitor. Idarucizumab is a humanized monoclonal antibody fragment that is FDA-approved for the reversal of the anticoagulant effects of dabigatran. It is indicated in the event of severe bleeding or when an urgent procedure is required. Given the patient's acute presentation with hematemesis and the need for rapid reversal of anticoagulation due to ongoing bleeding, immediate administration of idarucizumab is warranted.

Option B is incorrect because andexanet alfa is an intravenous factor Xa decoy protein that is approved for the reversal of factor Xa inhibitors, not direct thrombin inhibitors like dabigatran.

Option C is incorrect because four-factor prothrombin complex concentrate may partially reverse the effects of direct oral anticoagulants, but it is not the reversal agent of choice for dabigatran-induced bleeding. Idarucizumab is the specific reversal agent for dabigatran.

Option D is incorrect because while supportive measures are important, they are not sufficient in the setting of ongoing severe bleeding. The patient requires a specific reversal agent for dabigatran to address the immediate bleeding risk.

In cases of severe bleeding in patients taking dabigatran, idarucizumab, a humanized monoclonal antibody approved by the FDA, can be used for rapid reversal of the anticoagulant effects during severe bleeding or urgent procedures. Andexanet alfa, an injectable agent that mimics factor Xa, is authorized for reversing the effects of factor Xa inhibitors. Four-factor prothrombin complex concentrate can partially counteract the effects of these drugs. Supportive measures such as local control, packed red blood cells, and platelets may be sufficient until the direct oral anticoagulants (DOACs) have been eliminated, given their relatively short half-life of 10–12 hours with adequate renal function. Although warfarin has traditionally been used for a longer period around the time of cardioversion, there is significant evidence supporting the safety and effectiveness of each of the DOACs in this context. In a small prospective randomized trial evaluating rivaroxaban for cardioversion, the incidence of stroke was minimal and comparable to warfarin when administered for a minimum of 3-4 weeks before cardioversion. DOACs offer the advantage of achieving stable anticoagulation faster than warfarin before elective cardioversion. Left atrial appendage occluders, such as the Watchman and Amulet devices, are useful in preventing strokes in individuals with a high risk of bleeding who cannot undergo long-term anticoagulation. However, they may not be as effective as warfarin in preventing ischemic strokes. Surgical occlusion of the left atrial appendage during cardiac surgery provides additional protection against ischemic stroke in addition to continued use of oral anticoagulants.

Direct Oral Anticoagulants (DOACs)

The DOACs, which include dabigatran (direct thrombin inhibitor), rivaroxaban, apixaban, and edoxaban (factor Xa inhibitors), have emerged as alternatives to warfarin for stroke prevention in non-valvular atrial fibrillation. They offer several advantages over warfarin:

- Rapid onset and offset of action
- More predictable pharmacokinetics
- Fewer food and drug interactions
- No routine coagulation monitoring required

Efficacy and Safety

Large randomized controlled trials have demonstrated that DOACs are at least as effective as warfarin for stroke prevention in AF, with a similar or lower risk of major bleeding. Some key trial data:

- RE-LY trial showed dabigatran 150mg bid was superior to warfarin for preventing stroke/systemic embolism in AF patients.
- ROCKET-AF trial found rivaroxaban was non-inferior to warfarin for preventing stroke/systemic embolism.
- ARISTOTLE trial showed apixaban was superior to warfarin in preventing stroke/systemic embolism, with less bleeding.
- ENGAGE AF-TIMI 48 trial demonstrated edoxaban's non-inferiority to warfarin, with lower rates of bleeding.

Specific reversal agents are available for dabigatran (idarucizumab) and factor Xa inhibitors (andexanet alfa) in cases of life-threatening bleeding or urgent surgery. These provide an advantage over warfarin, which requires vitamin K and prothrombin complex concentrates for reversal. DOACs have been shown to be safe and effective alternatives to warfarin for patients undergoing electrical or pharmacological cardioversion. They achieve therapeutic anticoagulation faster than warfarin. For AF patients with contraindications to long-term oral anticoagulation, percutaneous left atrial appendage occlusion with devices like the Watchman and Amulet can reduce stroke risk. This is an option for those at high bleeding risk.

Syed YY et al. Idarucizumab: A Review as a Reversal Agent for Dabigatran. Am J Cardiovasc Drugs. 2016 Aug;16(4):297-304. PMID: 27388764

7.10 Atrial Fibrillation and Recurrent Gastrointestinal Bleeding

Case 109

A 76-year-old woman with a history of non-valvular atrial fibrillation presents to the clinic for a follow-up visit. She has a CHA2DS2-VASc score of 5 and a history of recurrent gastrointestinal bleeding, which has necessitated multiple hospital admissions and blood transfusions. Her bleeding episodes have been attributed to angiodysplasia. She has been on warfarin for stroke prevention, but given her bleeding history, long-term anticoagulation is deemed high risk. Her echocardiogram shows normal left ventricular function and no valvular abnormalities. She is not a surgical candidate due to multiple comorbidities.
Which of the following is the most appropriate next step in the management of this patient's stroke risk?

- A. Discontinue warfarin and start aspirin.
- B. Continue warfarin with closer INR monitoring.
- C. Refer for percutaneous left atrial appendage occlusion.
- D. Initiate a direct oral anticoagulant (DOAC) with a lower bleeding profile.

The correct answer is C. Refer for percutaneous left atrial appendage occlusion. This patient has a high risk of stroke due to her non-valvular atrial fibrillation, as indicated by her CHA2DS2-VASc score of 5. However, her history of recurrent gastrointestinal bleeding and hospitalizations for blood transfusions makes long-term anticoagulation with warfarin a high-risk strategy. Left atrial appendage occlusion devices, such as the Watchman and Amulet, have been shown to provide protection against stroke in patients who are unsuitable for long-term anticoagulation. This procedure is a non-pharmacological alternative that can reduce the risk of stroke without the increased bleeding risk associated with anticoagulants.

Option A is incorrect because aspirin alone is significantly less effective than anticoagulation for stroke prevention in atrial fibrillation and would not provide adequate protection for a patient with a high CHA2DS2-VASc score. Option B is incorrect because despite closer INR monitoring, the patient's history of significant bleeding episodes makes continued warfarin therapy a less favorable option. Option D is incorrect because, although DOACs generally have a lower bleeding profile compared to warfarin, the patient's severe and recurrent gastrointestinal bleeding episodes pose a high risk regardless of the anticoagulant used. Considering her high stroke risk due to atrial fibrillation and high bleeding risk due to gastrointestinal bleeding, a left atrial appendage occlusion (LAAO) could be an appropriate option for this patient. An LAAO is a device that can be inserted percutaneously to seal the left atrial appendage, thereby reducing the risk of thromboembolism. This option can be considered when oral anticoagulation is contraindicated or not tolerated due to an increased bleeding risk. In this patient's case, it would allow for stroke prevention while minimizing the risk of further bleeding episodes. Preventing strokes is a crucial objective in healthcare systems due to the associated morbidity and mortality. Various strategies have been developed and implemented for different patient groups at higher risk of stroke: oral anticoagulation (OAC) for individuals with atrial fibrillation, surgical and percutaneous revascularization for those with carotid artery disease, device closure for patients with patent foramen ovale, and more recently, left atrial appendage occlusion (LAAO) for specific individuals with non-valvular atrial fibrillation (NVAF). LAAO as an adjunctive therapy to OAC appears to be feasible and safe in patients with previous cardioembolic events despite optimal OAC therapy.

Holmes DR Jr et al.MA. Left atrial appendage occlusion. EuroIntervention. 2023 Feb 6;18(13):e1038-e1065. PMID: 36760206

Freixa X et al. Left Atrial Appendage Occlusion as Adjunctive Therapy to Anticoagulation for Stroke Recurrence. J Invasive Cardiol. 2019 Aug;31(8):212-216. PMID: 31088992

Table 7.3: Hemodynamically Stable Patient

Condition	Treatment	Details
Hemodynamically stable patient	No hospitalization usually necessary	This is if the patient has no symptoms, hemodynamic instability, or evidence of important precipitating conditions such as silent MI or ischemia, decompensated HF, PE, or hemodynamically significant valvular disease.
Atrial fibrillation	Managed accordingly	In most of these cases, atrial fibrillation is an unrecognized chronic or paroxysmal condition. For new-onset atrial fibrillation, thyroid function tests and echocardiography to assess for occult valvular or myocardial disease should be performed.
Strategy of rate control and anticoagulation	Appropriate	This is true whether the conditions that precipitated atrial fibrillation are likely to persist or might resolve spontaneously over a period of hours to days.
First-line agent for ventricular rate control	Beta-blocker or calcium channel blocker	The choice of agent is guided by the hemodynamic status of the patient, associated conditions, and the urgency of achieving rate control.
Beta-blockers	Metoprolol or esmolol	Metoprolol is administered as a 5 mg intravenous bolus, repeated twice at intervals of 5 minutes and then given as needed by repeat boluses or orally at total daily doses of 25–200 mg. Esmolol is given as 0.5 mg/kg intravenously, repeated once if necessary, followed by a titrated infusion of 0.05–0.2 mg/kg/min.
Calcium channel blockers	Diltiazem or verapamil	Diltiazem is the preferred calcium blocker if hypotension or LV dysfunction is present. Otherwise, verapamil may be used.
Cardioversion	Considered for symptomatic patients	If the onset of atrial fibrillation was more than 48 hours prior to presentation (or unknown), a transesophageal echocardiogram should be performed prior to cardioversion to exclude left atrial thrombus.
Anticoagulation	Follows cardioversion	Cardioversion should be followed by anticoagulation for at least 1 month unless there is a strong contraindication. Younger patients without HF, diabetes, hypertension, or other risk factors for stroke may not require long-term anticoagulation.

7.11 Management of Persistent Symptoms in a 63-Year-Old Man with AF

Case 110

A 63-year-old man with a history of hypertension and diabetes presents to the clinic with palpitations and fatigue. He was diagnosed with atrial fibrillation 6 months ago and has a CHA2DS2-VASc score of 3. He has been on rate control with metoprolol and anticoagulation with apixaban. Despite these measures, he reports persistent symptoms that are affecting his quality of life. His blood pressure is 135/85 mmHg, heart rate is irregularly irregular at 88 beats per minute, and his physical examination is otherwise unremarkable. A recent echocardiogram showed normal left ventricular function and no significant valvular disease. He has no history of heart failure or structural heart disease.
Which of the following is the most appropriate next step in the management of this patient's atrial fibrillation?

- A. Increase the dose of metoprolol for tighter rate control.
- B. Initiate an antiarrhythmic drug for rhythm control.
- C. Refer for catheter ablation for rhythm control.
- D. Discontinue anticoagulation as it is not improving symptoms.

The correct answer is B. Initiate an antiarrhythmic drug for rhythm control. This patient has symptomatic atrial fibrillation despite rate control and anticoagulation. Given that his atrial fibrillation is of recent onset (less than 1 year), and he is symptomatic, a rhythm control strategy may be beneficial. The EAST-AFNET 4 trial demonstrated that early rhythm control therapy was associated with a lower risk of cardiovascular outcomes in patients with recent-onset atrial fibrillation. Antiarrhythmic drugs are a reasonable first step in the rhythm control strategy, especially in patients without significant heart disease, as is the case here. Option A is incorrect because the patient is already on rate control medication and continues to have symptoms, suggesting that rate control alone is not sufficient for his quality of life. Option C is incorrect as the initial step because while catheter ablation is an option for rhythm control, it is generally considered after antiarrhythmic drugs have been tried or if the patient has a preference for a non-pharmacological approach after discussing the risks and benefits. Option D is incorrect because anticoagulation is indicated based on his CHA2DS2-VASc score to reduce the risk of stroke and should be continued regardless of its effect on symptoms. Anticoagulation is not intended to improve symptoms but to prevent thromboembolic complications. After assessing the risk of stroke and initiating anticoagulation as needed, two primary therapeutic strategies for the long-term management of atrial fibrillation are rate control and rhythm control, which are not mutually exclusive. Rate control is typically the initial approach recommended for most patients with atrial fibrillation, regardless of their potential future choice for rhythm restoration. It can also serve as the primary treatment for individuals with minimal or asymptomatic long-standing atrial fibrillation. The EAST-AFNET 4 trial revealed that patients with recent-onset atrial fibrillation (less than 1 year) who undergo rhythm management through antiarrhythmic medications or catheter ablation experience a decreased risk of cardiovascular mortality, stroke, or hospitalization for heart failure. The decision to pursue rhythm control is usually individualized, considering factors such as symptoms, the type of atrial fibrillation (paroxysmal or persistent), comorbidities (like heart failure), and overall health status. For initial intervention, it is generally recommended to proceed with elective cardioversion following an appropriate period of anticoagulation (minimum 3 weeks) or after confirming the absence of a left atrial thrombus via transesophageal echocardiography (TEE) in patients suspected of recent-onset atrial fibrillation or when a specific trigger is identified. Cardioversion is a viable option for patients who persistently experience symptoms related to the rhythm despite efforts to control heart rate. The EAST-AFNET 4 trial, also known as the Early Treatment of Atrial Fibrillation for Stroke Prevention Trial, compared a rhythm-control strategy with usual care (rate control in most cases) for patients recently diagnosed with atrial fibrillation (AF). The trial, conducted between July 2011 and December 2016, involved 2,789 patients randomized to either rhythm control or usual care. The primary outcome of cardiovascular death, stroke, hospitalization for heart failure, or acute coronary syndrome was significantly lower in the rhythm control group compared to usual care (3.9 vs. 5.0 per 100 person-years). The trial demonstrated that early rhythm control therapy, involving antiarrhythmic drugs or AF ablation, was superior to usual care in improving cardiovascular outcomes. Notably, sinus rhythm at 12 months explained a significant portion of the treatment effect of early rhythm control therapy compared to usual care. The results suggest that systematic and early rhythm control therapy can reduce cardiovascular events in patients with recently diagnosed AF, regardless of symptoms.

Kirchhof P et al. Early Rhythm-Control Therapy in Patients with Atrial Fibrillation. N Engl J Med. 2020 Oct 1;383(14):1305-1316. PMID: 32865375

7.12 Management of Newly Diagnosed Atrial Fibrillation

Case 111

A 58-year-old man with a history of hypertension and obesity presents to the emergency department with palpitations and mild dyspnea that started 12 hours ago. He has no history of heart failure or structural heart disease. His blood pressure is 150/90 mmHg, heart rate is 140 beats per minute, and he is in atrial fibrillation on the ECG with no evidence of ischemia. His echocardiogram shows normal left ventricular function and no valvular abnormalities. His CHA2DS2-VASc score is 2. He has no history of bleeding disorders and has not been on anticoagulation. A transesophageal echocardiogram (TEE) shows no evidence of left atrial thrombus. Which of the following is the most appropriate next step in the management of this patient's atrial fibrillation?

- A. Start anticoagulation with warfarin and schedule for elective cardioversion in 3 weeks.
- B. Administer intravenous ibutilide and perform immediate cardioversion, then start anticoagulation.
- C. Initiate oral amiodarone and schedule for elective cardioversion in 4 weeks.
- D. Begin anticoagulation with a direct oral anticoagulant (DOAC) and perform immediate cardioversion.

The correct answer is D. Begin anticoagulation with a direct oral anticoagulant (DOAC) and perform immediate cardioversion. This patient presents with recent-onset atrial fibrillation (less than 48 hours) and has a TEE that shows no left atrial thrombus, making him a candidate for immediate cardioversion. Since his CHA2DS2-VASc score is 2, he should be started on anticoagulation to reduce the risk of thromboembolic events. DOACs have a rapid onset of action and are suitable for initiating anticoagulation in this setting. Immediate cardioversion can be considered in this scenario to restore sinus rhythm and potentially alleviate his symptoms. Option A is incorrect because elective cardioversion typically requires a minimum of 3 weeks of anticoagulation to reduce the risk of thromboembolic events, but this patient's atrial fibrillation onset is within 48 hours, and he has no evidence of a thrombus on TEE, allowing for immediate cardioversion. Option B is incorrect because while intravenous ibutilide can be used for pharmacologic cardioversion, anticoagulation should be initiated before or at the time of cardioversion to reduce the risk of thromboembolic events, regardless of the cardioversion strategy. Option C is incorrect because although amiodarone can be used for rhythm control, it is not typically used for immediate cardioversion. Additionally, amiodarone has a slower onset of action and is more commonly used for long-term rhythm management rather than acute cardioversion. Elective cardioversion can be achieved through either pharmacological agents or electrical shock. Pharmacologic cardioversion involves the use of intravenous ibutilide (1 mg over 10 minutes, with a possible repeat dose in 10 minutes) or procainamide (15 mg/kg over 30 minutes), with continuous ECG monitoring for at least 4-6 hours post-administration.

Administering 1-2 grams of intravenous magnesium before ibutilide administration can help prevent occasional occurrences of torsades de pointes. For patients requiring ongoing antiarrhythmic therapy to maintain sinus rhythm, cardioversion can be attempted with a medication under investigation for long-term use. Following the initiation of therapeutic anticoagulation, outpatient treatment with amiodarone can be started. The initial dose is 400 mg twice daily for 2 weeks, then reduced to 200 mg twice daily for at least 2 to 4 weeks, and finally a maintenance dose of 200 mg daily. It is important to note that amiodarone can affect prothrombin time in patients on warfarin and elevate digoxin levels, necessitating careful monitoring of anticoagulation and drug levels.

Other antiarrhythmic drugs suitable for extended maintenance therapy include propafenone, flecainide, dronedarone, dofetilide, and sotalol. Dofetilide, administered orally at a dosage of 125–500 mcg twice daily, should be initiated in a hospital setting due to the risk of torsades de pointes and the need for dose adjustment in patients with renal impairment. Propafenone (150–300 mg orally every 8 hours) and flecainide (50–150 mg orally twice daily) should be avoided in patients with structural heart disease (such as coronary artery disease, systolic dysfunction, or significant left ventricular hypertrophy). These medications should be used in conjunction with an AV nodal blocking agent, especially in cases of atrial flutter. Sotalol should be started at a dose of 80–160 mg orally twice daily in hospitalized patients with structural heart disease to prevent torsades de pointes. While not highly effective for converting atrial fibrillation, sotalol can aid in maintaining sinus rhythm post-cardioversion. Dronedarone is contraindicated in individuals with recent decompensated heart failure or persistent atrial fibrillation.

Approximately 30-50% of individuals on long-term antiarrhythmic therapy will sustain sinus rhythm. Due to the high likelihood of arrhythmia recurrence, the decision to continue long-term anticoagulation should be based on individual risk factors.

Bansal N et al. Management of Adults with Newly Diagnosed Atrial Fibrillation with and without CKD. J Am Soc Nephrol. 2022 Feb;33(2):442-453. PMID: 34921110

7.13 Medication Management in a 72-Year-Old Man with AF and Heart Failure

Case 112

A 72-year-old man with a history of chronic atrial fibrillation, heart failure with reduced ejection fraction (HFrEF), and chronic kidney disease stage III is seen in the clinic for follow-up. He has been on warfarin for stroke prevention with a target INR of 2-3 and digoxin for rate control. Despite optimal medical therapy for heart failure, he continues to have symptomatic atrial fibrillation with frequent exacerbations of heart failure. His current medications include warfarin, digoxin, an ACE inhibitor, a beta-blocker, and a loop diuretic. His recent echocardiogram shows an ejection fraction of 30%. His current INR is 2.5, and his digoxin level is within the therapeutic range. After a thorough discussion of the risks and benefits, a decision is made to initiate amiodarone for rhythm control.
Which of the following is the most appropriate next step in the management of this patient's medications?

- A. Start amiodarone without changing the current doses of warfarin and digoxin.
- B. Reduce the dose of warfarin before starting amiodarone and monitor INR closely.
- C. Discontinue digoxin before starting amiodarone to avoid toxicity.
- D. Start amiodarone and reduce the dose of digoxin, and monitor digoxin levels closely.

The correct answer is D. Start amiodarone and reduce the dose of digoxin, and monitor digoxin levels closely. Amiodarone is a potent inhibitor of the cytochrome P450 system and can increase the serum levels of drugs metabolized by this pathway, including warfarin and digoxin. When initiating amiodarone in a patient already on warfarin, careful monitoring of the INR is required, but an immediate dose reduction of warfarin is not always necessary; instead, the INR should be monitored closely and the warfarin dose adjusted as needed. However, because amiodarone can significantly increase digoxin levels, leading to toxicity, it is prudent to reduce the dose of digoxin when starting amiodarone and to monitor digoxin levels closely. Option A is incorrect because starting amiodarone without adjusting the doses of warfarin and digoxin could lead to increased INR and digoxin toxicity due to drug interactions. Option B is incorrect because although amiodarone can increase the INR in patients taking warfarin, immediate dose reduction is not always necessary; instead, the INR should be monitored closely after initiation of amiodarone, and the warfarin dose should be adjusted based on INR values. Option C is incorrect because it is not necessary to discontinue digoxin altogether, as it can be beneficial for rate control in atrial fibrillation, especially in patients with heart failure. Instead, the dose of digoxin should be reduced and levels monitored to avoid toxicity. Digitalis glycosides have demonstrated efficacy in improving heart failure symptoms through various multicenter trials. These studies have revealed that discontinuing digoxin can result in exacerbated symptoms, increased hospitalizations, and reduced exercise tolerance in heart failure patients. Digoxin is a viable option for individuals with heart failure who continue to experience symptoms despite treatment with diuretics and ACE inhibitors. It is also recommended for heart failure patients with atrial fibrillation requiring rate control. However, concerns exist regarding the safety of digoxin in individuals with atrial fibrillation, especially when digoxin levels are elevated.

With a half-life of 24–36 hours and primarily renal excretion, the recommended oral maintenance dose of digoxin ranges from 0.125 mg three times weekly to 0.5 mg daily. Dosage adjustments are necessary for those with renal impairment, elderly patients, and individuals with reduced lean body mass.

An initial oral loading dose of 0.75–1.25 mg over 24–48 hours may be considered for a more rapid response, although most chronic heart failure patients can initiate treatment with the standard maintenance dose of 0.125–0.25 mg daily. Drugs such as amiodarone, quinidine, propafenone, and verapamil have the potential to increase digoxin levels. Monitoring serum digoxin levels is crucial, with blood level testing recommended 7-14 days after the last dose administration, ensuring a minimum 6-hour interval between medication intake and testing. The target serum digoxin levels typically range from 0.7 to 1.2 ng/mL. Digoxin may precipitate ventricular arrhythmias, especially in the presence of low potassium levels or myocardial ischemia. In cases of significant intoxication, the administration of digoxin-specific antibodies (digoxin immune Fab DigiFab) is warranted.

Pincus M. Management of digoxin toxicity. Aust Prescr. 2016 Feb;39(1):18-20. PMID: 27041802

7.14 Persistent Atrial Fibrillation Refractory to Antiarrhythmic Drugs

Case 113

A 55-year-old woman with symptomatic persistent atrial fibrillation refractory to multiple antiarrhythmic drugs, including sotalol and flecainide, presents to the cardiology clinic. She has no significant structural heart disease, but her quality of life is severely impacted by her symptoms, which include palpitations, dyspnea on exertion, and fatigue. Her current medications include warfarin with a therapeutic INR and a beta-blocker for rate control. She has no history of heart failure and her left ventricular ejection fraction is normal. She is interested in pursuing non-pharmacologic options for symptom relief.
Which of the following is the most appropriate next step in the management of this patient's atrial fibrillation?

- A. Increase the dose of the beta-blocker for tighter rate control.
- B. Refer for catheter ablation of the atrial fibrillation.
- C. Schedule for surgical ablation via thoracotomy.
- D. Proceed with radiofrequency ablation of the AV node and permanent pacemaker implantation.

The correct answer is B. Refer for catheter ablation of the atrial fibrillation. This patient has symptomatic persistent atrial fibrillation that is refractory to at least two antiarrhythmic drugs and is impacting her quality of life. Catheter ablation is a reasonable next step for patients with symptomatic atrial fibrillation refractory to pharmacologic therapy, especially in the absence of significant structural heart disease. The CABANA trial showed that while there was no difference in the primary endpoint of death, disabling stroke, serious bleeding, or cardiac arrest, catheter ablation did improve the quality of life for patients with symptomatic atrial fibrillation. Option A is incorrect because the patient is already on a beta-blocker for rate control and has persistent symptoms, indicating that rate control alone is not sufficient for her quality of life. Option C is incorrect because surgical ablation is more invasive and typically reserved for patients undergoing other cardiac surgeries or when catheter ablation is not feasible or has failed. Option D is incorrect because AV node ablation and pacemaker implantation are usually considered a last resort when other therapies, including catheter ablation, have failed or are contraindicated. This patient has not yet tried catheter ablation, which is less invasive and can preserve the physiological pacing of the heart. Atrial fibrillation is considered refractory when it persists, causing chronic symptoms or limiting activity despite attempts to manage heart rate or rhythm. If antiarrhythmic or rate control medications prove ineffective in symptom relief, catheter ablation targeting the pulmonary veins to isolate the triggers responsible for initiating and sustaining atrial fibrillation may be a viable option. This approach is recommended for individuals with symptomatic paroxysmal or persistent atrial fibrillation unresponsive to drug therapy, particularly for specific patients (those under 65 years old or with concurrent heart failure) as an initial treatment. Catheter ablation generally leads to an improvement in quality of life. The CABANA trial revealed no significant difference in the primary outcomes of death, debilitating stroke, major hemorrhage, or cardiac arrest between patients undergoing catheter ablation and those receiving medical therapy as the initial treatment for symptomatic atrial fibrillation. Successful ablation rates range from approximately 50-70%, with up to 20% of patients requiring repeat procedures. The procedure is commonly performed in the electrophysiology laboratory using a catheter-based approach, with minimal adverse events when conducted by experienced operators. Surgical ablation can be performed via a subxiphoid route, thoracoscopically through thoracotomy, or via median sternotomy in the operating room either as a standalone procedure or in conjunction with other surgeries.

For symptomatic patients with inadequate rate control who are not suitable candidates for pulmonary vein isolation, radiofrequency ablation of the AV node coupled with permanent pacing can help achieve rate control and enhance response to physical activity. This intervention is typically considered after other treatment modalities have proven unsuccessful.

The incidence of stroke or transient ischemic attack after catheter ablation for atrial fibrillation is relatively low. Studies have shown that the risk of stroke or transient ischemic attack post-ablation is around 0.49% to 0.64% in patients undergoing catheter ablation, with some studies reporting rates as low as 0.1% to 0.8%. Factors such as recurrent atrial fibrillation, old age (above or 60 years old), non-paroxysmal atrial fibrillation, larger left atrium size, specific echocardiographic findings, and late recurrence after ablation have been associated with an increased risk of ischemic stroke following the procedure. After undergoing catheter ablation for atrial fibrillation, it is recommended to follow up with specific care to prevent stroke or transient ischemic attack. During the 6-month follow-up period post-procedure, monitoring for stroke or transient ischemic attack is crucial. Additionally, extended follow-up for up to 3 years after ablation is advised to ensure ongoing vigilance against these potential complications. Regular monitoring and appropriate management of anticoagulation therapy are essential components of post-ablation care to reduce the risk of stroke.

Kistler PM et al. Persistent atrial fibrillation in the setting of pulmonary vein isolation-Where to next? J Cardiovasc Electrophysiol. 2020 Jul;31(7):1857-1860.PMID: 31778259

7.15 Acute Management of Atrial Flutter

Case 114

A 67-year-old man with a history of hypertension and diabetes presents to the emergency department with palpitations and shortness of breath that began 6 hours ago. He has a history of paroxysmal atrial fibrillation and is currently on oral anticoagulation with apixaban. His blood pressure is 145/85 mmHg, heart rate is 150 beats per minute, and he is in atrial flutter on the ECG. There is no evidence of ischemia, and his echocardiogram shows normal left ventricular function with no valvular abnormalities. His CHA2DS2-VASc score is 3. He denies any history of mitral valve disease.
Which of the following is the most appropriate next step in the management of this patient's atrial flutter?

- A. Administer intravenous ibutilide and prepare for possible electrical cardioversion.
- B. Increase the dose of apixaban and continue to monitor the patient.
- C. Schedule for immediate catheter ablation of the atrial flutter.
- D. Administer a class I antiarrhythmic agent and monitor for conversion to sinus rhythm.

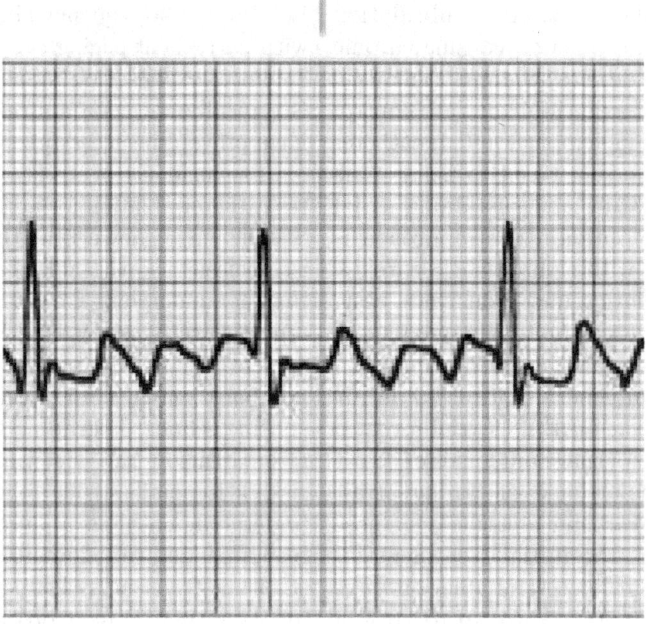

Figure 7.5: Atrial Flutter

The correct answer is A. Administer intravenous ibutilide and prepare for possible electrical cardioversion. This patient presents with new-onset atrial flutter of less than 48 hours' duration. Intravenous ibutilide is a class III antiarrhythmic agent that has been shown to be effective in converting atrial flutter to sinus rhythm, with a success rate of 50-70%. Given the patient's stable hemodynamic status and the recent onset of symptoms, chemical cardioversion with ibutilide is an appropriate first step. Additionally, preparations should be made for possible electrical cardioversion if chemical cardioversion is unsuccessful or if the patient becomes hemodynamically unstable. Option B is incorrect because while the patient is already on anticoagulation, which is appropriate for his CHA2DS2-VASc score, simply increasing the dose of apixaban will not address the immediate issue of atrial flutter and associated symptoms. Option C is incorrect because while catheter ablation is the treatment of choice for long-term management of atrial flutter, it is not typically the first-line treatment for acute management in the emergency department setting. Option D is incorrect because class I antiarrhythmic agents are not generally preferred for conversion of atrial flutter due to the risk of slowing the atrial flutter rate and potentially causing 1:1 AV conduction, which can lead to hemodynamic collapse. Atrial flutter can manifest as either paroxysmal or chronic, with clinical presentation varying based on the ventricular rate, typically falling within the range of 120 to 150 due to 2:1 AV conduction. However, instances of 1:1 AV conduction can lead to very high rates that are poorly tolerated clinically, necessitating prompt intervention. In atrial fibrillation, the lack of coordinated atrial and ventricular contraction coupled with rapid ventricular rates can result in symptoms like low blood pressure, chest pain, heart failure, fainting, or palpitations, prompting patients to seek medical attention. Atrial flutter may sometimes be asymptomatic for extended periods, with sustained rapid heartbeats potentially causing systolic ventricular dysfunction and heart failure known as tachycardiomyopathy. While restoration of sinus rhythm can lead to improved ventricular function and atrial size normalization, arrhythmia recurrence may induce dysfunction and elevate the risk of sudden death. For symptomatic patients with a rapid ventricular rate, rate control should be the initial therapeutic strategy. Achieving this goal in flutter can be challenging, and medications targeting AV node conduction (such as digoxin, beta-blockers, and calcium antagonists) may prove ineffective, necessitating cardioversion to restore sinus rhythm. Dofetilide and ibutilide, classified as pure class III antiarrhythmics, are effective in terminating flutter with minimal risk of QT prolongation and torsades de pointes. Class IA and IC antiarrhythmic agents are less effective and may pose issues if they lead to a slow atrial flutter rate of 200/min with 1:1 AV conduction resulting in QRS widening resembling ventricular tachycardia. While amiodarone is not highly successful in acute sinus rhythm restoration, it aids in controlling ventricular rate.

Radiofrequency catheter ablation of the cavotricuspid isthmus (CTI) has emerged as a standard treatment for typical flutter. Complete ablation of the CTI along a line extending from the tricuspid ring (TR) to the inferior vena cava (IVC) is essential for successful treatment.

Thomas D et al. Typical atrial flutter: Diagnosis and therapy. Herzschrittmacherther Elektrophysiol. 2016 Mar;27(1):46-56. PMID: 26846223

7.16 Managing Arrhythmia in a Patient with Severe COPD: A Case Study

Case 115

A 68-year-old woman with a history of severe chronic obstructive pulmonary disease (COPD) presents to the emergency department with palpitations and shortness of breath. She reports that her symptoms started abruptly while at rest. On examination, her blood pressure is 130/80 mmHg, heart rate is 125 beats per minute, and respiratory rate is 22 breaths per minute. Her oxygen saturation is 92% on room air. Lung auscultation reveals diffuse wheezing. The ECG shows an irregularly irregular rhythm with varying P wave morphologies and different PP intervals. There is no evidence of ischemia or previous infarction. Her medications include inhaled bronchodilators and oral corticosteroids for COPD management.
Which of the following is the most appropriate next step in the management of this patient's arrhythmia?

- A. Administer intravenous adenosine to attempt conversion to sinus rhythm.
- B. Start intravenous beta-blockers to control the ventricular rate.
- C. Treat the underlying COPD exacerbation and consider oral verapamil for rate control.
- D. Initiate long-term anticoagulation with warfarin due to the risk of thromboembolism.

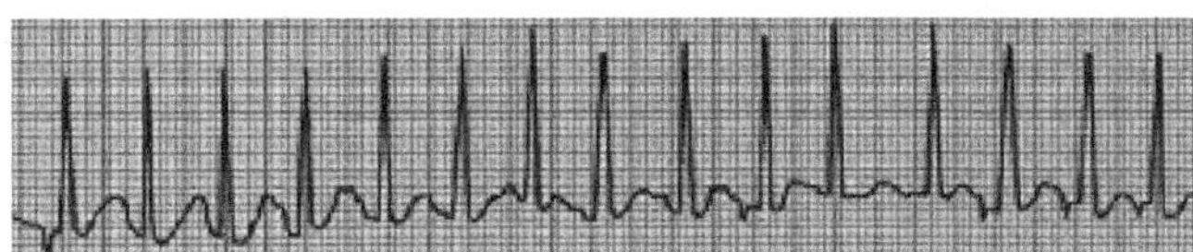

Figure 7.6: MAT

The correct answer is C. Treat the underlying COPD exacerbation and consider oral verapamil for rate control. The patient's ECG findings are consistent with multifocal atrial tachycardia (MAT), which is often seen in patients with severe COPD. MAT is characterized by an irregularly irregular rhythm with at least three distinct P wave morphologies, indicating multiple ectopic atrial foci. The primary treatment for MAT is to address the underlying condition, which in this case is COPD. Management of the COPD exacerbation may include increasing the dose of inhaled bronchodilators, administering systemic corticosteroids, and providing supplemental oxygen if needed. Verapamil is a calcium channel blocker that can be effective in controlling the ventricular rate in patients with MAT, and it can be considered once the acute exacerbation of COPD is being managed.

Option A is incorrect because adenosine is generally less effective in terminating atrial tachycardias, especially MAT, and is more commonly used for the diagnosis and treatment of supraventricular tachycardias (SVTs) with a reentrant mechanism.

Option B is incorrect because beta-blockers can potentially exacerbate COPD by causing bronchoconstriction and should be used with caution in patients with severe COPD. Option D is incorrect because long-term anticoagulation is not indicated in MAT unless there is coexistent atrial fibrillation or atrial flutter, or other risk factors for thromboembolism. The management of atrial tachycardia initially follows a similar approach to other forms of paroxysmal supraventricular tachycardia (PSVT), although vagal maneuvers and intravenous adenosine are often less effective. Hemodynamically stable patients can be treated with intravenous beta-blockers or calcium channel blockers, with a transition to oral formulations for long-term management. Patients experiencing persistent symptomatic episodes may consider antiarrhythmic medications or catheter ablation as treatment options. Long-term anticoagulation is generally not recommended unless concurrent atrial fibrillation or atrial flutter is present. Addressing underlying conditions such as COPD is essential for patients with multifocal atrial tachycardia. Verapamil, administered orally at a dose of 240–480 mg daily in divided doses, may offer benefits for certain individuals. The success rate of catheter ablation for atrial tachycardia is approximately 81% . Some studies have shown that the success rates for different types of arrhythmias vary, with accessory pathways or flutter having a success rate of 92% and AVNRT or atrioventricular node ablation having a success rate of 99% . Additionally, other sources state that the overall success rate for atrial tachycardia ablation ranges from 75-85%

Harvey M. Challenges in diagnosing and managing multifocal atrial tachycardia. HeartRhythm Case Rep. 2023 Feb 15;9(2):129-130. PMID: 36860743

7.17 Wide-Complex Tachycardia in a Patient with Ischemic Cardiomyopathy

Case 116

A 72-year-old man with a history of ischemic cardiomyopathy and a previous myocardial infarction presents to the emergency department with palpitations and lightheadedness. He has a documented history of a left bundle branch block on prior ECGs. His current medications include aspirin, a beta-blocker, an ACE inhibitor, and a statin. On examination, his blood pressure is 110/70 mmHg, heart rate is 170 beats per minute, and he appears alert but anxious. The ECG shows a wide-complex tachycardia with a QRS duration of 0.16 seconds, left axis deviation, and no visible P waves. There are occasional beats with a narrower QRS complex that appear to be regularly interspersed with the wide complexes.
Which of the following is the most appropriate next step in the management of this patient's tachycardia?

- A. Administer intravenous adenosine to attempt to terminate the tachycardia.
- B. Perform immediate synchronized electrical cardioversion.
- C. Administer intravenous amiodarone to stabilize the rhythm.
- D. Obtain an electrophysiology study to determine the origin of the tachycardia.

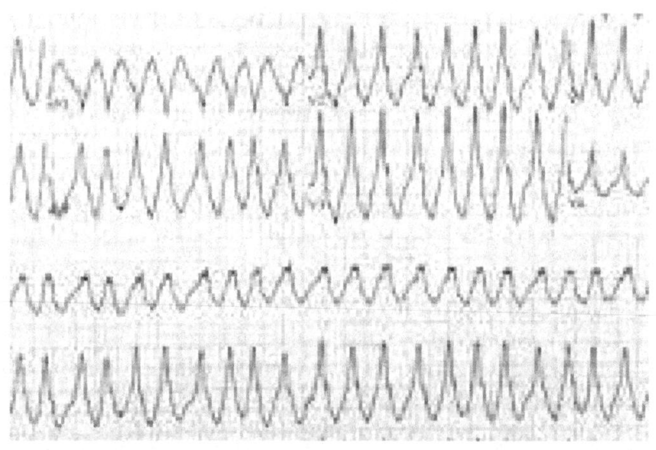

Figure 7.7: wide-complex tachycardia

The correct answer is B. Perform immediate synchronized electrical cardioversion. The patient presents with a wide-complex tachycardia and a history of structural heart disease, which makes ventricular tachycardia (VT) more likely than supraventricular tachycardia (SVT) with aberrancy. The presence of a QRS duration exceeding 0.14 seconds and left axis deviation are findings that favor a ventricular origin. Additionally, the presence of occasional narrower beats suggests the presence of capture beats, which are also indicative of VT. Given the patient's symptoms of palpitations and lightheadedness, along with the hemodynamic stability but potential for deterioration, immediate synchronized electrical cardioversion is the most appropriate next step to restore sinus rhythm and prevent hemodynamic collapse. Option A is incorrect because adenosine is typically used to help diagnose or terminate SVT and is less effective in VT. Moreover, in the setting of VT and structural heart disease, adenosine could potentially worsen the hemodynamic situation. Option C is incorrect because while intravenous amiodarone can be used to treat VT, the acute presentation with symptoms suggests that immediate cardioversion is more appropriate to rapidly restore sinus rhythm. Option D is incorrect because while an electrophysiology study can be useful in determining the origin of a tachycardia, it is not the appropriate immediate step in the acute management of a symptomatic wide-complex tachycardia where VT is highly suspected. Distinguishing between ventricular tachycardia and SVT with aberrant conduction on a 12-lead ECG can pose a challenge in individuals presenting with wide-complex tachycardia. This differentiation is crucial due to the distinct prognosis and therapeutic implications associated with each condition. Key characteristics supporting a ventricular origin include: (1) AV dissociation; (2) QRS duration exceeding 0.14 seconds; (3) presence of sinus capture or fusion beats; (4) left axis deviation with right bundle branch block morphology; (5) monophasic (R) or biphasic (qR, QR, or RS) complexes in V1; and (6) a qR or QS complex in V6. On the other hand, features indicative of a supraventricular origin include: (1) a characteristic right or left bundle branch block morphology; (2) QRS duration less than 0.14 seconds; and (3) history of preexcitation syndrome or its presence on prior ECGs. In cases of broad complex tachycardia with uncertainty in diagnosis, particularly in patients with underlying cardiac conditions, ventricular tachycardia should be assumed.

The management of acute ventricular tachycardia depends on the degree of hemodynamic compromise and the duration of the arrhythmia. Individuals with structurally normal hearts generally have a favorable prognosis and infrequently experience syncope. Episodes often originate from activity in the right ventricular or left ventricular outflow tract. Immediate intervention with a short-acting injectable beta-blocker or verapamil can effectively terminate the episode. In the presence or suspicion of structural heart disease, assessing hemodynamic stability aids in determining the need for immediate direct current cardioversion. Synchronized direct current cardioversion at 120–200 J should be promptly performed if ventricular tachycardia leads to hypotension, heart failure, or myocardial ischemia. Intravenous amiodarone should be administered for recurrent episodes, following a bolus dose of 150 mg and subsequent infusions to establish rhythm stability. Caution is advised to prevent rapid infusions of amiodarone leading to significant hypotension. Hemodynamically stable individuals with sustained ventricular tachycardia may be managed with intravenous amiodarone, lidocaine, or procainamide. If tachycardia persists or symptoms worsen, consideration should be given to direct current cardioversion. Intravenous magnesium replacement at 1-2 g may be beneficial, especially for treating polymorphic ventricular tachycardia. To prevent further episodes, increasing heart rate via isoproterenol infusion (up to 20 mcg/min) or atrial pacing with temporary pacemaker support (at 90–120 beats/min) can effectively reduce the QT interval. Patients with polymorphic ventricular tachycardia may require implantation of an implantable cardioverter-defibrillator (ICD), either subcutaneously or transvenously, when pacing is not indicated.

Kashou AH et al. Wide Complex Tachycardia Differentiation: A Reappraisal of the State-of-the-Art. J Am Heart Assoc. 2020 Jun 2;9(11):e016598. PMID: 32427020

Case 116B

A 56-year-old man with a history of ischemic cardiomyopathy and left ventricular ejection fraction of 30% presents to the clinic with recurrent episodes of palpitations and dizziness. He has an implantable cardioverter-defibrillator (ICD) in place for primary prevention of sudden cardiac death. Interrogation of the ICD reveals multiple appropriate shocks for episodes of sustained ventricular tachycardia (VT) over the past month. He is currently on optimal medical therapy including a beta-blocker, ACE inhibitor, and spironolactone. His electrolytes are within normal limits, and there is no evidence of acute ischemia. He reports adherence to his medication regimen and has no recent changes in medications.
Which of the following is the most appropriate next step in the management of this patient's recurrent ventricular tachycardia?

- A. Increase the dose of the beta-blocker to maximum tolerated levels.
- B. Initiate therapy with amiodarone to reduce the frequency of ICD shocks.
- C. Refer the patient for catheter ablation of ventricular tachycardia.
- D. Replace the ICD with a biventricular pacemaker/defibrillator to improve cardiac function.

The correct answer is B. Perform immediate synchronized electrical cardioversion. The correct answer is C. Refer the patient for catheter ablation of ventricular tachycardia. This patient with ischemic cardiomyopathy and reduced ejection fraction has an ICD in place for primary prevention and is experiencing recurrent ICD shocks due to sustained VT, despite being on optimal medical therapy. Catheter ablation is an important treatment option for patients with recurrent VT who do not respond to or are intolerant of medical therapy. Given the patient's recurrent VT and the fact that he is already on a beta-blocker, the next appropriate step would be to consider catheter ablation to reduce the burden of VT and the number of ICD shocks, which can significantly impact the quality of life. Option A is incorrect because the patient is already on optimal medical therapy, which includes a beta-blocker. Increasing the dose may not prevent recurrent VT and could lead to adverse effects, especially if the patient is already on the maximum tolerated dose. Option B is incorrect because while amiodarone may reduce the frequency of ICD shocks, it has not been shown to lower mortality in patients with structural heart disease and carries a risk of significant side effects. Given the patient's recurrent VT despite optimal medical therapy, a more definitive treatment like catheter ablation should be considered. Option D is incorrect because there is no indication that the patient's cardiac function would improve with a biventricular pacemaker/defibrillator (cardiac resynchronization therapy) if he is already appropriately managed with an ICD and there is no mention of a specific indication for resynchronization therapy, such as left bundle branch block with a wide QRS complex. Common causes of ventricular tachycardia include various heart-related issues and external factors. These causes can lead to faulty heart signaling, resulting in a rapid heartbeat in the lower heart chambers (ventricles). Some common causes are:

1. Structural Heart Disease: Conditions like heart attack, cardiomyopathy, heart failure, myocarditis, and valvular heart disease can create abnormal electrical pathways in the ventricles, leading to ventricular tachycardia.
2. Coronary Artery Disease: Poor blood flow to the heart muscle due to blockages in the coronary arteries can result in ventricular tachycardia.
3. Genetic Conditions: Inherited conditions like long QT syndrome or Brugada syndrome can predispose individuals to ventricular tachycardia.
4. Electrolyte Imbalance: Changes in the levels of body minerals such as potassium, sodium, calcium, and magnesium can disrupt heart signaling and trigger ventricular tachycardia.
5. Medications and Stimulants: Side effects of certain medications, anti-arrhythmic drugs, or the use of stimulants like cocaine or methamphetamine can also contribute to ventricular tachycardia.
6. Idiopathic Causes: In some cases, the exact cause of ventricular tachycardia cannot be determined, leading to idiopathic ventricular tachycardia.
7. Other Factors: Conditions like sarcoidosis (inflamed tissues), changes in blood chemistry (e.g., low potassium levels), and ischemic heart disease can also play a role in triggering ventricular tachycardia

Persistent ventricular tachycardia (VT) poses a significant risk for morbidity and mortality in individuals with cardiac conditions. Implantable cardioverter-defibrillators (ICDs) play a crucial role in terminating VT events, thereby reducing the likelihood of sudden cardiac death. Following ICD placement post an episode of persistent VT, recurrent VT is observed in 40% to 60% of patients. Within 3 to 5 years post-ICD implantation for primary prevention in high-risk populations, around 20% experience their first VT episode. However, ICD shocks can impact quality of life and are associated with increased mortality risk. Antiarrhythmic drugs like amiodarone or sotalol are used to reduce VT occurrences, yet their side effects and efficacy may be suboptimal. Catheter ablation has shown effectiveness in decreasing VT episodes and can be life-saving for cases of persistent VT. Idiopathic ventricular tachycardias, occurring in individuals without underlying heart abnormalities, rarely lead to sudden death. Electrophysiological studies with catheter ablation are often required to confirm the diagnosis, provide evidence of the absence of ventricular scarring or other issues, and offer treatment for the arrhythmia. Ablation is a viable option for patients experiencing symptomatic nonsustained VT and frequent ventricular ectopy.

Konstantino Y et al. Successful ablation of a wide complex tachycardia with distinct intracardiac electrograms. J Cardiovasc Electrophysiol. 2022 Sep;33(9):2107-2110.PMID: 35930619

7.18 Recurrent Ventricular Arrhythmias in a Post-Cardiac Arrest

Case 117

A 63-year-old man with a history of hypertension and hyperlipidemia is brought to the emergency department after experiencing a witnessed cardiac arrest at home. His wife performed immediate cardiopulmonary resuscitation (CPR) and emergency medical services defibrillated him from ventricular fibrillation. On arrival, he is post-cardiac arrest but hemodynamically stable with a blood pressure of 125/80 mmHg and a heart rate of 78 beats per minute. The patient is intubated and sedated. An ECG shows ST-segment elevations in the anterior leads. His initial troponin I level is elevated. He is started on targeted temperature management protocol. Coronary angiography reveals a 90% occlusion of the left anterior descending artery, which is successfully revascularized with a drug-eluting stent.
Which of the following is the most appropriate next step in the management of this patient's risk for recurrent ventricular arrhythmias?

- A. Immediate implantation of a permanent transvenous ICD.
- B. Initiate antiarrhythmic drug therapy with amiodarone.
- C. Prescribe a wearable cardioverter defibrillator upon discharge.
- D. Perform an electrophysiology study to assess for inducible ventricular tachycardia.

The correct answer is C. Prescribe a wearable cardioverter defibrillator upon discharge. This patient has experienced a sudden cardiac arrest likely secondary to acute myocardial ischemia, as evidenced by the ST-segment elevations and successful coronary revascularization. Immediate post-myocardial infarction (MI) period is associated with a transiently increased risk of arrhythmias, and implantation of a prophylactic ICD during this time is not recommended due to a trend toward worse outcomes. Instead, the patient should be managed with a wearable cardioverter defibrillator until recovery of ventricular function can be assessed by echocardiogram at a later date (6–12 weeks following MI or coronary intervention). If at that time the ejection fraction (EF) remains less than or equal to 35%, a permanent ICD should be considered.

Option A is incorrect because immediate implantation of a permanent transvenous ICD is not recommended in the immediate post-MI period due to the potential for recovery of ventricular function and the associated increased risk of complications and mortality.

Option B is incorrect because while antiarrhythmic drugs like amiodarone may be used in the acute setting to manage recurrent ventricular arrhythmias, they are not a substitute for definitive therapy with an ICD in patients at high risk for sudden cardiac death.

Option D is incorrect because an electrophysiology study is not routinely performed immediately after MI for risk stratification of future ventricular arrhythmias. The decision to implant an ICD is based on the assessment of left ventricular function and clinical stability after the acute phase of MI. Survivors of sudden cardiac arrest often experience a high rate of recurrence, making the use of an Implantable Cardioverter Defibrillator (ICD) typically recommended. In cases of sudden cardiac arrest during acute ischemia or infarction, immediate coronary revascularization is strongly advised. However, the practice of preemptively implanting an ICD in individuals following a heart attack has been associated with suboptimal outcomes. Instead, individuals in this scenario may benefit from utilizing a wearable cardioverter defibrillator until their ventricular function can be assessed via echocardiography 6-12 weeks post-heart attack or coronary intervention. For those with reduced ventricular function (EF under or 35%), the recommendation is to consider implanting a permanent subcutaneous ICD (if pacing is unnecessary) or a transvenous ICD. For individuals with a low ventricular function (EF unsder or 35%), the recommended treatment options include:

1. The ACC/AHA guidelines suggest ICD placement for primary prevention of sudden cardiac death in patients with non-ischemic dilated cardiomyopathy and an EF under or 35%
2. For symptomatic heart failure (NYHA II-III) with LVEF under or 35%, despite optimal medical therapy, CRT (Cardiac Resynchronization Therapy) is recommended.
3. Coronary artery bypass grafting (CABG), angioplasty, or percutaneous coronary intervention (PCI) may be indicated for patients with heart failure and angina, along with suitable coronary anatomy.
4. In cases where symptoms persist and BNP levels remain elevated despite optimal medical and device therapy, adding dapagliflozin is recommended/
5. Lifestyle changes such as increasing physical activity, weight loss, smoking cessation, reduced alcohol intake, and dietary adjustments can help improve heart function and overall health.
6. Continuous monitoring of heart function through imaging tests is essential to track progress and adjust treatment plans accordingly.

Madhavan M et al. Implantable cardioverter-defibrillator therapy in patients with ventricular fibrillation out of hospital cardiac arrest secondary to acute coronary syndrome. J Am Heart Assoc. 2015 Feb 23;4(2):e001255. PMID: 25713292

7.19 Syncope and Seizure-like Episodes in a Patient with Prolonged QTc Interval

Case 118

A 44-year-old woman with a history of syncope presents to the emergency department after experiencing a witnessed seizure-like episode. Her family reports that she had a similar episode a year ago, but no diagnosis was made at that time. Her medications include sertraline for depression and no known drug allergies. On examination, she is alert and oriented with no focal neurological deficits. Her blood pressure is 130/85 mmHg, heart rate is 68 beats per minute, and her ECG shows a QTc interval of 500 milliseconds. Laboratory tests including electrolytes are within normal limits. She denies any recent illness or fever.
Which of the following is the most appropriate next step in the management of this patient?

- A. Discontinue sertraline and start intravenous magnesium sulfate.
- B. Initiate treatment with a Class Ia antiarrhythmic medication.
- C. Implant a permanent pacemaker to prevent recurrent episodes.
- D. Start intravenous beta-blocker therapy and consult cardiology for possible ICD placement.

The correct answer is A. Discontinue sertraline and start intravenous magnesium sulfate. This patient's presentation is suggestive of torsades de pointes (TdP), a type of polymorphic ventricular tachycardia that occurs in the setting of a prolonged QT interval. Sertraline is known to prolong the QT interval and could be contributing to her arrhythmia. The first step in managing TdP is to remove any offending agents that prolong the QT interval. Intravenous magnesium sulfate is the treatment of choice for acute episodes of TdP, even if serum magnesium levels are normal. Option B is incorrect because Class Ia antiarrhythmic medications prolong the QT interval and could exacerbate TdP. These should be avoided in patients with long QT syndrome. Option C is incorrect because a permanent pacemaker is not the treatment of choice for TdP. Pacing may be used as a temporary measure in the acute setting if TdP is recurrent and refractory to medical therapy, but it does not address the underlying issue of QT prolongation. Option D is incorrect because while intravenous beta-blockers may be effective in treating electrical storm due to long QT syndrome, the immediate concern is to terminate the TdP and remove any QT-prolonging agents. Consultation with a cardiologist is advisable, with consideration for ICD placement following stabilization and evaluation of the arrhythmia's recurrence pattern and the patient's risk of sudden cardiac death. The clinical presentation varies, encompassing asymptomatic cases, palpitations, prolonged tachyarrhythmia, syncope, or sudden cardiac arrest. Syncope in young individuals can sometimes be misinterpreted as a primary seizure disorder. Thorough evaluation of personal and family medical history is essential. Conducting a 12-lead ECG with meticulous attention to ST segment, T wave, and QT interval abnormalities is crucial. A prolonged QT interval exceeding 500 milliseconds on consecutive ECGs without an identifiable secondary cause (such as medication or electrolyte imbalance) indicates a high-risk group for long QT syndrome. Ambulatory ECG monitoring is valuable for assessing ventricular arrhythmias and dynamic changes in the QT interval or T wave. Exercise electrocardiogram (ECG) testing may be performed on suspected long QT syndrome patients to assess QT interval adaptation at increased heart rates. Genetic testing, ideally by a multidisciplinary genetics team, is recommended when hereditary sudden cardiac arrest is suspected to aid in diagnosis and identify at-risk family members.

Management of polymorphic ventricular tachycardia (e.g., torsades de pointes) with a prolonged QT interval differs from other ventricular tachycardia types. It is crucial to avoid or discontinue Class Ia or III antiarrhythmics that can further prolong the QT interval in individuals with long QT syndrome. Intravenous beta-blockers can be effective in managing electrical storms associated with long QT syndrome or catecholaminergic polymorphic ventricular tachycardia. Increasing heart rate using beta-agonists like dopamine or isoproterenol, or temporary atrial or ventricular pacing, can successfully disrupt and prevent irregular cardiac rhythms.

Shah SR et al.Long QT Syndrome: A Comprehensive Review of the Literature and Current Evidence. Curr Probl Cardiol. 2019 Mar;44(3):92-106. PMID: 29784533

Case 118A

A 19-year-old female college athlete with no significant past medical history presents to the clinic after experiencing a syncopal episode during a track meet. She reports a brief period of palpitations followed by lightheadedness before passing out. She regained consciousness within a minute and denies any confusion or incontinence during the event. Her family history is notable for her father who died suddenly at the age of 32 during a recreational basketball game. On examination, her vital signs are within normal limits, and her physical examination is unremarkable. An ECG performed in the clinic shows a QTc interval of 480 milliseconds. Serum electrolytes, including potassium, calcium, and magnesium, are within normal limits. Which of the following is the most appropriate next step in the evaluation of this patient?

- A. Start a beta-blocker to prevent recurrent syncopal episodes.
- B. Perform ambulatory ECG monitoring to evaluate for ventricular arrhythmias.
- C. Refer for genetic counseling and consider genetic testing for inherited arrhythmia syndromes.
- D. Prescribe an antiepileptic drug to prevent potential seizure activity.

The correct answer is C. Refer for genetic counseling and consider genetic testing for inherited arrhythmia syndromes. This young patient has experienced a syncopal episode during exertion, which raises concern for an underlying cardiac arrhythmia, particularly in the context of her family history of sudden cardiac death at a young age. The ECG finding of a prolonged QTc interval further supports the possibility of an inherited arrhythmia syndrome, such as long QT syndrome. Before initiating treatment, it is important to establish a definitive diagnosis, which can be aided by genetic testing. Genetic counseling is essential to discuss the implications of the test results, the potential for identifying at-risk family members, and the management of the condition. Option A is incorrect because while beta-blockers are the mainstay of treatment for long QT syndrome, starting a beta-blocker before confirming the diagnosis with genetic testing may not be appropriate. It is important to first establish the diagnosis and then tailor the therapy accordingly. Option B is incorrect because although ambulatory ECG monitoring can be useful to evaluate for ventricular arrhythmias and dynamic changes to the QT interval or T wave, the patient's history and family background strongly suggest an inherited syndrome, which requires a more definitive evaluation. Option D is incorrect because there is no evidence to suggest that the patient's syncopal episode was due to seizure activity. Antiepileptic drugs would not be indicated in this scenario without further evidence of seizure, and they could potentially mask the underlying cardiac issue. Genetic testing plays a crucial role in diagnosing Long QT Syndrome (LQTS). It helps confirm the diagnosis and identify specific genetic mutations associated with the condition. A genetic test for LQTS is available to confirm the diagnosis, although it's important to note that genetic tests can't detect all inherited cases of LQTS. The three major genes responsible for most cases of LQTS are KCNQ1, KCNH2, and SCN5A, which collectively account for approximately 75% of the disorder. Additionally, there are ten minor LQTS-susceptibility genes that contribute to less than 5% of LQTS cases The genetic testing process involves detecting single nucleotide and copy number variants in genes associated with LQTS, such as CACNA1C, CALM1, CALM2, CALM3, KCNE1, KCNH2, KCNJ2, KCNQ1, SCN5A, and TRDN. Genetic testing is recommended for individuals with a strong clinical suspicion of LQTS or persistent QT abnormalities. It aids in establishing a diagnosis, guiding treatment decisions, assessing prognosis, facilitating familial screening, and providing genetic counseling for affected individuals and their families.

Case 118B

After genetic counseling, the 19-year-old female college athlete undergoes genetic testing which confirms a diagnosis of Long QT Syndrome (LQTS). She is started on a beta-blocker as recommended by current guidelines. She understands the need to avoid competitive sports and is compliant with her medication. Despite this, she reports experiencing palpitations and a near-syncopal episode while climbing stairs. She denies any medication noncompliance or use of QT-prolonging drugs. Her repeat ECG in the clinic shows a QTc interval of 470 milliseconds on the beta-blocker.
Which of the following is the most appropriate next step in managing this patient's LQTS?

- A. Increase the dose of the beta-blocker.
- B. Add a sodium channel blocker to her treatment regimen.
- C. Implant a loop recorder to monitor for arrhythmias.
- D. Refer for implantable cardioverter-defibrillator (ICD) placement.

The correct answer is D. Refer for implantable cardioverter-defibrillator (ICD) placement. In patients with LQTS who experience syncope or near-syncope despite beta-blocker therapy, the risk of sudden cardiac death is increased. An ICD is indicated in LQTS patients who are symptomatic on beta-blockers, as it can provide life-saving defibrillation in the event of a ventricular arrhythmia. Given this patient's symptoms despite appropriate medical therapy and her significant family history of sudden cardiac death, an ICD is the most appropriate next step to prevent sudden cardiac death.

Option A is incorrect because simply increasing the dose of the beta-blocker may not be sufficient in a patient who has had a breakthrough event while on therapy, especially with a history of near-syncope during exertion.

Option B is incorrect because sodium channel blockers are not typically used in the treatment of LQTS and can actually worsen the condition, particularly in LQTS type 3.

Option C is incorrect because while a loop recorder can monitor for arrhythmias, it does not provide any therapeutic intervention. Given the patient's breakthrough symptoms on a beta-blocker, a more proactive approach is warranted. The long-term management of individuals with inherited arrhythmia syndromes relies on the identification of high-risk characteristics. For patients with long QT syndrome or catecholaminergic polymorphic ventricular tachycardia, beta-blockers, specifically propranolol or nadolol, are the primary treatment. Patients who do not respond to or cannot tolerate beta-blockers should consider undergoing surgical cervicothoracic sympathectomy. No effective drug is available for treating Brugada syndrome. Prevention of arrhythmias in inherited arrhythmia syndromes involves promptly addressing aggravating factors, especially fever. It is crucial to avoid antiarrhythmic drugs in patients with inherited arrhythmia syndromes, except for specific diagnosed genetic anomalies under the guidance of a professional. ICD implantation is typically advised for patients with an inherited arrhythmia syndrome who experience sudden cardiac arrest as their first symptom. An Implantable Cardioverter Defibrillator (ICD) should be explored for patients who experience repeated persistent ventricular arrhythmias or syncope while receiving medical treatment. The primary treatment options for patients with long QT syndrome or catecholaminergic polymorphic ventricular tachycardia (CPVT) include:

1. Beta-blockers: Beta-blockers, such as propranolol or nadolol, are the cornerstone of therapy for patients with long QT syndrome or CPVT.
2. Flecainide: Sodium channel blockers, specifically flecainide, have an additive role in treating CPVT.
3. Cardiac sympathetic denervation (CSD): Left cardiac sympathetic denervation (LCSD) is a surgical procedure that can help suppress arrhythmias and symptoms in some patients with CPVT
4. Implantable Cardioverter-Defibrillator (ICD): ICD implantation is typically advised for patients with an inherited arrhythmia syndrome who experience sudden cardiac arrest as their first symptom or for those who have recurrent persistent ventricular arrhythmias or syncope despite medical treatment.
5. Electrolyte correction: In cases of electrolyte imbalances, such as hypokalemia or hypomagnesemia, correcting the abnormality may be necessary for successful cardioversion.
6. Other antiarrhythmic medications: In some cases, medications like magnesium sulfate, isoproterenol, or pacing may be used to treat polymorphic VT with QT prolongation.
7. Genetic counseling and family screening: Genetic testing and counseling can help identify at-risk family members and guide appropriate management strategies.

Shah SR et al.Long QT Syndrome: A Comprehensive Review of the Literature and Current Evidence. Curr Probl Cardiol. 2019 Mar;44(3):92-106. PMID: 29784533

7.20 A Syncopal Episode While Climbing Stairs case

Case 119

A 72-year-old man with a history of hypertension and hypercholesterolemia presents to the emergency department after experiencing a syncopal episode while climbing stairs. He reports no prodromal symptoms such as dizziness or palpitations. He also mentions that he has had episodes of exertional chest pain and shortness of breath over the past few months, which he attributed to aging. On examination, he has a systolic murmur that is loudest at the right upper sternal border and radiates to the carotids. His blood pressure is 145/90 mmHg, and his pulse is 68 beats per minute and regular. An ECG shows left ventricular hypertrophy with no ST or T wave changes. Chest X-ray is unremarkable.
Which of the following is the most appropriate next step in the diagnosis of this patient?

- A. Immediate cardiac catheterization.
- B. Transthoracic echocardiogram.
- C. 24-hour Holter monitoring.
- D. Head-up tilt table testing.

The correct answer is B. Transthoracic echocardiogram. This patient's clinical presentation, including exertional symptoms and a systolic murmur that radiates to the carotids, is suggestive of aortic stenosis (AS). AS can lead to syncope, especially during exertion when the fixed obstruction from the stenotic aortic valve prevents an adequate increase in stroke volume to meet the body's demands. A transthoracic echocardiogram is the diagnostic test of choice to evaluate for AS, as it can assess the aortic valve anatomy, measure the severity of stenosis, and evaluate the impact on left ventricular function. Option A is incorrect because immediate cardiac catheterization is not the initial diagnostic test for suspected AS. It may be used later for coronary artery evaluation prior to surgical intervention if significant stenosis is confirmed by echocardiography. Option C is incorrect because while 24-hour Holter monitoring is useful for detecting arrhythmias as a cause of syncope, this patient's history and physical examination findings are more suggestive of a structural heart problem such as AS. Option D is incorrect because head-up tilt table testing is typically used to diagnose vasovagal syncope, which is usually accompanied by a prodrome and is not consistent with the patient's exertional symptoms and physical examination findings indicative of AS. Cardiac syncope can result from issues related to the heart's autonomic function, problems with electrical conduction, or rapid abnormal heart rhythms. A resting electrocardiogram (ECG) is recommended for individuals being evaluated for syncope, with high-risk findings including non-sinus rhythm, left bundle branch block, and voltage criteria suggestive of left ventricular hypertrophy. Patients with a normal initial assessment, including a non-significant medical history and physical examination, absence of heart disease, and a normal baseline ECG, may not need further testing initially. However, continuous ambulatory ECG monitoring or wearable/implantable cardiac monitors are options if a cardiac arrhythmia is suspected.

Treatment for syncope caused by cardiac arrhythmias may involve cardiac pacing, implantable cardioverter-defibrillators (ICDs), or catheter ablation. Cardiac pacing can be effective in specific cases like carotid sinus syndrome and documented bradycardia. Catecholaminergic polymorphic ventricular tachycardia (CPVT) is an inherited arrhythmia syndrome that often requires pharmacological therapies like beta-blockers and sodium channel blockers. Left cardiac sympathetic denervation can also play a role in managing arrhythmias in CPVT patients.

Syncope, commonly known as fainting, can be a symptom of various conditions ranging from harmless to life-threatening. It can be caused by factors like low blood pressure or serious heart conditions such as bradycardia or tachycardia. An initial evaluation for syncope includes a detailed medical history, physical exam, and tests like an ECG to determine the cause. Older adults are at higher risk of syncope related to serious heart conditions like sick sinus syndrome or atrial fibrillation.

In summary, diagnosing and treating syncope involves thorough evaluations, including ECGs and monitoring for cardiac arrhythmias. Treatment options vary depending on the underlying cause of syncope, with considerations for cardiac pacing or pharmacological therapies in specific conditions like CPVT. The diagnostic tests for cardiac syncope include:

1. Electrocardiogram (ECG): This test can identify various arrhythmias, such as Wolff-Parkinson-White syndrome, Brugada syndrome, atrial flutter, or atrioventricular (AV) blocks. It can also reveal conditions like ischemic cardiac events, which may indicate a preceding myocardial infarction.
2. Echocardiogram: This imaging test can directly identify structural abnormalities in the heart, such as those seen in hypertrophic cardiomyopathy or arrhythmogenic right ventricular cardiomyopathy.
3. Long-term rhythm monitoring: This can be employed if ECG and echocardiogram do not provide a definitive diagnosis.
4. Exercise stress testing: This test can reveal the diagnosis in cases of exertional syncope.
5. Holter monitor: A Holter monitor is an outpatient test that can detect arrhythmias over a longer period.
6. Head-up tilt-table test: This test is useful for confirming autonomic dysfunction and can generally be safely arranged on an outpatient basis.
7. Chest radiography: This imaging test may be helpful in evaluating certain etiologies of syncope, such as pneumonia or congestive heart failure.
8. Ambulatory external or implantable cardiac monitor: These devices may be required if the initial evaluation suggests cardiac vascular abnormalities or if the patient has experienced multiple instances of fainting due to heart problems.
9. Tilt test: If the initial evaluation is unclear, a tilt test may be useful to assess for other cardiac causes.
10. Cardiac pacing, implantable cardioverter-defibrillators, and catheter ablation: These treatments are used for syncope caused by cardiac arrhythmias, depending on the specific diagnosis and individual patient needs.

Numeroso F et al. Evaluation of the current prognostic role of cardiogenic syncope. Intern Emerg Med. 2013 Feb;8(1):69-73. PMID: 23247682

7.21 Evaluation of Syncope in a Hypertensive and Diabetic Patient

Case 120

A 60-year-old man with a history of hypertension and diabetes mellitus presents to the clinic with a single episode of syncope. He reports that he felt lightheaded upon standing up from a sitting position and then lost consciousness for a few seconds. He had no convulsions and recovered quickly with no residual symptoms. His medications include lisinopril, metformin, and atorvastatin. On examination, his blood pressure is 140/85 mmHg while seated and 130/80 mmHg after standing. His heart rate is 78 beats per minute and regular in both positions. Cardiac examination reveals no murmurs, rubs, or gallops, and carotid auscultation is unremarkable. A resting ECG shows normal sinus rhythm with no evidence of left ventricular hypertrophy, bundle branch block, or ischemic changes.
Which of the following is the most appropriate next step in the evaluation of this patient?

- A. Carotid ultrasound.
- B. Continuous ambulatory ECG monitoring.
- C. Electrophysiologic study.
- D. Tilt-table testing.

The correct answer is B. Continuous ambulatory ECG monitoring. This patient experienced syncope upon standing, which may suggest orthostatic hypotension; however, the blood pressure measurements do not support a significant drop upon standing. Given the absence of cardiac disease signs on examination and a normal ECG, the syncope could be due to a transient arrhythmic event. Continuous ambulatory ECG monitoring is a reasonable next step to detect intermittent arrhythmias that may not have been present during the initial ECG. Option A is incorrect because there is no clinical indication for carotid ultrasound in this scenario. The patient does not have bruits on auscultation or other signs suggestive of carotid stenosis. Option C is incorrect because electrophysiologic studies are generally not indicated in the initial evaluation of syncope in patients without structural heart disease, a history of arrhythmias, or a high suspicion for arrhythmic etiology. Option D is incorrect because tilt-table testing is more appropriate for patients with recurrent episodes of syncope where vasovagal syncope is suspected, particularly when the diagnosis remains unclear after an initial evaluation. This patient had a single episode with a clear trigger (standing up), and there is no description of recurrent episodes. Syncope is a transient loss of consciousness characterized by a sudden and temporary inability to maintain postural tone, often leading to falls. It affects approximately 30% of adults and accounts for about 3% of emergency department visits. During the initial evaluation, a specific cause is identified in around 50% of syncope cases. The prognosis for syncope is generally favorable unless there is underlying heart disease. Recurrent syncope or near-syncope in many individuals is not primarily attributed to arrhythmias, especially when there are no indications of associated heart conditions based on medical history, physical examination, routine ECG, or noninvasive tests. A thorough medical history is essential in determining the underlying cause of syncope during assessment.

- Reflex syncope, also known as neurally mediated syncope, can stem from either increased vagal tone or dysfunction in reflex regulation of peripheral circulation. The most common form is vasovagal syncope, often triggered by stressful or uncomfortable situations. Carotid sinus hypersensitivity and post-micturition syncope result from heightened vagal tone causing low blood pressure, potentially leading to vagally-induced bradycardia, sinus arrest, and AV block, culminating in syncope.
- Orthostatic hypotension, or postural hypotension, is a common cause of vasodepressor syncope. It is prevalent in elderly individuals, those with diabetes or autonomic neuropathy, individuals experiencing blood loss or hypovolemia, and patients using certain medications like vasodilators, diuretics, and adrenergic blockers. Additionally, chronic idiopathic orthostatic hypotension is frequently observed in older males where the typical vasoconstrictive response upon standing upright may be impaired.

Runser LA et al. A. Syncope: Evaluation and Differential Diagnosis. Am Fam Physician. 2017 Mar 1;95(5):303-312. PMID: 28290647

7.22 Management of Recurrent Syncope in a Woman with No Cardiac History

Case 121

A 54-year-old woman presents to the clinic with a history of recurrent syncope. She reports several episodes over the past year, often occurring with prolonged standing or in crowded, warm places. She describes a sensation of warmth and lightheadedness prior to the episodes, with rapid recovery after lying down. She has no history of heart disease, and her only medication is a multivitamin. Physical examination, including orthostatic blood pressure measurements, is unremarkable. A resting ECG shows normal sinus rhythm with no conduction abnormalities. She has performed counterpressure maneuvers such as leg crossing and squatting, which have not prevented her syncopal episodes. She is concerned about the impact of her condition on her daily activities, including driving.
Which of the following is the most appropriate management step for this patient?

- A. Start midodrine.
- B. Implant a permanent pacemaker.
- C. Begin fludrocortisone therapy.
- D. Advise the patient not to drive for 3–6 months.

The correct answer is A. Start midodrine. This patient's clinical presentation is consistent with vasovagal syncope, characterized by recurrent episodes often triggered by standing or warm environments and associated with prodromal symptoms. Since she has not had success with conservative measures such as counterpressure maneuvers, pharmacotherapy with midodrine, an alpha-agonist that increases peripheral vasoconstriction and decreases venous pooling, is a reasonable next step. Midodrine has been shown in small randomized trials to reduce the frequency of syncopal episodes in patients with vasovagal syncope. Option B is incorrect because permanent pacemaker implantation is generally not indicated in patients with vasovagal syncope, except for a subset of older patients with documented prolonged asystole, which this patient does not have. Option C is incorrect because fludrocortisone, while used in the treatment of vasovagal syncope, is generally considered after trying other measures such as midodrine, especially given its minimal benefit and potential side effects. Option D is incorrect because the patient's syncope is thought to be due to vasovagal episodes, which are not typically associated with ventricular tachycardia or aborted sudden death. Driving restrictions are more stringent for patients with syncope due to arrhythmias or other cardiac conditions that pose a high risk for recurrence and sudden incapacitation. This patient does not fit that category, and such a long driving restriction is not warranted based on the information provided. Tilt-table testing can be valuable for patients suspected of having vasovagal syncope when the diagnosis remains uncertain following the initial evaluation, especially in cases of recurrent syncope. The hemodynamic response to tilting determines whether there is a cardioinhibitory, vasodepressor, or mixed reaction. The test's efficacy is heightened when there is a strong suspicion of neurally mediated syncope before conducting the test, as its sensitivity and specificity are only moderate in the general population. Electrophysiological studies have a limited role in evaluating syncope, particularly in patients without structural heart abnormalities or specific scenarios where an arrhythmic etiology is less likely. However, electrophysiological assessment can aid in identifying the underlying cause of syncope and guiding treatment decisions in patients with ischemic heart disease, left ventricular dysfunction, established conduction abnormalities, or arrhythmias. Approximately 50% of patients with structural heart disease exhibit positive diagnostic findings. The sensitivity of tilt-table testing in diagnosing vasovagal syncope has been found to be around 71% to 92% when potentiated with nitroglycerin and clomipramine, respectively. Specificity data is limited, but tilt-table testing is known to have limitations in terms of specificity, often being positive in patients without syncope.The test is more useful in establishing a diagnosis of reflex syncope, particularly when reflex syncope is suspected or when differentiating reflex syncope from orthostatic hypotension for specific therapy.The latest guidelines recommend TTT for specific clinical scenarios, emphasizing its role in diagnosing reflex syncope and guiding therapy decisions

Case 121B

Six months after starting midodrine for recurrent vasovagal syncope, a 54-year-old woman returns to the clinic for a follow-up visit. She reports a decrease in the frequency of her syncopal episodes but still experiences occasional lightheadedness with prolonged standing. She has been adherent to her medication regimen and has implemented lifestyle modifications including increased fluid and salt intake. She denies any side effects from the midodrine. Her blood pressure today is 132/84 mmHg, and her heart rate is 72 beats per minute. She is not taking any other medications that could contribute to her symptoms.
Which of the following is the most appropriate next step in managing this patient's vasovagal syncope?

- A. Increase the dose of midodrine.
- B. Add fludrocortisone to her treatment regimen.
- C. Prescribe waist-high support stockings.
- D. Discontinue midodrine and begin a beta-blocker.

The correct answer is C. Prescribe waist-high support stockings. The patient has experienced a decrease in the frequency of her syncopal episodes with midodrine, which suggests that her treatment is effective but may need additional support. Waist-high support stockings with a minimum of 30 mmHg ankle counterpressure can help decrease venous pooling and prevent syncopal episodes by improving venous return . This non-pharmacological intervention can be a useful adjunct to her current treatment with midodrine. Option A is incorrect because there is no indication that the dose of midodrine needs to be increased, especially since the patient has reported a decrease in the frequency of her episodes and no side effects. Option B is incorrect because adding fludrocortisone, a mineralocorticoid that increases sodium retention and expands plasma volume, may be considered if the patient had not responded to midodrine or if she had contraindications to compression stockings. Since the patient has partially responded to midodrine and there are no contraindications mentioned, it is more appropriate to try additional non-pharmacological measures before adding another medication. Option D is incorrect because there is no indication to discontinue midodrine, which has been effective for the patient. Beta-blockers are not typically first-line for vasovagal syncope and are generally considered when other treatments have failed or are contraindicated. Treatment for vasovagal syncope primarily involves patient education about the benign nature of the condition and advising them to avoid triggers. Counterpressure techniques, such as squatting, leg-crossing, and abdominal contraction, can help alleviate or prevent episodes. Medical therapy is only considered for patients who continue to experience symptoms despite these measures. Midodrine, an alpha-agonist, can improve peripheral vasoconstriction and reduce venous pooling during vasovagal episodes, which has been shown to decrease the frequency of syncopal episodes in small randomized trials.

Fludrocortisone and beta-blockers are sometimes employed, but their benefits are often limited. Selective serotonin reuptake inhibitors (SSRIs) have demonstrated efficacy in specific patients. Pacemaker implantation is generally not recommended for patients with vasovagal syncope, except for individuals over 40 years old who experience prolonged (greater than 3 seconds) symptomatic episodes of asystole confirmed with ambulatory monitoring. Pacemaker insertion should not be based solely on tilt-table-induced asystolic (cardioinhibitory) response, as it is rarely necessary. Cardioneuroablation, which involves catheter ablation of ganglionated plexi, is a promising therapy option for those with vasovagal syncope and vagal hyperactivity. Patients with vasovagal syncope can manage their symptoms through several non-pharmacological and pharmacological interventions. Here are some strategies:

1. Avoiding triggers: Patients should avoid conditions that trigger vasovagal reflexes, such as a hot environment, humid atmosphere, prolonged standing, and reduced water intake. They should also discontinue hypotensive drug treatment for concomitant conditions, especially in older patients.
2. Increasing salt intake and hydration: Substitution of salt and intake of isotonic drinks can expand the circulating blood volume and improve venous return, potentially reducing the risk of vasovagal syncope.
3. Identifying prodromals and early symptoms: Patients should be motivated to identify prodromals of syncope, such as weakness, lightheadedness, yawning, nausea, diaphoresis, hyperventilation, blurred vision, or impaired hearing. Lying or sitting down

when initial symptoms appear may avert or attenuate syncope or traumatic falls.

4. Counterpressure maneuvers: Hand-grip and leg crossing can increase venous return and delay or even prevent vasovagal syncope.
5. Tilt training: Orthostatic training, such as twice-a-day training sessions of 40-minute tilt positioning at home, can improve symptoms in adolescents with neurocardiogenic syncope.
6. Pharmacological therapy: Several drugs have been tested in the treatment of vasovagal syncope, including beta-blockers, disopyramide, scopolamine, theophylline, ephedrine, etilefrine, midodrine, clonidine, and serotonin reuptake inhibitors (SRI). However, no convincing data exist to support the use of one over another as a first-line therapy, and there is limited data from placebo-controlled trials.
7. Counseling and observation: A conservative, non-drug approach is appropriate for patients with infrequent occurrences and recognizable prodromal symptoms.
8. Pacing: The role of cardiac pacing in the management of vasovagal syncope is unclear at present.
9. Compression hose and pacemakers: The use of compression hose and pacemakers has been recommended for some patients with vasovagal syncope.
10. Hydration and salt intake: Increasing hydration and salt intake, especially in warm weather, can help prevent vasovagal syncope.

8 HEART FAILURE

8.1 Acute Heart Failure Exacerbation in a Geriatric Patient

Case 122

A 77-year-old woman with a history of hypertension and type 2 diabetes mellitus presents to the clinic with worsening shortness of breath, orthopnea, and bilateral lower extremity edema over the past two weeks. She has a history of chronic atrial fibrillation and is on rate control and anticoagulation therapy. Her medications include metoprolol, lisinopril, furosemide, and warfarin. On physical examination, her blood pressure is 150/90 mm Hg, heart rate is irregularly irregular at 110 beats per minute, and jugular venous pressure is elevated. Lung auscultation reveals bibasilar crackles, and there is 2+ pitting edema up to the mid-shins. An echocardiogram shows left ventricular hypertrophy (LVH), left atrial enlargement, and preserved left ventricular ejection fraction (LVEF) of 55%. Echocardiogram: LVH, left atrial enlargement, preserved LVEF (55%). Physical Examination: Irregularly irregular heart rate, elevated jugular venous pressure, bibasilar crackles, 2+ pitting edema.
What is the most appropriate next step in the management of this patient?

- A) Increase the dose of furosemide
- B) Initiate amiodarone therapy for rhythm control
- C) Start treatment with a sodium-glucose cotransporter 2 (SGLT2) inhibitor
- D) Perform cardiac catheterization

The correct answer is A) Increase the dose of furosemide. This patient is presenting with signs and symptoms of heart failure with preserved ejection fraction (HFpEF), which is characterized by symptoms of heart failure, preserved LVEF, and evidence of diastolic dysfunction. The patient's symptoms of shortness of breath, orthopnea, and edema, along with physical findings of elevated jugular venous pressure and bibasilar crackles, suggest volume overload. Increasing the dose of furosemide, a loop diuretic, is appropriate to reduce fluid retention and relieve symptoms of congestion. Option B) Initiate amiodarone therapy for rhythm control is not the most appropriate next step as the patient's primary issue is volume overload, and there is no indication that she is symptomatic from atrial fibrillation (AF) beyond what rate control can manage. Option C) Start treatment with a sodium-glucose cotransporter 2 (SGLT2) inhibitor could be considered in the management of heart failure, as recent studies have shown benefits in patients with HF-pEF. However, the immediate concern is to address the patient's volume overload, which is best managed with diuretics. Option D) Perform cardiac catheterization is not indicated at this time as there is no suggestion of acute coronary syndrome or ischemic heart disease that would necessitate this invasive procedure. The patient's symptoms are more consistent with volume overload secondary to HFpEF. Heart failure is a prevalent illness that is on the rise. It predominantly affects older adults, with more than 75% of both current and new cases happening in people over the age of 65. Seventy-five percent of people with heart failure have a history of hypertension. HF prevalence increases from around 1% in persons under 60 years old to almost 10% in those over 80 years old.

Heart failure can manifest on the left side, right side, or bilaterally. Left heart failure often presents with symptoms related to decreased cardiac output and elevated pulmonary vein pressure, with shortness of breath being a primary indicator. Conversely, signs of fluid retention are typically prominent in right-sided heart failure. Many patients exhibit features of both right and left heart failure, with left ventricular dysfunction commonly driving right ventricular failure. Approximately half of heart failure cases involve preserved left ventricular systolic function alongside some degree of diastolic impairment. Distinguishing between reduced and preserved systolic function based solely on clinical presentation can be challenging.

In developed countries, coronary artery disease leading to myocardial infarction and ischemic cardiomyopathy is a primary cause of systolic heart failure. Systemic hypertension significantly contributes to heart failure and exacerbates cardiac dysfunction in patients with conditions like coronary artery disease in the United States. Dilated or congestive cardiomyopathy can present in various forms, characterized by left ventricular or biventricular dilation and overall systolic dysfunction. Common types include alcoholic cardiomyopathy, viral myocarditis (including HIV infections), and idiopathic dilated cardiomyopathies. Less common etiologies encompass infiltrative diseases like hemochromatosis, sarcoidosis, amyloidosis, as well as infectious agents, metabolic abnormalities, cardiotoxins, and drug-induced toxicity.

Valvular heart diseases such as degenerative aortic stenosis and chronic aortic or mitral regurgitation are frequent contributors to heart failure. Persistent rapid heart rates, often accompanied by atrial arrhythmias, can lead to impaired cardiac contraction that may be reversible through rate control strategies. Diastolic dysfunction is associated with aging, myocardial stiffness, left ventricular hypertrophy (LVH) often due to hypertension. Conditions like hypertrophic or restrictive cardiomyopathy, diabetes, and pericardial disease may present with similar clinical features. Atrial fibrillation, with or without rapid ventricular response, can impede left ventricular filling.

Heidenreich PA et al. 2022 AHA/ACC/HFSA Guideline for the Management of Heart Failure: A Report of the American College of Cardiology/American Heart Association Joint Committee on Clinical Practice Guidelines. Circulation. 2022 May 3;145(18):e895-e1032. PMID: 35363499

Case Note

In conclusion, the most appropriate next step is to increase the dose of furosemide to manage the patient's volume overload and improve her heart failure symptoms. This approach is consistent with the management of acute decompensated heart failure with preserved ejection fraction.

8.2 Managing a Patient with Left Ventricular Hypertrophy

Case 123

A 58-year-old woman with a history of hypertension and obesity presents for a routine follow-up visit. She is currently taking hydrochlorothiazide and has no complaints. She denies any chest pain, palpitations, dyspnea, orthopnea, or lower extremity edema. Her blood pressure in the clinic is 142/88 mm Hg. Her body mass index (BMI) is 32 kg/m^2. A recent echocardiogram revealed left ventricular hypertrophy (LVH) with normal left ventricular systolic function and no valvular abnormalities. Her electrocardiogram (ECG) shows left ventricular strain pattern but no other abnormalities.
Diagnostic Test Results:

1. Echocardiogram: LVH with normal systolic function.
2. ECG: Left ventricular strain pattern.
3. Physical Examination: Blood pressure 142/88 mm Hg, BMI 32 kg/m^2.

What is the most appropriate next step in the management of this patient?

- A) Start an angiotensin-converting enzyme (ACE) inhibitor
- B) Refer for bariatric surgery consultation
- C) Initiate a beta-blocker
- D) Prescribe a statin

The correct answer is A) Start an angiotensin–converting enzyme (ACE) inhibitor. This patient is in Stage B of heart failure, which includes patients with structural heart disease but without symptoms of heart failure. She has hypertension, which is a risk factor for developing heart failure, and evidence of structural heart disease in the form of left ventricular hypertrophy (LVH). ACE inhibitors have been shown to be effective in reducing the progression to symptomatic heart failure in patients with structural heart disease, such as LVH, and they also provide additional blood pressure control, which is needed in this patient.

Option B) Refer for bariatric surgery consultation may be considered for long-term management of obesity, but it is not the immediate next step in the prevention of heart failure in a patient who is currently asymptomatic with controlled blood pressure and no diabetes or other obesity-related complications that would warrant immediate surgical intervention.

Option C) Initiate a beta-blocker could be considered for additional blood pressure control and for the management of LVH. However, ACE inhibitors are generally the first choice in patients with LVH due to their proven benefit in reducing cardiovascular events and preventing heart failure in this patient population.

Option D) Prescribe a statin is indicated for the management of dyslipidemia and the prevention of coronary artery disease. While statins are important in the overall cardiovascular risk management, they are not specifically indicated in this scenario for the prevention of progression to heart failure in a patient with LVH and without evidence of ischemic heart disease. Heart failure can be effectively prevented through the timely identification of high-risk individuals and the initiation of prompt interventions. The importance of these strategies is highlighted by US guidelines that have established a four-stage classification system for heart failure. Stage A includes individuals at risk of developing heart failure, such as those with hypertension. Implementing measures like strict hypertension management, addressing coronary risk factors, and reducing excessive alcohol intake can prevent heart failure in this group. Stage B comprises patients with structural heart disease but no current or prior symptoms of heart failure, including those with a history of myocardial infarction, reduced systolic function, left ventricular hypertrophy, or asymptomatic valvular disease. While ACE inhibitors and beta-blockers are effective in preventing heart failure in the first two categories, more aggressive hypertension treatment and early surgical intervention are beneficial for the latter two. Stages C and D encompass patients with established heart failure and those who are unresponsive to standard therapies, respectively. In summary, the recommended course of action involves initiating ACE inhibitor therapy to address hypertension more aggressively and provide cardioprotective benefits in the presence of left ventricular hypertrophy, thereby reducing the risk of progressing to symptomatic heart failure.

Heidenreich PA et al. 2022 AHA/ACC/HFSA Guideline for the Management of Heart Failure: A Report of the American College of Cardiology/American Heart Association Joint Committee on Clinical Practice Guidelines. Circulation. 2022 May 3;145(18):e895-e1032. PMID: 35363499

8.3 Acute Respiratory Symptoms in a Hypertensive Patient with CKD

Case 124

A 60-year-old male with a history of hypertension and chronic kidney disease presents with shortness of breath, leg swelling, and fatigue. He reports a recent upper respiratory infection that has since resolved. His current medications include lisinopril and furosemide. On physical examination, his heart rate is 69 bpm, blood pressure is 196/92 mm Hg, respiratory rate is 24/min, and oxygen saturation is 91% on 10 liters of oxygen. Jugular venous pressure is elevated at 5 cm at a 45-degree angle. Cardiac examination reveals a regular rate and rhythm with an S4 gallop, but no murmurs. Lung auscultation shows bilateral crackles, and the abdomen is soft and non-tender with audible bowel sounds. Extremities show 2+ pitting edema around his ankles. Laboratory tests reveal a hemoglobin of 12.7 g/dL, white cell count of 9.5, normal liver function tests, BUN/Creatinine of 29/1.4 mg/dL, and a troponin level of ¡0.01 ng/mL. An NT-proBNP level is 90 pg/mL, and a chest X-ray shows infiltrates consistent with pneumonia. What is the most appropriate next step in the management of this patient?

- A) Increase the dose of furosemide
- B) Initiate treatment with a beta-blocker
- C) Start broad-spectrum antibiotics
- D) Refer for urgent coronary angiography

The correct answer is C) Start broad-spectrum antibiotics The patient presents with signs and symptoms suggestive of acute decompensated heart failure (ADHF) in the context of recent pneumonia. The elevated jugular venous pressure, bilateral crackles on lung auscultation, and pitting edema are consistent with fluid overload, a common feature of ADHF . However, the presence of infiltrates on the chest X-ray and a recent upper respiratory infection point towards pneumonia as a precipitating factor for the decompensation. The NT-proBNP level is not significantly elevated , which may be due to the chronic nature of the patient's heart failure or the influence of other factors such as obesity or renal dysfunction. Given the clinical picture and the diagnostic findings, the most appropriate next step is to address the underlying infection with broad-spectrum antibiotics to treat the pneumonia, which is likely contributing to the patient's heart failure exacerbation. Option A) Increase the dose of furosemide would be appropriate if the patient's primary issue was volume overload without an infectious precipitant. While diuretics are a mainstay of treatment for ADHF, the presence of pneumonia must be addressed concurrently. Option B) Initiate treatment with a beta-blocker is not indicated in the acute setting of ADHF, especially when there is a potential infectious cause. Beta-blockers are typically used in the chronic management of heart failure to improve survival but are not first-line for acute exacerbations. Option D) Refer for urgent coronary angiography would be indicated if there was a suspicion of acute coronary syndrome, which is not supported by the patient's normal troponin levels and the presence of pneumonia on the chest X-ray. Heart failure patients' laboratory test results can provide valuable insights into their condition and prognosis. Anemia and a high red-cell distribution width (RDW) detected in a blood test are associated with a poor prognosis in chronic heart failure, although the underlying mechanisms are not well understood. Kidney function tests can indicate if heart failure is linked to reduced kidney function, which may suggest inadequate kidney blood flow. Chronic kidney disease (CKD) is a negative prognostic factor for heart failure and can limit treatment options. Serum electrolyte levels can reveal hypokalemia, which increases the risk of arrhythmias; hyperkalemia, which can restrict the use of renin-angiotensin system inhibitors; or hyponatremia, indicating significant activation of the renin-angiotensin system and a negative prognostic indicator. Thyroid function should be evaluated for hidden hyperthyroidism or hypothyroidism, and iron levels should be examined for hemochromatosis. Appropriate biopsies can lead to a diagnosis of amyloidosis in cases where the cause is unknown. Myocardial biopsy can rule out some causes of dilated cardiomyopathy, but it rarely uncovers specific treatable conditions.

Serum BNP is a potent prognostic indicator that enhances clinical evaluation in distinguishing dyspnea caused by heart failure from noncardiac origins. Two markers, BNP and NT-proBNP, offer comparable diagnostic and prognostic data. Brain natriuretic peptide (BNP) is primarily produced in the ventricles and its levels increase in response to high ventricular filling pressures. It is highly sensitive in individuals with symptomatic heart failure, regardless of whether it is caused by systolic or diastolic dysfunction, but less specific in older patients, women, and patients with chronic obstructive pulmonary disease. Research suggests that BNP can assist in emergency department triage for diagnosing acute decompensated heart failure. An NT-proBNP level below 300 pg/mL or BNP level below 100 pg/mL, along with a normal ECG, suggests that heart failure is unlikely. BNP is less accurate in diagnosing heart failure in a long-term setting due to its reduced sensitivity and specificity. BNP can assist in determining the appropriate level of diuretic medication and ensuring a more regular application of disease-modifying treatments like ACE inhibitors and beta-blockers for the treatment of chronic heart failure. Neprilysin inhibitors elevate BNP levels as neprilysin breaks down BNP, but not NT-proBNP. NT-proBNP remains reliable, but BNP is not suitable for monitoring heart failure severity in patients on sacubitril/valsartan treatment. If dyspnea or weight gain worsens and is accompanied by an increase in BNP levels, consider increasing the diuretic dosage.

Serial natriuretic peptide measures do not have established usefulness in guiding therapy, as demonstrated in the GUIDE-IT experiment. Serum troponin levels, particularly high-sensitivity troponin, are frequently elevated in both chronic and acute heart failure, and are linked to a greater likelihood of negative outcomes. In conclusion, the patient's presentation is consistent with ADHF precipitated by pneumonia, and the most appropriate management step is to start broad-spectrum antibiotics to treat the underlying infection. This approach addresses the precipitating cause of the heart failure exacerbation and is likely to improve the patient's symptoms and clinical status.

Jobs A et al. Pneumonia and inflammation in acute decompensated heart failure: a registry-based analysis of 1939 patients. Eur Heart J Acute Cardiovasc Care. 2018 Jun;7(4):362-370.PMID: 28357890

8.4 Optimizing Treatment for a Patient with HFrEF

Case 125

A 68-year-old male with a history of heart failure with reduced ejection fraction (HFrEF) presents to the clinic for a routine follow-up. He is currently on an ACE inhibitor, beta-blocker, and loop diuretic. His most recent echocardiogram showed a left ventricular ejection fraction (LVEF) of 30%. He reports improved exercise tolerance and no recent hospitalizations. His blood pressure is 122/76 mmHg, heart rate is 68 bpm, and he has no signs of volume overload on examination. His serum potassium level is 4.5 mEq/L, and his serum creatinine is 1.2 mg/dL, with an estimated glomerular filtration rate (eGFR) of 55 mL/min/1.73m^2. He has no history of diabetes mellitus. Which of the following is the most appropriate next step in the management of this patient?

- A. Initiate spironolactone 25 mg daily and monitor potassium and renal function in 1 week.
- B. Increase the dose of the loop diuretic to improve LVEF.
- C. Start eplerenone 50 mg daily without the need for further potassium monitoring.
- D. Add digoxin to improve symptoms and reduce hospitalizations.

The correct answer is A. Initiate spironolactone 25 mg daily and monitor potassium and renal function in 1 week. According to the RALES trial, the addition of spironolactone in patients with advanced heart failure (class IV) who are already on ACE inhibitors and diuretics can significantly reduce mortality.

Although this patient is not in class IV heart failure, the EMPHASIS-HF trial has shown benefits of aldosterone antagonism with eplerenone in patients with mild to moderate heart failure, which can be extrapolated to spironolactone. Given the patient's stable condition, normal potassium levels, and adequate renal function, it is appropriate to initiate spironolactone to further reduce morbidity and mortality associated with HFrEF. Close monitoring of potassium and renal function is necessary after initiation of therapy to avoid hyperkalemia, especially since the patient is already on an ACE inhibitor. Option B is not appropriate because there is no evidence of volume overload, and increasing the loop diuretic dose does not directly improve LVEF. Option C is incorrect because, even though eplerenone is indicated for mild to moderate HF, potassium levels must still be monitored closely after initiation, particularly in a patient on an ACE inhibitor. Option D is not the best choice because, while digoxin may help with symptoms and reduce hospitalizations, it does not have the same mortality benefit in HFrEF as aldosterone antagonists, and this patient's symptoms are currently well-managed. The management of heart failure aims to alleviate symptoms, improve functional capacity, and reduce mortality and hospitalizations. Many interventions have limited evidence of efficacy in reducing death, hospitalization, and sudden cardiac death, particularly in individuals with heart failure and a reduced left ventricular ejection fraction (LVEF of 40% or less). Notably, SGLT2 inhibitors are the sole treatment shown to decrease heart failure hospitalizations in patients with preserved ejection fraction, contrary to the typical pattern. Patients with a mildly reduced ejection fraction (41–49%) may benefit from treatment with a mineralocorticoid receptor antagonist and an angiotensin receptor-neprilysin inhibitor (ARNI) like sacubitril/valsartan. Managing heart failure with preserved left ventricular ejection fraction focuses on symptom relief and addressing concurrent health issues. Achieving the target dose or maximum tolerated dose is crucial to realizing the proven benefits of these medications as demonstrated in clinical trials.

Oral potassium-sparing agents are commonly used alongside loop diuretics and thiazides, with preferred choices being the aldosterone inhibitors spironolactone (12.5–100 mg daily) or eplerenone (25–100 mg daily). Elevated aldosterone levels are common in heart failure. These agents prevent potassium loss, exhibit diuretic effects (especially at higher doses), and improve clinical outcomes, including survival. Spironolactone has a quicker onset of action compared to other potassium-sparing agents but may lead to side effects like gynecomastia and hyperkalemia.

Combining potassium supplements or ACE inhibitors with potassium-sparing drugs can increase the risk of hyperkalemia, although they have been safely used in individuals with persistent hypokalemia. Patients with refractory edema may benefit from a combination of a loop diuretic and thiazide-like agents. Metolazone is particularly effective when combined with chronic kidney disease due to its sustained efficacy. Caution is advised when employing this approach as it can result in significant diuresis and electrolyte imbalances. Adding 2.5 mg of metolazone orally to the current loop diuretic dose is common practice, often requiring weekly adjustments, although doses up to 10 mg per day have been utilized in specific cases.

Romero-González G et al. The "FIFTY SHADOWS" of the RALES Trial: Lessons about the Potential Risk of Dietary Potassium Supplementation in Patients with Chronic Kidney Disease. J Clin Med. 2022 Jul 8;11(14):3970.PMID: 35887733

Case Note

Close monitoring of potassium and renal function is necessary after initiation of therapy to avoid hyperkalemia, especially since the patient is already on an ACE inhibitor.

8.5 Management of Chronic Heart Failure with Reduced EF

Case 126

A 56-year-old woman with a history of chronic heart failure with reduced ejection fraction (HFrEF) presents to the clinic for a follow-up visit. She is currently on lisinopril 20 mg daily, furosemide 40 mg daily, and has been recently started on carvedilol 3.125 mg twice daily. She reports no recent episodes of acute decompensated heart failure and has been compliant with her medications. She denies any symptoms of dizziness or hypotension. Her blood pressure is 110/70 mmHg, heart rate is 68 bpm, and physical examination is notable for an S3 heart sound without rales or peripheral edema. Her laboratory tests show a serum potassium of 4.2 mEq/L and a serum creatinine of 1.0 mg/dL. Her most recent echocardiogram showed an LVEF of 25Which of the following is the most appropriate next step in the management of this patient?

- A. Increase carvedilol to 6.25 mg twice daily and reassess in 2 weeks.
- B. Discontinue carvedilol due to the risk of worsening heart failure.
- C. Add short-acting metoprolol tartrate to further improve LVEF.
- D. Increase lisinopril to the maximum tolerated dose before adjusting carvedilol.

The correct answer is A. Increase carvedilol to 6.25 mg twice daily and reassess in 2 weeks. The patient is stable on her current regimen of heart failure medications, including a low starting dose of carvedilol, and she has no symptoms of hypotension or dizziness, which are common side effects of beta-blockers. Given her stability and lack of contraindications, it is appropriate to up-titrate the dose of carvedilol to improve her heart function further. The COPERNICUS trial showed that carvedilol is effective in reducing mortality and heart failure hospitalizations, even in patients with severe symptoms, provided they are free of fluid retention at the time of initiation. The patient should be reassessed in 2 weeks to ensure she remains stable and free of side effects before considering further dose increases.

Option B is incorrect because the patient is stable and there is no indication that carvedilol is causing worsening heart failure. In fact, beta-blockers are a cornerstone of HFrEF management and should be continued unless contraindicated. Option C is not appropriate because short-acting metoprolol tartrate has not been shown to reduce mortality in chronic heart failure, and the patient is already on carvedilol, which is preferred. Option D is not the best next step because the patient's current dose of lisinopril may be adequate, and the priority at this visit is to optimize beta-blocker therapy, which has been shown to improve LVEF and outcomes in HFrEF. The ACE inhibitor dose can be re-evaluated after carvedilol is titrated to the target or maximum tolerated dose. Beta-blockers play a crucial role in the management of chronic heart failure due to their life-saving benefits. While the exact mechanism behind this advantage is not fully elucidated, it is likely that prolonged exposure to catecholamines and heightened sympathetic nervous system activity contributes to gradual myocardial damage, resulting in decreased left ventricular function and enlargement. A key supporting factor for this hypothesis is the consistent improvement in ejection fraction (EF) by an average of 10% and reduction in left ventricular size and mass observed over a 3-6 month period with beta-blocker therapy. Three medications with robust evidence for reducing mortality in heart failure are carvedilol, a nonselective beta-1- and beta-2-receptor blocker, metoprolol succinate, a beta-1-selective extended-release formulation (as opposed to short-acting metoprolol tartrate), and bisoprolol, a beta-1-selective agent. It is strongly recommended that patients with stable heart failure, regardless of severity, receive beta-blocker therapy unless contraindicated by noncardiac reasons. Carvedilol has demonstrated excellent tolerability and remarkable efficacy in reducing mortality and heart failure hospitalizations in patients with severe symptoms, as evidenced by the COPERNICUS study. Close monitoring for fluid retention is essential when initiating treatment. The COPERNICUS trial showed that one life was saved for every 13 patients treated for a year, highlighting its significant impact comparable to the most influential pharmacological therapies in cardiovascular medicine history. In the COMET study, carvedilol was compared to short-acting metoprolol tartrate and exhibited substantial reductions in all-cause mortality and cardiovascular mortality. Patients with chronic heart failure are recommended to receive extended-release metoprolol succinate, bisoprolol, or carvedilol instead of short-acting metoprolol tartrate for optimal management of their condition. Initiation of beta-blockers must be done gradually and with great care due to the risk of deterioration in apparently stable patients. Carvedilol is started at a dose of 3.125 mg orally twice a day and can be raised to 6.25, 12.5, and 25 mg twice day every 2 weeks. The regimen for sustained-release metoprolol began with a daily oral dose of 12.5 or 25 mg, which was increased every 2 weeks until reaching a daily goal dose of 200 mg using the Toprol XL sustained-release formulation. Bisoprolol was given orally at doses of 1.25, 2.5, 3.75, 5, 7.5, and 10 mg per day, with adjustments made every 1 to 4 weeks. A slower increase in dosage is typically more convenient and may be more accepted. Patients should be advised to regularly check their weight at home to track fluid retention and promptly report any symptoms or weight changes. Prior to each dosage escalation, patients should have a thorough examination to confirm the absence of fluid retention or deterioration of symptoms. Worsening HF can often be addressed by increasing diuretic dosages and postponing additional increases in beta-blocker doses, with potential need for reducing or stopping the medication. Carvedilol may lead to dizziness or low blood pressure due to its beta-blocking properties. This can typically be controlled by decreasing the doses of other vasodilators and moderating the rate of dose increments.

Cleland JGF et al. Beta-blockers in Heart Failure Collaborative Group. Beta-blockers for heart failure with reduced, mid-range, and preserved ejection fraction: an individual patient-level analysis of double-blind randomized trials. Eur Heart J. 2018 Jan 1;39(1):26-35. PMID: 29040525

8.6 Patient with HFpEF, CKD, and Persistent AF

Case 127

A 72-year-old man with a history of chronic heart failure with preserved ejection fraction (HFpEF), chronic kidney disease stage 3, and persistent atrial fibrillation presents to the clinic for follow-up. He reports increasing dyspnea on exertion and fatigue over the past few months. His current medications include furosemide 40 mg daily, lisinopril 10 mg daily, and warfarin with an INR maintained around 2.5. His blood pressure is 135/85 mmHg, heart rate is irregularly irregular at 110 bpm, and his physical examination is notable for a 2+ pitting edema in the lower extremities. An EKG confirms atrial fibrillation with a rapid ventricular response. His serum creatinine is 1.8 mg/dL (stable from previous measurements), and his potassium is 4.8 mEq/L. His echocardiogram shows an LVEF of 55% with left atrial enlargement. Which of the following is the most appropriate next step in the management of this patient?

- A. Initiate digoxin 0.125 mg daily to control heart rate and improve symptoms.
- B. Increase the dose of furosemide to manage volume overload. C. Start amiodarone for rhythm control in atrial fibrillation. D. Discontinue lisinopril due to potential for worsening renal function.

The correct answer is A. Initiate digoxin 0.125 mg daily to control heart rate and improve symptoms. This patient with HFpEF and atrial fibrillation with a rapid ventricular response is symptomatic with dyspnea on exertion and fatigue, which may be attributed to inadequate rate control. Digoxin is effective for rate control in atrial fibrillation, particularly in the setting of heart failure, and can improve symptoms. Given the patient's chronic kidney disease, a lower dose of digoxin is appropriate to minimize the risk of toxicity, and serum levels should be monitored after initiation to ensure they are within the therapeutic range.

Option B is not the most appropriate next step because, although the patient has signs of volume overload, the primary issue seems to be the uncontrolled heart rate, which can contribute to symptoms of heart failure. Diuretic adjustment may be considered but would not address the primary issue of rate control. Option C is not the best choice at this time because amiodarone is typically used for rhythm control, not rate control, and carries a higher risk of side effects, especially in a patient with chronic kidney disease. Additionally, rhythm control is not always necessary in patients with HFpEF and atrial fibrillation. Option D is incorrect because there is no indication that lisinopril is worsening the patient's renal function; ACE inhibitors are a mainstay of treatment in HFpEF and provide renal protection over the long term. However, close monitoring of renal function is warranted in this patient.

Several multicenter trials have confirmed the efficacy of digitalis glycosides in alleviating symptoms of heart failure (HF). These studies have also demonstrated that discontinuing digoxin can worsen HF symptoms and signs, increase hospitalizations for decompensation, and reduce exercise tolerance. Digoxin should be considered for patients with persistent symptoms despite diuretic and ACE inhibitor therapy, as well as those with HF and atrial fibrillation requiring rate control. However, the safety of digoxin in atrial fibrillation patients remains uncertain, especially with higher digoxin concentrations. With a half-life of 24–36 hours, digoxin is predominantly eliminated by the kidneys. The recommended daily oral maintenance dose is 0.5 mg or 0.125 mg three times weekly. Dosage adjustments are necessary for the elderly, individuals with renal impairment, and those with a lower lean body mass index. For rapid onset of action, an oral loading dose of 0.75–1.25 mg (based on lean body weight) over 24–48 hours can be considered. In most chronic HF cases, initiating treatment with the expected maintenance dose (usually 0.125–0.25 mg daily) is sufficient. Certain medications like amiodarone, quinidine, propafenone, and verapamil can significantly increase digoxin levels by up to 100%. Monitoring blood levels 7–14 days after the last dose administration and at least 6 hours later is recommended. Target serum digoxin concentrations should fall between 0.7 and 1.2 ng/mL. Digoxin may precipitate ventricular arrhythmias, especially in the presence of hypokalemia or myocardial ischemia.

Digoxin, a therapeutic agent frequently employed in the management of heart failure, is associated with a spectrum of potential adverse effects. These may encompass gastrointestinal disturbances such as nausea, vomiting, and persistent diarrhea, neurological manifestations like confusion, and physical debility characterized by weakness and loss of appetite. Cardiac irregularities and visual disturbances are also reported side effects. Furthermore, certain populations are subject to specific warnings associated with digoxin use. For instance, in pediatric patients, an overdose may manifest as symptoms including weight loss, failure to thrive, abdominal discomfort, lethargy, and alterations in behavior. Hypersensitivity reactions to digoxin may present with dermatological symptoms such as skin rash and hives, pruritus, facial or lip swelling, and respiratory distress. Moreover, individuals with certain health conditions are advised against the use of digoxin. Specifically, those with ventricular fibrillation or Wolff-Parkinson-White syndrome may experience exacerbation of their conditions with digoxin therapy.

Abdul-Rahim AH et al. Efficacy and safety of digoxin in patients with heart failure and reduced ejection fraction according to diabetes status: An analysis of the Digitalis Investigation Group (DIG) trial. Int J Cardiol. 2016 Apr 15;209:310-6. PMID: 26913372

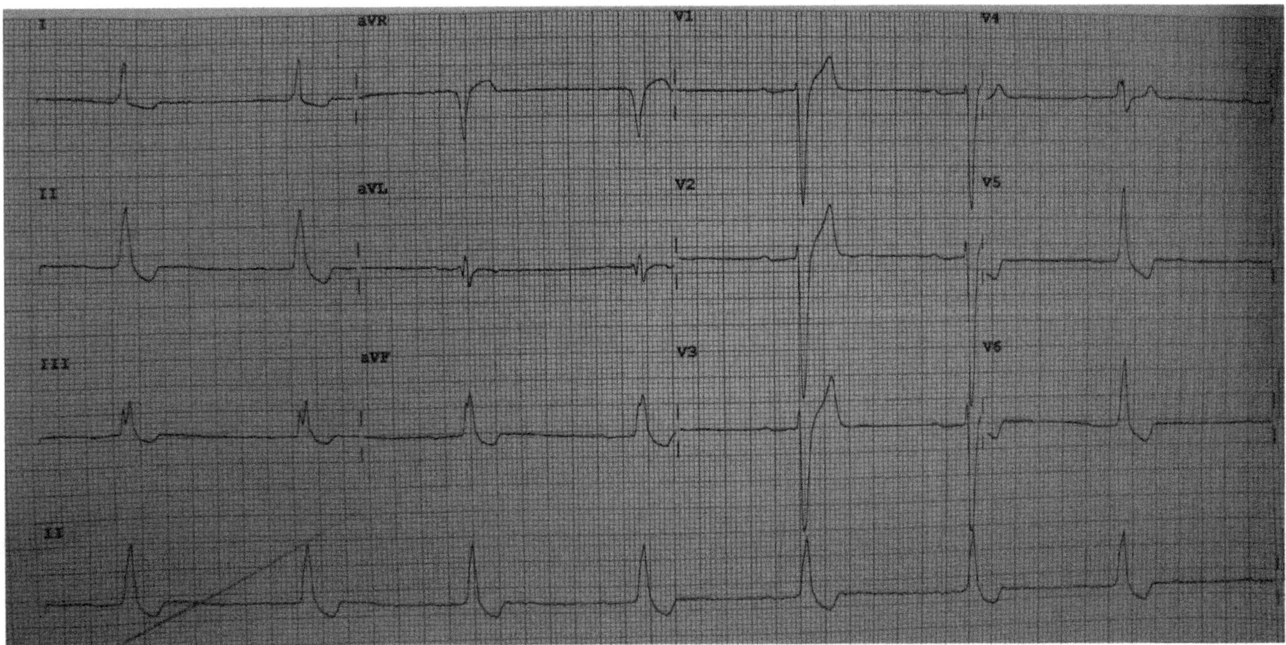

Figure 8.1: Digoxin Toxicity ECG

8.7 Heart Failure: A Case of Persistent Symptoms Despite Optimal Therapy

Case 128

A 63-year-old woman with a history of chronic systolic heart failure due to non-ischemic cardiomyopathy presents to the outpatient clinic for a routine follow-up. She reports persistent fatigue and mild dyspnea on exertion despite optimal medical therapy, which includes enalapril 20 mg twice daily, carvedilol 25 mg twice daily (the maximum tolerated dose due to hypotension with higher doses), and spironolactone 25 mg daily. Her blood pressure is 100/60 mmHg, heart rate is 78 bpm, and she is in sinus rhythm. Physical examination reveals no jugular venous distension, clear lungs, and no peripheral edema. Her laboratory tests show a serum potassium of 4.5 mEq/L, serum creatinine of 1.1 mg/dL, and an NT-proBNP of 800 pg/mL. An echocardiogram shows a left ventricular ejection fraction (LVEF) of 30% with no valvular abnormalities. Which of the following is the most appropriate next step in the management of this patient?

- A. Initiate ivabradine to reduce heart rate and improve symptoms.
- B. Increase the dose of carvedilol to improve beta-blockade.
- C. Add digoxin to improve symptoms of heart failure.
- D. Refer for cardiac resynchronization therapy (CRT).

The correct answer is A. Initiate ivabradine to reduce heart rate and improve symptoms. This patient has chronic systolic heart failure with a reduced ejection fraction (HFrEF) and remains symptomatic despite being on a maximally tolerated dose of beta-blocker, an ACE inhibitor, and an aldosterone antagonist. Her heart rate is above 70 bpm, which makes her a candidate for ivabradine according to both US and European guidelines. Ivabradine specifically targets the If channel in the sinus node, leading to a reduction in heart rate without affecting blood pressure or myocardial contractility. This can improve heart failure symptoms and has been shown to reduce hospitalizations for heart failure. Option B is incorrect because the patient is already on the maximum tolerated dose of carvedilol, and further increase may lead to hypotension and worsening of symptoms. Option C is not the best choice as digoxin may be considered for symptom control, but it is not the primary agent for patients who are symptomatic despite optimal therapy and have a heart rate above 70 bpm in sinus rhythm. Option D, referral for CRT, is not indicated in this scenario as the patient is in sinus rhythm and there is no mention of a left bundle branch block (LBBB) or QRS prolongation, which are criteria for CRT. Additionally, CRT is typically considered after optimizing medical therapy, which in this case would include the addition of ivabradine. By blocking the If channel in the sinus node, ivabradine causes a specific decrease in the sinus rate. The FDA has approved the use of ivabradine for stable heart failure (HF) patients with a heart rate of 70 beats per minute who are on maximum beta-blocker therapy or cannot tolerate beta-blockers. The European Medicines Agency allows its use in patients with a heart rate above 75 beats per minute. Patients in sinus rhythm with a heart rate of 70 beats per minute or higher, an ejection fraction (EF) of 35% or less, and persistent symptoms despite optimal treatment with beta-blockers, ACE inhibitors (or ARBs), and aldosterone antagonists (or ARBs) receive a class IIa recommendation from both US and European guidelines. A clinical trial in chronic angina patients showed that ivabradine did not significantly reduce cardiovascular events. In fact, symptomatic angina patients may have experienced more events while on ivabradine compared to a placebo.

Ivabradine is contraindicated in heart failure patients with certain conditions, including severe hepatic impairment, sick sinus syndrome, sinoatrial block, second- or third-degree atrioventricular block, clinically significant bradycardia, acute decompensated heart failure, and pacemaker dependence. Additionally, it should not be used in patients with a resting heart rate less than 60 bpm before treatment.

The potential side effects of drug interactions with ivabradine can include an increased risk of irregular or rapid heartbeat (atrial fibrillation or heart rhythm problems), slow heart rate (bradycardia), increased blood pressure, and temporary brightness in part of the field of vision. These side effects may manifest in symptoms such as palpitations, chest pressure, worsened shortness of breath, near fainting or fainting, dizziness, fatigue, lack of energy, feeding problems, and blue lips or fingernails. It is essential to monitor for these symptoms and seek medical attention if they occur.

Abdin A et al. Efficacy of ivabradine in heart failure patients with a high-risk profile (analysis from the SHIFT trial). ESC Heart Fail. 2023 Oct;10(5):2895-2902. PMID: 37427483

8.8 Exacerbation of Heart Failure: The Impact of NSAID Use

Case 129

A 58-year-old man with a history of heart failure with reduced ejection fraction (HFrEF) and type 2 diabetes mellitus presents to the emergency department with increasing shortness of breath, orthopnea, and lower extremity edema over the past week. His medications include metformin 1000 mg twice daily, lisinopril 20 mg daily, carvedilol 25 mg twice daily, and spironolactone 25 mg daily. He also reports that he recently started taking ibuprofen for chronic knee pain. On examination, his blood pressure is 150/90 mmHg, heart rate is 88 bpm, and he has rales halfway up both lung fields and 2+ pitting edema up to his shins. Laboratory tests reveal a serum creatinine of 1.5 mg/dL (baseline 1.2 mg/dL), serum potassium of 5.2 mEq/L, and a BNP of 900 pg/mL. An echocardiogram shows an LVEF of 30Which of the following is the most appropriate next step in the management of this patient?

- A. Add a thiazolidinedione to improve glycemic control.
- B. Discontinue ibuprofen and optimize diuretic therapy.
- C. Start a calcium channel blocker for better blood pressure control.
- D. Introduce an ARB in addition to the current regimen for synergistic effects.

The correct answer is B. Discontinue ibuprofen and optimize diuretic therapy. This patient with HFrEF is presenting with signs and symptoms of acute decompensated heart failure, likely precipitated by the use of ibuprofen, a nonsteroidal anti-inflammatory drug (NSAID). NSAIDs can cause sodium and water retention, leading to worsening heart failure, and can also impair renal function. The patient's increased serum creatinine and potassium levels may be due to the combination of NSAID use and his current regimen of an ACE inhibitor and an aldosterone blocker, which can affect renal function and potassium balance. The immediate discontinuation of ibuprofen and optimization of diuretic therapy to relieve volume overload are the most appropriate next steps. Option A is incorrect because thiazolidinediones (glitazones) can cause fluid retention and exacerbate heart failure, and therefore should be avoided in patients with HFrEF. Option C is not appropriate because most calcium channel blockers, except amlodipine and felodipine, are contraindicated in HFrEF due to their negative inotropic effects, which can worsen heart failure. Option D is incorrect because the combination of an ACE inhibitor, ARB, and aldosterone blocker significantly increases the risk of hyperkalemia and renal impairment, as evidenced by the patient's current laboratory values, and should be avoided. Between thirty to fifty percent of hospitalized heart failure (HF) patients face readmission within three to six months, highlighting the need for proactive measures to prevent such occurrences. Strategies like tailored diuretic regimens, comprehensive case management, home monitoring of weight and clinical status, and other preventive interventions play a crucial role in averting clinical deterioration and reducing rehospitalizations. These interventions should be integrated into the management of advanced HF, emphasizing the importance of a multidisciplinary team approach and in-person communication for optimal outcomes.

Initiating life-saving medications during hospitalization for HF and ensuring prompt titration post-discharge are essential steps to enhance patient prognosis. Patients are advised to adhere to a moderate salt restriction diet (2–2.5 g sodium or 5–6 g salt daily), as overly strict sodium limitations are often impractical given the effectiveness of potent diuretics.

Exercise training is beneficial in improving activity tolerance by addressing peripheral abnormalities associated with HF and deconditioning. While strict activity restriction may temporarily improve symptoms in severe HF cases, structured exercise programs have shown mixed results in terms of mortality and hospital admissions despite enhancing functional status and symptom management. Therefore, a gradual increase in physical activity or a consistent exercise routine is recommended for stable HF patients, as it correlates with symptom reduction and notable improvements in physical capacity. Exercise training helps in increasing activity tolerance, reversing peripheral abnormalities associated with heart failure and deconditioning, and improving overall physical capacity. It has been found to enhance quality of life, increase exercise capacity (measured by VO2peak), and positively impact health-related outcomes.

Rotunno R et al. NSAIDs and heart failure: A dangerous relationship. Monaldi Arch Chest Dis. 2018 Jun 7;88(2):950. PMID: 29877658

8.9 Managing Hypertension and Diastolic Dysfunction in a Diabetic Patient

Case 130

A 65-year-old woman with a history of hypertension and type 2 diabetes mellitus presents with exertional dyspnea and fatigue. She denies chest pain. Her medications include metformin, lisinopril, and hydrochlorothiazide. On physical examination, her blood pressure is 145/90 mmHg, heart rate is 78 bpm, and her BMI is 32 kg/m^2. Lung auscultation reveals bibasilar crackles, and there is 1+ pitting edema in her ankles. An EKG shows left ventricular hypertrophy with strain pattern but no ischemic changes. A chest X-ray indicates mild pulmonary congestion. An echocardiogram reveals a left ventricular ejection fraction (LVEF) of 55%, left ventricular hypertrophy, and diastolic dysfunction with a normal-sized left atrium and no significant valvular disease. Which of the following is the most appropriate next step in the management of this patient?

- A. Initiate treatment with a beta-blocker to improve diastolic function.
- B. Perform a stress test to evaluate for myocardial ischemia. C. Refer for cardiac MRI to assess for myocardial scar or infiltrative disease.
- D. Increase the dose of lisinopril to achieve better blood pressure control.

The correct answer is D. Increase the dose of lisinopril to achieve better blood pressure control. This patient presents with signs and symptoms suggestive of heart failure with preserved ejection fraction (HFpEF), which is often associated with hypertension and diabetes. The echocardiogram shows diastolic dysfunction and left ventricular hypertrophy, which are common in HFpEF, especially in the context of poorly controlled hypertension. The most immediate and appropriate step is to optimize blood pressure control, which can improve diastolic function and symptoms of heart failure. Lisinopril, an ACE inhibitor, not only lowers blood pressure but also has beneficial effects on the heart's structure and function, particularly in the setting of HFpEF. New data has shown that ACE although effective treatments for the comorbidity of hypertension, inhibitors of the renin–angiotensin–aldosterone system (ACE inhibitors and ARBs) have not been demonstrated to enhance outcome in patients with heart failure and preserved LVEF. Although sacubitril/valsartan appears to improve outcome for patients with marginally reduced LVEF (41–50%), it does not significantly improve outcome in patients with HF and preserved LVEF. In a large trial involving patients with HF and preserved LVEF, spironolactone did not enhance prognosis. However, patients enrolled in the Americas who had more precisely defined HF may have benefited from its use. Spironolactone ought to continue to be considered as a viable therapeutic alternative, particularly for patients co-occurring with hypertension. Option A is not the most appropriate next step because, while beta-blockers can be beneficial in the treatment of HFpEF, the priority in this patient is to achieve better blood pressure control, which can have a direct impact on diastolic function. Option B, performing a stress test, may be considered if there is a suspicion of myocardial ischemia contributing to the patient's symptoms, but there is no current evidence of ischemic heart disease, and the patient denies chest pain. Option C, referral for cardiac MRI, is not indicated at this point as the echocardiogram did not suggest infiltrative disease or myocardial scar, and the patient's symptoms can be explained by poorly controlled hypertension and diastolic dysfunction. SGLT2 inhibitors, such as dapagliflozin or empagliflozin, stand out as the sole treatments proven to reduce cardiovascular mortality or heart failure hospitalization in a population where a significant portion of heart failure cases occur in patients with normal LVEF, often accompanied by diastolic dysfunction. The use of SGLT2 inhibitors and effective fluid management are crucial in the treatment of heart failure with preserved EF to prevent diuretic overload and address associated conditions like hypertension, diabetes, and arrhythmias.

Reversible risk factors like hypotension, pericardial disease, and atrial tachycardias can contribute to myocardial infarction in individuals with preserved LVEF. Managing tachycardia becomes essential due to its impact on diastolic filling time. Considering effective therapeutic options for familial and wild-type transthyretin amyloid cardiomyopathy may be beneficial for patients with puzzling heart failure and preserved EF.

Diuretic therapy remains vital for alleviating fluid retention symptoms in patients with heart failure and preserved LVEF, akin to its role in systolic heart failure symptom management. Unlike those with reduced LVEF, patients with preserved LVEF do not derive benefits from ICDs or resynchronization devices. Revascularization decisions should be guided by similar considerations for both patient groups to optimize outcomes.

SGLT2 inhibitors, like dapagliflozin or empagliflozin, play a unique role in preventing diuretic overload in heart failure patients. These inhibitors offer cardiovascular benefits that include reducing heart failure events, making them a valuable addition to treatment strategies. By incorporating SGLT2 inhibitors and effective fluid management, healthcare providers can address heart failure with preserved EF more efficiently. This approach helps prevent excessive diuretic use, manages comorbidities such as hypertension, diabetes, and arrhythmias, and optimizes patient outcomes in this specific population.

Goldstein D et al. Diastolic Heart Failure: A Review of Current and Future Treatment Options Cardiol Rev. 2021 PMID: 32101908

8.10 Managing Chronic Heart Failure with Ischemic Cardiomyopathy

Case 131

A 72-year-old man with a history of chronic heart failure presents to the clinic with worsening dyspnea on exertion and orthopnea over the past two weeks. He has a known history of ischemic cardiomyopathy with a left ventricular ejection fraction (LVEF) of 25% on his last echocardiogram six months ago. His current medications include lisinopril 20 mg daily, carvedilol 25 mg twice daily, furosemide 40 mg daily, and spironolactone 25 mg daily. On examination, his blood pressure is 110/70 mmHg, heart rate is 88 bpm, and he has an elevated jugular venous pressure of 10 cm H2O at a 45-degree angle. Auscultation of the lungs reveals bibasilar crackles, and there is 2++ pitting edema up to his mid-shins. The liver is palpable 3 cm below the right costal margin and is tender. A positive hepatojugular reflux is noted. The cardiac examination reveals a laterally displaced apical impulse, an S3 gallop, and a holosystolic murmur at the apex radiating to the axilla. Which of the following is the most appropriate next step in the management of this patient?

- A. Increase the dose of furosemide to manage volume overload.
- B. Initiate amiodarone for rhythm control.
- C. Perform a right heart catheterization to measure hemodynamics.
- D. Refer for implantable cardioverter-defibrillator (ICD) evaluation.

The correct answer is A. Increase the dose of furosemide to manage volume overload. This patient with chronic heart failure and reduced ejection fraction (HFrEF) is presenting with clinical signs of volume overload, as evidenced by elevated jugular venous pressure, bibasilar crackles, hepatic congestion with a positive hepatojugular reflux, and peripheral edema. The immediate priority is to address the volume overload to alleviate symptoms and prevent further decompensation. Increasing the dose of furosemide, a loop diuretic, is appropriate to enhance diuresis and reduce fluid accumulation. Option B is incorrect because there is no mention of arrhythmia in the clinical scenario, and amiodarone is primarily used for rhythm control in the context of arrhythmias such as atrial fibrillation or ventricular tachycardia, not for the management of volume overload. Option C, performing a right heart catheterization, may be useful in certain cases to measure hemodynamics, but it is not the first step in the management of a patient with clear clinical signs of volume overload who can be managed with diuretic therapy. Option D, referral for ICD evaluation, may be appropriate for a patient with HFrEF to prevent sudden cardiac death, but it is not the immediate next step in the management of acute decompensated heart failure due to volume overload. Diauretics—For HF with preserved or reduced LVEF, diuretics are the most effective therapeutic agents for symptomatic alleviation in patients with moderate to severe HF who also have dyspnea and fluid overload. Fluid retention symptoms or indications can be optimally managed in a minority of patients. prevented the use of a diuretic. Nevertheless, excessive diuresis may result in the activation of neurohormones and an electrolyte imbalance. Initiating treatment for symptomatic heart failure with reduced LVEF typically involves a combination of a diuretic and an ACE inhibitor or ARNI, along with a beta-blocker and SGLT2 inhibitor in a timely manner. For patients with more severe heart failure, oral loop diuretics are often recommended, such as torsemide (20–200 mg daily), furosemide (20–320 mg daily), and bumetanide (1–8 mg daily), known for their rapid onset of action and relatively short duration. Multiple daily doses are preferred in patients with preserved kidney function over a single larger dose, especially in uncertain gastrointestinal absorption or acute scenarios where intravenous administration may be necessary.

Torsemide, due to its longer half-life and better absorption profile, may offer advantages over furosemide, although clinical outcomes from a large randomized trial showed no significant difference between the two diuretics. In cases of severe renal impairment, higher doses (up to 500 mg of furosemide or equivalent) may be required. Adverse effects like hypotension, prerenal azotemia, and intravascular volume depletion are common, with hypokalemia posing a significant risk, particularly when combined with digitalis therapy.

Less frequent adverse effects include skin rashes, gastrointestinal disturbances, and ototoxicity, the latter being more associated with ethacrynic acid and potentially less so with bumetanide. It is essential to monitor patients closely for these adverse effects and adjust treatment accordingly to optimize therapeutic outcomes.

Beta-blockers and SGLT2 inhibitors play crucial roles in managing heart failure symptoms by targeting different aspects of the condition. Beta-blockers work by reducing the strength of heart contractions and slowing the heart rate, which can slow the progression of heart failure and potentially strengthen the heart muscle. They are also known to reduce the risk of death and other long-term events related to worsening heart failure. Commonly prescribed beta-blockers for heart failure include metoprolol succinate and carvedilol.

SGLT2 inhibitors, such as dapagliflozin and empagliflozin, have emerged as a new class of drugs for heart failure treatment. These medications were initially developed to treat hyperglycemia in patients with type 2 diabetes, but their potential benefits in heart failure management were discovered through clinical trials. SGLT2 inhibitors reduce the risk of cardiovascular events, hospitalization, and mortality by inhibiting the tubular reabsorption of glucose, leading to a reduction in blood pressure and an improvement in endothelial function. They also lower interstitial volume, which can contribute to improved outcomes in heart failure patients, regardless of their diabetic status.

Felker GM et al. Diuretic Therapy for Patients With Heart Failure: JACC State-of-the-Art Review. J Am Coll Cardiol. 2020 Mar 17;75(10):1178-1195. PMID: 32164892

8.11 Chronic Heart Failure with Preserved Ejection Fraction and CKD

Case 132

A 73-year-old woman with a history of chronic heart failure with preserved ejection fraction (HFpEF) presents to the clinic with worsening dyspnea on exertion and fatigue. She has a history of chronic kidney disease (stage 3) and hypertension. Her current medications include amlodipine, furosemide, and spironolactone. On examination, her blood pressure is 160/90 mmHg, heart rate is 102 bpm, and she has 2+ pitting edema in her lower extremities. Laboratory findings reveal a serum creatinine of 2.1 mg/dL (increased from a baseline of 1.8 mg/dL), serum potassium of 5.5 mEq/L, BNP of 550 pg/mL, and hemoglobin of 10.5 g/dL with an RDW of 15.5%. An ECG shows left ventricular hypertrophy with no acute ischemic changes. Which of the following is the most appropriate next step in the management of this patient?

- A. Initiate therapy with sacubitril/valsartan to improve heart failure symptoms.
- B. Increase the dose of spironolactone to enhance diuresis and potassium excretion.
- C. Start oral iron supplementation for suspected iron-deficiency anemia.
- D. Adjust antihypertensive therapy to achieve better blood pressure control.

The correct answer is D. Adjust antihypertensive therapy to achieve better blood pressure control. This patient with HFpEF and chronic kidney disease presents with poorly controlled hypertension, which can exacerbate heart failure symptoms and further impair kidney function. Achieving better blood pressure control is essential in the management of HFpEF and can lead to symptomatic improvement. Adjusting her antihypertensive regimen, potentially by adding or substituting medications that do not raise potassium levels, is warranted given her elevated blood pressure and hyperkalemia.

Option A is incorrect because sacubitril/valsartan, while beneficial in HFrEF, is not indicated in HFpEF, especially in the context of elevated potassium levels and worsening renal function. Additionally, sacubitril/valsartan can increase serum potassium, which is already high in this patient. Option B is not appropriate because increasing the dose of spironolactone, a potassium-sparing diuretic, could exacerbate hyperkalemia. Option C, starting oral iron supplementation, may be considered if iron-deficiency anemia is confirmed with additional iron studies, but it is not the most immediate concern given the patient's hypertension, hyperkalemia, and worsening renal function. The anemia may also be related to her chronic kidney disease, and the RDW alone is not sufficient to diagnose iron-deficiency anemia. Four significant clinical trials, two involving patients with preserved LVEF and heart failure, and two focusing on patients with preserved LVEF, have highlighted the effectiveness of dapagliflozin and empagliflozin, SGLT2 inhibitors, in reducing the risk of cardiovascular death and heart failure hospitalization in individuals with preserved LVEF, heart failure, and diabetes. These medications are typically prescribed at a daily dose of 10 mg each, offering rapid benefits within two weeks of initiation while being well-tolerated in terms of renal function and blood pressure management. Notably, the progression of kidney disease was also observed to be slowed with the use of SGLT2 inhibitors, with clinical trials including patients with an eGFR as low as 20 mL/min/1.73 m2. SGLT-2 inhibitors have emerged as a crucial therapy for heart failure (HF) patients with preserved left ventricular ejection fraction (LVEF) and diabetes, offering several benefits:

1. Reduction in HF Hospitalizations: Clinical trials have shown a significant decrease in HF hospitalizations with the use of SGLT-2 inhibitors, such as empagliflozin and dapagliflozin
2. Cardiovascular Risk Reduction: These inhibitors not only reduce blood glucose levels but also lower the risk of cardiovascular events, stroke, cardiovascular death, and renal failure in patients with known cardiovascular disease or at high risk.
3. Improved Endothelial Function: SGLT-2 inhibitors lead to a reduction in blood pressure and an enhancement in endothelial function, contributing to improvements in hospitalization rates and mortality.
4. Multi-System Effects: Beyond their glucose-lowering effects, SGLT-2 inhibitors offer benefits across various systems, including the cardiovascular system, making them valuable in managing HF and associated conditions.
5. Potential Cardioprotective Effects: Experimental studies suggest a cardioprotective effect of SGLT-

2 inhibitors post-myocardial infarction, indicating broader implications beyond diabetes management.

6. Weight Loss and Renal Protection: These inhibitors cause significant weight loss and have renoprotective effects, making them beneficial for patients with T2DM at high risk for cardiovascular events.

Vaduganathan M et al. SGLT-2 inhibitors in patients with heart failure: a comprehensive meta-analysis of five randomised controlled trials. Lancet. 2022 Sep 3;400(10354):757-767 PMID: 36041474

8.12 Preoperative Cardiac Risk Assessment for Elective Hip Arthroplasty

Case 133

A 70-year-old man with a history of controlled hypertension and type 2 diabetes mellitus is scheduled for elective total hip arthroplasty due to severe osteoarthritis. He has no history of heart failure or coronary artery disease, but he has a 10-pack-year smoking history and quit smoking 5 years ago. His current medications include metformin, lisinopril, and atorvastatin. On physical examination, his blood pressure is 138/82 mmHg, heart rate is 78 bpm, and his cardiovascular examination is unremarkable with no murmurs, rubs, or gallops. His preoperative workup includes a normal ECG and a chest X-ray without any cardiopulmonary abnormalities. Given his age and comorbidities, you consider further preoperative cardiac risk assessment. Which of the following is the most appropriate next step in the preoperative evaluation of this patient?

- A. Order a preoperative BNP or NT-proBNP level.
- B. Schedule a dobutamine stress echocardiogram.
- C. Proceed with surgery without further cardiac testing.
- D. Refer for coronary angiography.

The correct answer is A. Order a preoperative BNP or NT-proBNP level. According to the Canadian Cardiovascular Society and European Society of Cardiology guidelines, measuring BNP or NT-proBNP levels prior to major noncardiac surgery is recommended in patients older than 65 years and those with cardiovascular disease (CVD) or CVD risk factors. This patient is over 65 and has risk factors for CVD, including hypertension, diabetes, and a history of smoking. Elevated BNP or NT-proBNP levels would indicate an increased risk for perioperative cardiac complications and may influence the perioperative management strategy. Option B is incorrect because a dobutamine stress echocardiogram is typically reserved for patients with poor functional capacity who have at least one clinical risk factor and are undergoing high-risk surgery. This patient's surgery is not high-risk, and there is no indication from the clinical scenario that he has poor functional capacity or known coronary artery disease. Option C, proceeding with surgery without further cardiac testing, may be considered if the patient had no risk factors for CVD, but in this case, the patient's age and comorbidities warrant further risk assessment. Option D, referral for coronary angiography, is not indicated in the absence of symptoms or signs suggestive of coronary artery disease and would expose the patient to unnecessary risks associated with an invasive procedure. Delaying elective surgery until decompensated heart failure (HF) is effectively managed is recommended, indicated by clinical signs such as a third heart sound, elevated jugular venous pressure, or signs of pulmonary edema. The risk of perioperative cardiac complications is similar in patients with compensated HF, regardless of whether they have ischemic or nonischemic cardiomyopathy. However, HF with reduced ejection fraction (EF) may pose a higher risk compared to HF with preserved EF. Guidelines suggest preoperative echocardiography to evaluate left ventricular function in patients with unexplained dyspnea or those experiencing clinical deterioration despite known HF.

Prior to surgery, it is essential to assess serum electrolyte and digoxin levels in patients on diuretics and digoxin, as imbalances can heighten the risk of perioperative arrhythmias. Careful consideration is advised when administering diuretics, especially in patients with depleted intraoperative volume who are more susceptible to hypotension. Informing the surgical and anesthesia teams about the presence and severity of left ventricular dysfunction is crucial for tailored intraoperative monitoring and perioperative fluid management decisions.

Halvorsen S et al. 2022 ESC guidelines on cardiovascular assessment and management of patients undergoing non-cardiac surgery: developed by the task force for cardiovascular assessment and management of patients undergoing non-cardiac surgery. Eur Heart J. 2022;43:3826. PMID: 36017553

8.13 Managing Worsening Dyspnea and Fatigue in Nonischemic Cardiomyopathy

Case 134

A 67-year-old male with a history of nonischemic cardiomyopathy presents to the clinic with worsening dyspnea on exertion and fatigue. He has a history of hypertension and type 2 diabetes mellitus. His medications include lisinopril, metoprolol, spironolactone, and furosemide. He reports compliance with his medication regimen and dietary restrictions. On physical examination, his blood pressure is 130/85 mmHg, heart rate is 78 beats per minute, and he has a 2+ pitting edema in his lower extremities. His chest auscultation reveals bibasilar crackles. An ECG shows a left bundle branch block (LBBB) with a QRS duration of 150 msec. An echocardiogram indicates a left ventricular ejection fraction (LVEF) of 30% with evidence of left ventricular dilation and global hypokinesis.
Which of the following is the most appropriate next step in the management of this patient's heart failure?

- A. Optimize medical therapy by increasing the dose of metoprolol.
- B. Refer for implantation of an implantable cardioverter-defibrillator (ICD).
- C. Refer for cardiac resynchronization therapy (CRT) with a biventricular pacemaker.
- D. Initiate treatment with an angiotensin receptor-neprilysin inhibitor (ARNI).

The correct answer is C. Refer for cardiac resynchronization therapy (CRT) with a biventricular pacemaker This patient has heart failure with reduced ejection fraction (HFrEF) and is symptomatic despite being on guideline-directed medical therapy. He has a wide QRS complex due to LBBB, which is associated with dyssynchronous ventricular contractions. CRT has been shown to improve symptoms, exercise tolerance, and survival in patients with HFrEF, particularly in those with a QRS duration of 120 msec or more and LBBB, as seen in this patient. Therefore, referral for CRT is indicated to improve his heart failure symptoms and potentially reduce mortality and hospitalization.

Option A is incorrect because while optimizing medical therapy is important in heart failure management, this patient already has a wide QRS complex and symptoms despite being on a beta-blocker, which suggests that he may benefit more from a device-based intervention like CRT.

Option B is incorrect because while an ICD may be indicated for primary prevention of sudden cardiac death in patients with HFrEF, the patient's wide QRS and LBBB make CRT the more appropriate intervention at this time. An ICD could be considered in conjunction with CRT if the patient meets criteria for both.

Option D is incorrect because although ARNI therapy is recommended for patients with HFrEF to reduce morbidity and mortality, the patient's wide QRS and LBBB suggest that CRT would address the dyssynchrony and potentially provide more immediate symptomatic relief and long-term benefit.

In a significant proportion of heart failure (HF) patients with systolic dysfunction, an abnormal intraventricular conduction pattern leads to dyssynchronous contractions, resulting in inefficient cardiac function. The efficacy of "multisite" pacing, utilizing leads to stimulate both the right ventricle (RV) from the apex and the left ventricle (LV) from the lateral wall via the coronary sinus, has been investigated in various studies. These studies focused on patients with wide QRS complexes (typically 120 msec or longer), reduced ejection fractions (EFs), and symptoms ranging from moderate to severe. Clinical trials with follow-up periods of up to two years have shown promising results, including improvements in exercise tolerance and symptoms, increased EF, and reductions in mortality and hospitalization rates. Patients with widened QRS complexes, left bundle branch block, and nonischemic cardiomyopathy tend to respond most positively to cardiac resynchronization therapy. Conversely, individuals with narrow QRS complexes and non-left bundle branch block patterns exhibit less favorable outcomes. Therefore, resynchronization therapy is recommended in line with the 2013 European guidelines for patients with ambulatory class IV HF, classes II and III HF, an EF of 35% or less, and a left bundle branch block pattern with a QRS duration of 120 msec or longer. Consideration may also be given to patients with a non-left bundle branch block pattern accompanied by a prolonged QRS duration. In patients with heart failure caused by systolic dysfunction, abnormal intraventricular conduction patterns are frequently observed. This conduction abnormality leads to dyssynchronous contractions, resulting in inefficient cardiac function. Studies have explored the effectiveness of "multisite" pacing, which involves stimulating the right ventricle (RV) from the apex and the left ventricle (LV) from the lateral wall via the coronary sinus. Patients with wide QRS complexes (typically 120 msec or longer), reduced ejection fractions (EFs), and moderate to severe symptoms have been the focus of these investigations. Research has shown that delayed intraventricular conduction, as detected on electrocardiograms (ECGs), is a common clinical abnormality associated with adverse outcomes in heart disease patients. Prolonged QRS duration, particularly due to left bundle branch block (LBBB) or intraventricular conduction disturbance (IVCD), has been linked to increased mortality and higher risks for adverse events. Patients with acute heart failure (AHF) and delayed intraventricular conduction, especially nonspecific intraventricular conduction disturbance (NICD), have shown an increased risk of mortality. In contrast, patients with narrow QRS complexes and non-left bundle branch block patterns tend to have less favorable outcomes. Overall, the relationship between intraventricular conduction abnormalities and heart failure caused by systolic dysfunction underscores the importance of assessing these conduction patterns in patients with HF to predict prognosis and guide treatment decisions effectively.

Boriani G et al. Cardiac Resynchronization Therapy: An Overview on Guidelines. Heart Fail Clin. 2017 Jan;13(1):117-137.PMID: 27886918

8.14 Management of Ischemic Cardiomyopathy in a Patient with a History of MI

Case 135

A 58-year-old male with a history of ischemic cardiomyopathy presents to the outpatient clinic for a routine follow-up. He had a myocardial infarction two years ago and underwent successful percutaneous coronary intervention to his left anterior descending artery. His current medications include aspirin, atorvastatin, lisinopril, carvedilol, and spironolactone. He has no complaints and has been adherent to his medication regimen. He has completed a cardiac rehabilitation program and has been following a heart-healthy diet. On examination, his blood pressure is 125/80 mmHg, heart rate is 60 beats per minute, and he has no signs of fluid overload. A recent echocardiogram showed an ejection fraction of 25% with no significant valvular disease. He has no history of ventricular arrhythmias and his ECG is normal except for Q-waves in the anterior leads. Which of the following is the most appropriate next step in the management of this patient?

- A. Continue current medical therapy without any changes.
- B. Refer for implantation of an implantable cardioverter-defibrillator (ICD).
- C. Initiate amiodarone therapy for arrhythmia prophylaxis.
- D. Perform a stress test to evaluate for residual ischemia.

The correct answer is B. Refer for implantation of an implantable cardioverter-defibrillator (ICD). According to the findings from the second Multicenter Automatic Defibrillator Implantation Trial (MADIT II), patients with a history of myocardial infarction and an ejection fraction of less than 30% have a significantly reduced mortality risk when treated with an ICD. This patient has ischemic cardiomyopathy with a significantly reduced ejection fraction (25%) despite optimal medical therapy and lifestyle modification. He is at high risk for sudden cardiac death due to ventricular arrhythmias, and an ICD would provide a survival benefit by preventing this outcome. The Centers for Medicare and Medicaid Services also provide coverage for ICD implantation in patients with similar profiles to this patient.

Option A is incorrect because while the patient is stable and asymptomatic on current medical therapy, the low ejection fraction significantly increases his risk for sudden cardiac death, which could be mitigated by an ICD.

Option C is incorrect because there is no indication for amiodarone therapy in this patient, as he has no history of ventricular arrhythmias. Amiodarone has significant long-term side effects and is not indicated solely for prophylaxis in patients without arrhythmias.

Option D is incorrect because while a stress test can evaluate for residual ischemia, this patient has no symptoms suggestive of ischemia, and the primary concern in this scenario is the prevention of sudden cardiac death due to his low ejection fraction.

Patients with chronic heart failure (HF) and left ventricular (LV) systolic dysfunction undergoing modern HF therapies, including beta-blockers, are considered candidates for implantable cardioverter-defibrillators (ICDs), alongside those with symptomatic or asymptomatic arrhythmias. In the second Multicenter Automatic Defibrillator Implantation Trial (MADIT II), 1232 patients with a history of myocardial infarction and an EF below 30% were randomized into either the control group or the ICD group. The study revealed a 31% reduction in mortality among those with ICDs, translating to nine lives saved per hundred patients fitted with the device over a three-year period.

Furthermore, the Centers for Medicare and Medicaid Services have expanded coverage to include patients with chronic HF and ischemic or nonischemic cardiomyopathy, having an ejection fraction (EF) of 35% or lower. This highlights the significant impact of ICD therapy in improving outcomes and reducing mortality rates in high-risk HF populations. Patients with chronic heart failure and ischemic or non-ischemic cardiomyopathy with an ejection fraction (EF) of 35% or lower fall into the category of heart failure with reduced ejection fraction (HFrEF). For these patients, treatment focuses on controlling blood pressure using beta-blockers, ACE inhibitors, or ARBs, diuretics to relieve symptoms of volume overload, and addressing risk factors and comorbidities Revascularization may be considered in patients where ischemia contributes to heart failure symptoms. Additionally, lifestyle modifications like smoking cessation, exercise, and diet changes are beneficial for managing ischemic cardiomyopathy. In terms of perioperative management for patients with heart failure undergoing surgery, it is recommended to delay elective surgery for at least three months for newly diagnosed HFrEF to allow medical stabilization and optimization of treatment. For patients with decompensated heart failure or new onset heart failure, delaying elective surgery for one month is advised to optimize therapy and stabilize clinical status. In cases where semi-urgent surgery is needed for patients with decompensated heart failure, a delay of a couple of days is recommended for clinical optimization. It is crucial to assess stability and severity of heart failure before proceeding with elective surgery.

Baman JR et al. Primary Prevention Implantable Cardioverter-Defibrillator Therapy in Heart Failure with Recovered Ejection Fraction. J Card Fail. 2021 May;27(5):585-596.PMID: 33636331

8.15 Anticoagulation in Heart Failure with Reduced Ejection Fraction

Case 136

A 72-year-old female with a history of heart failure with reduced ejection fraction (HFrEF) presents to the clinic for a routine follow-up. She has a history of hypertension and diabetes mellitus, both well-controlled with medication. She is currently on enalapril, metoprolol, and spironolactone. She has no history of atrial fibrillation or thromboembolic events. A recent echocardiogram showed an ejection fraction of 20%, with no evidence of intracardiac thrombus. She is active, with no recent hospitalizations, and reports no symptoms of dyspnea, chest pain, or palpitations. Her current medications do not include any anticoagulants.
Which of the following is the most appropriate next step in the management of this patient?

- A. Initiate anticoagulation with a direct oral anticoagulant (DOAC).
- B. Initiate anticoagulation with warfarin.
- C. Continue current management without anticoagulation.
- D. Obtain a cardiac MRI to further evaluate for left ventricular thrombus.

The correct answer is C. Continue current management without anticoagulation. In patients with heart failure and reduced ejection fraction, the risk of thromboembolism is increased, particularly in those with atrial fibrillation, a history of thromboembolic events, or evidence of an intracardiac thrombus. However, in the absence of these risk factors, routine anticoagulation is not recommended. This patient does not have atrial fibrillation, has not had a thromboembolic event, and her echocardiogram did not show evidence of a left ventricular thrombus. Therefore, there is no indication for anticoagulation in her case, and her current heart failure management should be continued without the addition of anticoagulation.

Option A is incorrect because DOACs are not indicated for primary prevention of thromboembolic events in patients with HFrEF without atrial fibrillation, prior thromboembolic events, or evidence of intracardiac thrombus.

Option B is incorrect for the same reason as Option A; warfarin is not indicated in this scenario for the same reasons that DOACs are not indicated.

Option D is incorrect because there is no clinical suspicion of a left ventricular thrombus based on the echocardiogram, and the patient is asymptomatic with no history suggestive of a thromboembolic event. Cardiac MRI is an additional imaging modality that could be used to evaluate for the presence of a thrombus, but it is not indicated in this patient without clinical suspicion.

Patients with impaired EF and LV failure have a marginally increased risk of developing systemic arterial emboli and intracardiac thrombi. However, this risk seems to be concentrated among patients with atrial fibrillation, thromboemboli, or thrombus in the left ventricle. DOACs appear to be equally efficacious in treating patients with LV thrombus as warfarin. The risk factors for thromboembolism in heart failure patients with reduced ejection fraction (HFrEF) include atrial fibrillation, a history of thromboembolic events, or evidence of an intracardiac thrombus. Patients with HFrEF are at an increased risk of developing systemic arterial emboli and intracardiac thrombi, particularly those with atrial fibrillation or a history of thromboembolic events. Additionally, patients with chronic heart failure have a higher risk of venous thromboembolism (VTE). Other contributing factors may include stasis of blood in the legs and heart, hypercoagulability, and endothelial dysfunction. Patients with HFrEF are at an increased risk of developing systemic arterial emboli and intracardiac thrombi, particularly those with atrial fibrillation or a history of thromboembolic events. It is important to note that routine anticoagulation is not recommended in the absence of these risk factors.

Beggs SAS et al. Anticoagulation therapy in heart failure and sinus rhythm: a systematic review and meta-analysis. Heart. 2019 Sep;105(17):1325-1334. PMID: 30962190

8.16 Management of Multi-Vessel Coronary Disease in a Patient with CHF

Case 137

A 69-year-old male with a history of chronic heart failure due to ischemic cardiomyopathy presents to the cardiology clinic. He has an ejection fraction of 30% and has been experiencing Canadian Cardiovascular Society (CCS) class II angina despite optimal medical therapy including high-dose beta-blockers, ACE inhibitors, statins, and aspirin. He has a history of diabetes mellitus and hypertension. A recent coronary angiogram revealed three-vessel coronary artery disease, including 70% stenosis in the proximal left anterior descending artery, 60% stenosis in the left circumflex artery, and 75% stenosis in the right coronary artery. There is no evidence of left main coronary artery disease. His left ventricular end-diastolic pressure is elevated. He has no history of ventricular arrhythmias and has a normal sinus rhythm on ECG.
Which of the following is the most appropriate next step in the management of this patient?

- A. Continue optimal medical therapy for angina and heart failure.
- B. Refer for percutaneous coronary intervention (PCI).
- C. Refer for coronary artery bypass grafting (CABG).
- D. Initiate therapy with a calcium channel blocker for angina.

The correct answer is C. Refer for coronary artery bypass grafting (CABG). This patient has ischemic cardiomyopathy with a reduced ejection fraction and is experiencing angina despite optimal medical therapy. He has significant multivessel coronary artery disease, which is likely contributing to his symptoms and heart failure. The STICH trial initially did not show a survival benefit at 5 years with CABG in patients with heart failure and reduced ejection fraction, but longer-term follow-up indicated a benefit at 10 years. Given the patient's more severe angina and significant multivessel disease, revascularization with CABG is warranted to potentially improve symptoms and prevent progression of heart failure. CABG is generally preferred over PCI in patients with diabetes and multivessel coronary artery disease because it has been associated with better long-term outcomes in this patient population.

Option A is incorrect because the patient is already on optimal medical therapy and continues to have angina, indicating that medical therapy alone is not sufficient to manage his symptoms or the underlying ischemic disease.

Option B is incorrect because while PCI could be considered for symptom relief, CABG is typically the preferred method of revascularization in patients with diabetes and multivessel coronary artery disease due to better long-term outcomes.

Option D is incorrect because the addition of a calcium channel blocker may not adequately address the underlying issue of significant coronary artery disease and may not provide the same potential for improved survival as revascularization. Additionally, some calcium channel blockers should be used with caution in patients with heart failure.

Given that coronary artery disease (CAD) underlies HF in the majority of patients, coronary revascularization has been hypothesized to prevent progression and alleviate symptoms. Although the STITCH trial did not demonstrate a superior overall survival outcome from coronary artery bypass grafting (CABG) for candidates with multivessel coronary disease, myocardium (HF), and LVEF (less than 35 percent) at 5 years, there was evidence of a benefit at 10 years of follow-up. Therefore, it seems that certain patients with heart failure, such as those with severe angina or left main coronary disease (which were precluded from the STITCH trial), do require revascularization. The significance of multivessel coronary artery disease (MVD) in heart failure patients lies in its association with increased morbidity and mortality. MVD is defined as luminal stenosis of at least 70% in at least two major coronary arteries or in one major coronary artery and the left main coronary artery with a stenosis of 50% or more. This condition is both common and deadly, with a mortality hazard ratio of 3.14 compared to single-vessel disease. In patients with heart failure, especially those with reduced ejection fraction (HFrEF), the presence of MVD can exacerbate the underlying cardiac dysfunction. The most common cause of HFrEF in the industrialized world is coronary heart disease, which is often complicated by MVD. The progressive nature of left ventricular dysfunction in HFrEF, often accompanied by comorbidities such as hypertension, is further complicated by the presence of MVD, making the management of these patients particularly challenging. Revascularization, through coronary artery bypass grafting (CABG) or percutaneous coronary intervention (PCI), has been studied as a strategy to improve outcomes in patients with MVD. In patients with MVD and diabetes, CABG has been shown to be superior to PCI. However, decision-making in patients without diabetes is more nuanced. The SYNTAX trial, for example, showed that in patients with higher SYNTAX scores (indicating more complex coronary anatomy), CABG was associated with lower rates of major adverse cardiac or cerebrovascular events at 1 year compared with PCI. Furthermore, the presence of MVD alone is not an automatic indication for revascularization. The ISCHEMIA trial showed that stable MVD, even with moderate-to-severe ischemia, can be initially managed with optimal medical therapy as opposed to immediate revascularization.

Hassanabad A et al. Surgical Treatment for Ischemic Heart Failure (STICH) trial: A review of outcomes. J Card Surg. 2019 Oct;34(10):1075-1082. PMID: 31374589

8.17 Acute Management of Severe Heart Failure

Case 138

A 68-year-old male with a history of chronic heart failure with reduced ejection fraction presents to the emergency department with acute onset of severe dyspnea, orthopnea, and paroxysmal nocturnal dyspnea that began two hours ago. He has a history of hypertension and type 2 diabetes mellitus. On examination, he is tachypneic with a respiratory rate of 30 breaths per minute, blood pressure is 180/100 mmHg, heart rate is 110 beats per minute, and oxygen saturation is 85% on room air. He is sitting upright, anxious, and diaphoretic with bilateral rales halfway up both lung fields and 2+ pitting edema in the lower extremities. Chest X-ray shows pulmonary edema with cephalization of blood flow and Kerley B lines. The patient is placed on supplemental oxygen by mask, which improves his oxygen saturation to 92%.
Which of the following is the most appropriate next step in the management of this patient?

- A. Administer intravenous morphine for symptomatic relief.
- B. Initiate noninvasive positive pressure ventilation (NIPPV) and intravenous nitroglycerin.
- C. Start high-dose intravenous furosemide and intravenous nesiritide.
- D. Proceed with endotracheal intubation and mechanical ventilation.

The correct answer is B. Initiate noninvasive positive pressure ventilation (NIPPV) and intravenous nitroglycerin. This patient is presenting with signs and symptoms of acute pulmonary edema secondary to decompensated heart failure, as evidenced by severe hypertension, tachypnea, hypoxemia, and radiographic findings of pulmonary edema. The immediate goals are to improve oxygenation, reduce the work of breathing, and decrease ventricular filling pressures. NIPPV, such as continuous positive airway pressure (CPAP) or bilevel positive airway pressure (BiPAP), can improve oxygenation and ventilation, reduce the work of breathing, and decrease preload and afterload, which can be beneficial in acute pulmonary edema. Intravenous nitroglycerin is indicated to rapidly reduce preload and afterload, especially in the setting of hypertension, and can alleviate dyspnea before diuresis occurs. Option A is incorrect because, although morphine has been traditionally used for symptomatic relief in acute pulmonary edema, it can lead to CO2 retention and is associated with increased mortality. Current guidelines recommend caution with its use or avoiding it altogether in favor of other treatments. Option C is incorrect because, while intravenous furosemide is appropriate to initiate diuresis, the addition of nesiritide is not the first-line treatment and is reserved for patients who remain symptomatic after initial treatment with diuretics and vasodilators. Moreover, the risk of hypotension with nesiritide may be problematic in this acute setting. Option D is incorrect because, although the patient is in severe respiratory distress, immediate endotracheal intubation may not be necessary if he can be stabilized with NIPPV and medical therapy. Intubation would be the next step if the patient fails to improve or deteriorates on NIPPV. A patient with severe pulmonary edema should be positioned supine with their legs draped over the side of the bed; this will promote ventilation and decrease venous return. By means of a respirator, oxygen is administered in order to achieve an arterial PO2 above 60 mm Hg. While pharmacologic interventions are in effect, noninvasive pressure support ventilation may enhance oxygenation and prevent severe CO2 retention. In the event that respiratory distress persists at a severe level, mechanical ventilation and endotracheal intubation may be required. Morphine demonstrates significant effectiveness in treating pulmonary edema and can be beneficial for managing milder decompensations when the patient is anxious. An initial intravenous dose of 2–8 mg (subcutaneous administration is suitable for less severe cases) can be increased after 2–4 hours. Morphine acts by increasing venous capacitance, reducing left atrial pressure, and alleviating anxiety, which can hinder effective ventilation. However, it may lead to CO2 retention by suppressing respiratory effort. Patients with neurogenic or opioid-induced pulmonary edema, conditions that may respond well to opioid antagonists, should avoid morphine use.

Intravenous diuretic therapy (such as furosemide 40 mg or bumetanide 1 mg, with adjustments for long-term diuretic users) is typically recommended even in the absence of prior fluid retention evidence. These agents induce venodilation before diuresis initiation. The DOSE trial revealed that bolus furosemide doses are as effective as continuous infusion for acute decompensated heart failure (HF). Higher furosemide doses (2.5 times the previous daily dose) facilitate faster fluid removal without significantly increasing the risk of kidney impairment.

Nitrate therapy accelerates clinical improvement by reducing blood pressure and left ventricular filling pressures. Sublingual nitroglycerin, isosorbide dinitrate, topical nitroglycerin, or intravenous nitrates provide immediate relief of dyspnea before diuresis initiation, particularly beneficial for hypertensive patients.

Nesiritide, a recombinant human BNP administered intravenously, acts as a potent vasodilator enhancing cardiac output and reducing ventricular filling pressures. It exhibits hemodynamic effects comparable to intravenous nitroglycerin but with a longer duration of action and a more predictable dose-response curve. Nesiritide significantly improves dyspnea and hemodynamics in clinical trials but may lead to symptomatic hypotension as a primary adverse effect. Reserved for patients who remain symptomatic after initial diuretic and nitrate therapy due to the favorable response of most acute HF patients to conventional treatments.

The effectiveness of intravenous milrinone in preventing readmissions, prolonging hospital stays, or enhancing survival in patients admitted with decompensated heart failure (HF) without clear indications for inotropic therapy was inconclusive in a randomized, placebo-controlled trial involving 950 patients. Additionally, there was a notable increase in sustained hypotension and atrial fibrillation rates. Therefore, the use of positive inotropic agents should be reserved for individuals with refractory symptoms and signs of reduced cardiac output, particularly in cases where critical organ hypoperfusion poses a life-threatening risk, such as deteriorating kidney function. Dobutamine or milrinone may be considered to support patients awaiting cardiac transplantation under specific circumstances.

Bronchospasm can arise as a consequence of pulmonary edema, potentially exacerbating hypoxemia and dyspnea. While intravenous aminophylline and inhaled beta-adrenergic agonists may offer benefits, they carry the risk of provoking supraventricular arrhythmias and tachycardia.

Resolution of pulmonary edema typically responds promptly to treatment. Following patient recovery, identifying the underlying cause or triggering factor is crucial. Evaluation of patients without a history of myocardial infarction should include echocardiography and, often, coronary angiography and cardiac catheterization.

Management of acute decompensation in chronic HF involves therapy promoting euvolemia and optimizing medication regimens. Before discharge, initiating an oral diuretic and an ACE inhibitor is recommended, with confirmation of efficacy and tolerability. In selected patients, cautious but early initiation of low-dose beta-blockers should be considered.

Arrigo M et al Acute heart failure. Nat Rev Dis Primers. 2020 Mar 5;6(1):16. PMID: 32139695

8.18 HF and Worsening Renal Function Dilated Cardiomyopathy

Case 139

A 58-year-old male with a history of dilated cardiomyopathy is admitted to the hospital with decompensated heart failure. He is on optimal medical therapy including an ACE inhibitor, beta-blocker, and aldosterone antagonist. On physical examination, he is tachypneic with a respiratory rate of 28 breaths per minute, blood pressure is 90/60 mmHg, heart rate is 105 beats per minute, and oxygen saturation is 90% on 2 liters of nasal cannula oxygen. He has jugular venous distension, bilateral rales at the lung bases, and 3+ pitting edema in the lower extremities. Laboratory tests reveal a serum creatinine of 2.1 mg/dL (increased from a baseline of 1.3 mg/dL), and a B-type natriuretic peptide (BNP) level of 900 pg/mL. An echocardiogram shows a left ventricular ejection fraction of 20% with no valvular abnormalities. Despite intravenous diuretics, his renal function continues to worsen, and he remains hypotensive with signs of poor perfusion.
Which of the following is the most appropriate next step in the management of this patient?

- A. Initiate intravenous milrinone therapy.
- B. Increase the dose of intravenous diuretics.
- C. Start intravenous vasopressor therapy.
- D. Refer for urgent evaluation for advanced heart failure therapies, including the possibility of cardiac transplantation or mechanical circulatory support.

The correct answer is D. Refer for urgent evaluation for advanced heart failure therapies, including the possibility of cardiac transplantation or mechanical circulatory support. This patient has evidence of advanced heart failure with refractory symptoms, worsening renal function, and hypotension despite optimal medical therapy and intravenous diuretics, indicating low cardiac output and poor vital organ perfusion. These findings suggest that he may be a candidate for advanced heart failure therapies such as cardiac transplantation or mechanical circulatory support (e.g., left ventricular assist device). Early referral to a specialized heart failure center is crucial for these patients to assess their eligibility and optimize their outcomes. Option A is incorrect because, although milrinone is a positive inotropic agent that can improve hemodynamics in heart failure, the question stem references a study showing no benefit in survival or hospitalization outcomes with milrinone in patients without a definite indication for inotropic therapy. Moreover, milrinone can increase the risk of arrhythmias and hypotension, which this patient is already experiencing. Option B is incorrect because the patient has already received intravenous diuretics and continues to show signs of worsening renal function and hypotension. Increasing the dose of diuretics is unlikely to be beneficial and may exacerbate renal dysfunction. Option C is incorrect because while vasopressors can increase blood pressure, they may not improve cardiac output or organ perfusion in the setting of advanced heart failure and could increase myocardial oxygen demand, potentially worsening the underlying condition. The understanding of heart failure (HF) has evolved, with patients having dilated cardiomyopathy typically categorized under HF with reduced ejection fraction (EF), where the left ventricular ejection fraction (LVEF) is 40% or lower. About half of these patients exhibit left ventricular (LV) enlargement, defining dilated cardiomyopathy. This category encompasses a range of myocardial disorders characterized by reduced myocardial contractility in the absence of abnormal loading conditions like hypertension or valvular disease. In the United States, the median incidence rate is 36 cases per 100,000 individuals, contributing to approximately 10,000 deaths annually. Black patients have a threefold higher incidence compared to White patients, with a grim prognosis of a 50% mortality rate within five years of symptom onset.

Dilated cardiomyopathy has diverse causes, with 20%–35% having a familial origin. Hereditary factors often manifest initially as conduction system disease before reduced LVEF. While idiopathic factors contribute significantly, genetic variations likely play a role in many cases.

Various factors such as obesity, diabetes, thyroid disease, celiac disease, SLE, acromegaly, and growth hormone deficiency, along with inflammatory, metabolic, and endocrine influences contribute to the condition. Toxic, drug-induced, and inflammatory triggers are discussed alongside nutritional deficiencies like carnitine, selenium, and thiamine deficiency.

Prolonged tachycardia from supraventricular arrhythmias, frequent PVCs or RV pacing can also lead to dilated cardiomyopathy. Other associated conditions include HIV, Chagas disease, rheumatologic disorders, iron overload, sleep apnea, amyloidosis, sarcoidosis, chronic alcohol use, ESKD, or cobalt exposure (known as "Quebec beer-drinkers' cardiomyopathy"). Stress-induced disease like takotsubo and peripartum cardiomyopathy are also distinct entities within this spectrum.

Heymans S et al. Dilated cardiomyopathy: causes, mechanisms, and current and future treatment approaches. Lancet. 2023 Sep 16;402(10406):998-1011. PMID: 37716772

8.19 ST-segment Elevations and No Obstructive Coronary Artery Disease

Case 140

A 58-year-old post-menopausal woman presents to the emergency department with acute onset chest pain that began 2 hours ago while she was arguing with her son. She describes the pain as a pressure-like sensation across her chest with radiation to her left arm. She denies any previous history of similar pain, has no known coronary artery disease, and her only medical history is hypertension, for which she takes amlodipine. On examination, her blood pressure is 165/95 mm Hg, heart rate is 78 bpm, and respiratory rate is 16 breaths per minute. She appears anxious. Cardiac examination reveals no murmurs, rubs, or gallops. An electrocardiogram (ECG) shows ST-segment elevations in the anterior leads. Initial troponin I level is mildly elevated. An urgent coronary angiography reveals no obstructive coronary artery disease, but left ventriculography shows apical ballooning.
Question: What is the most appropriate next step in the management of this patient?

- A) Initiate high-dose statin therapy
- B) Start treatment with an ACE inhibitor and beta-blocker
- C) Begin immediate reperfusion with thrombolytic therapy
- D) Schedule elective placement of an implantable cardioverter-defibrillator (ICD)

The correct answer is B) Start treatment with an ACE inhibitor and beta-blocker. This patient has been diagnosed with Takotsubo syndrome (TTS), which is characterized by transient left ventricular dysfunction triggered by emotional or physical stress, presenting with symptoms and ECG changes similar to an acute myocardial infarction but without significant coronary artery obstruction. The management of TTS involves supportive care and treatment aimed at relieving symptoms and preventing complications. ACE inhibitors or angiotensin receptor blockers (ARBs) are often used to reduce the stress on the heart and improve remodeling, while beta-blockers help to control the heart rate and reduce the effects of catecholamine surge, which is thought to be a contributing factor in TTS. Option A) Initiate high-dose statin therapy is not the most appropriate next step as there is no evidence of obstructive coronary artery disease, which is the primary indication for statin therapy in the context of acute coronary syndromes. Option C) Begin immediate reperfusion with thrombolytic therapy is not indicated because the coronary angiography did not reveal an occlusive thrombus, and the use of thrombolytics without evidence of coronary thrombosis could increase the risk of bleeding without any benefit. Option D) Schedule elective placement of an implantable cardioverter-defibrillator (ICD) is not appropriate at this stage. ICDs are used for the primary prevention of sudden cardiac death in patients with significantly reduced left ventricular ejection fraction or specific hereditary conditions, which is not the case here. TTS is typically a reversible condition, and decisions regarding ICD placement would be premature without evidence of persistent ventricular arrhythmias or severe systolic dysfunction after recovery from the acute phase. Numerous case reports have linked excess catecholamines to various triggers, with isolated instances of pericarditis and tamponade documented. Recurrences have been noted, with a higher incidence among women (up to 90%), primarily postmenopausal in Western countries. Stress cardiomyopathy, compared to acute coronary syndrome (ACS) patients, shows a higher prevalence of neurologic and psychiatric disorders. Patients receiving beta-agonists for COPD, migraines, or affective disorders may face increased risks of adverse outcomes. Initially perceived as having a benign prognosis, recent studies reveal significantly higher short-term and long-term mortality rates than previously thought. Acute phase mortality for hospitalized patients ranges from 4% to 5%, akin to STEMI mortality pre-primary percutaneous coronary interventions. Approximately 10% of patients are expected to encounter cardiac and neurologic complications in the following year.

The stress response involves structures of the autonomic and central nervous systems. Acute stressors trigger brain activation, elevating cortisol and catecholamines. Adrenal medullary chromaffin cells release increased epinephrine and norepinephrine into circulation, while sympathetic nerve terminals locally release norepinephrine.

Various mechanisms contribute to catecholamine-induced myocardial damage in stress cardiomyopathy, including direct toxicity, adrenoceptor-mediated harm, coronary vasoconstriction/spasm, and increased cardiac workload. The prevalence among postmenopausal women suggests estrogen deprivation may play a role, possibly through endothelial dysfunction.

In managing Takotsubo syndrome, initiating treatment with an ACE inhibitor and beta-blocker is recommended to address acute myocardial stress and prevent further cardiac complications effectively. **International Takotsubo diagnostic criteria** (InterTAK diagnostic criteria)

1. Patients show transient a left ventricular dysfunction (hypokinesia, akinesia or dyskinesia) presenting as apical ballooning or midventricular, basal or focal wall motion abnormalities. Right ventricular involvement can be present. Besides these regional wall motion patterns, transitions between all types can exist. The regional wall motion abnormality usually extends beyond a single epicardial vascular distribution; however, rare cases can exist where the regional wall motion abnormality is present in the subtended myocardial territory of a single coronary artery (focal TTS).
2. An emotional, physical or combined trigger can precede the takotsubo syndrome event, but this is not obligatory.
3. Neurologic disorders (eg, subarachnoid haemorrhage, stroke/transient ischaemic attack or seizures) as well as pheochromocytoma may serve as triggers for takotsubo syndrome.
4. New ECG abnormalities are present (ST-segment elevation, ST-segment depression, T-wave inversion and QTc prolongation); however, rare cases exist without any ECG changes.
5. Levels of cardiac biomarkers (troponin and creatine kinase) are moderately elevated in most cases; significant elevation of brain natriuretic peptide is common.
6. Significant coronary artery disease is not a contradiction in takotsubo syndrome.
7. Patients have no evidence of infectious myocarditis.
8. Postmenopausal women are predominantly affected

Assad J et al. Takotsubo Syndrome: A Review of Presentation, Diagnosis and Management. Clin Med Insights Cardiol. 2022 Jan 4;16:11795468211065782. PMID: 35002350;

Case 140B

A 37-year-old male with a history of recreational drug use presents to the emergency department with chest pain, palpitations, and shortness of breath that started shortly after using cocaine. He is diaphoretic and appears anxious. His blood pressure is 160/100 mmHg, heart rate is 110 beats per minute, and respiratory rate is 22 breaths per minute. Physical examination reveals bilateral rales halfway up both lung fields, and an ECG shows ST-segment elevations in leads V1-V4. Troponin I levels are elevated. The patient is treated with aspirin, nitroglycerin, and a benzodiazepine. His chest pain resolves, but he remains tachycardic and hypertensive. An echocardiogram shows mild left ventricular systolic dysfunction with an ejection fraction of 45% and no wall motion abnormalities.

Which of the following is the most appropriate next step in the management of this patient?

- A. Administer a beta-blocker to control heart rate and blood pressure.
- B. Start a calcium channel blocker for suspected coronary artery spasm.
- C. Perform immediate coronary angiography to evaluate for myocardial infarction.
- D. Initiate high-dose corticosteroids for suspected myocarditis.

The correct answer is B. Start a calcium channel blocker for suspected coronary artery spasm. Cocaine can cause coronary artery spasm leading to myocardial ischemia and infarction, even in the absence of fixed atherosclerotic coronary artery disease. The use of calcium channel blockers is effective in relieving cocaine-induced coronary artery spasm. Given the patient's presentation with chest pain, ST-segment elevations, and elevated troponin after cocaine use, along with the resolution of chest pain after initial management, coronary artery spasm is a likely diagnosis. Calcium channel blockers are preferred over beta-blockers in this setting due to the risk of unopposed alpha-adrenergic receptor activity with beta-blockade, which can potentially worsen coronary spasm.

Option A is incorrect because beta-blockers can potentially worsen cocaine-induced coronary spasm by blocking beta-mediated vasodilation while leaving alpha-mediated vasoconstriction unopposed. Therefore, they are generally avoided in acute cocaine intoxication with evidence of coronary spasm.

Option C is incorrect because while coronary angiography is important in the evaluation of myocardial infarction, the patient's symptoms have resolved with initial management, suggesting that the chest pain may have been due to reversible coronary spasm rather than fixed obstruction. Calcium channel blockers are an appropriate next step before invasive procedures unless the patient's symptoms recur or do not respond to medical therapy.

Option D is incorrect because there is no clear evidence of myocarditis in this scenario. Corticosteroids are not the treatment of choice for cocaine-induced cardiotoxicity and could potentially have adverse effects. Cocaine use can lead to the development of myocarditis, arrhythmias, coronary artery spasm, and cardiomyopathy. There have been documented cases of amphetamine-induced cardiomyopathy as well. The inhibitory effect of cocaine on sympathetic nerve norepinephrine reuptake is believed to play a role in these processes, prompting the use of beta-blockers in patients with fixed stenosis. Nitrates and calcium channel blockers are considered effective in cases of confirmed coronary spasm. Standard treatment is necessary for symptomatic patients with conduction system disease or heart failure. Multiple case reports have associated myocarditis with the use of recreational drugs. Myocarditis is also linked to systemic disorders such as sarcoidosis, celiac disease, granulomatosis with polyangiitis, and giant cell myocarditis. Immunotherapy, particularly in cases of giant cell myocarditis, has shown potential benefits in observational studies focusing on T cells (e.g., muromonab-CD3). Eosinophilic myocarditis is managed by discontinuing the offending medication or addressing the underlying trigger in addition to high-dose corticosteroids. While HIV is indirectly associated with HIV cardiomyopathy, factors like opportunistic infections, gp120 protein, and adverse reactions to antiretroviral therapy are more commonly implicated. Some patients have shown the presence of herpes simplex and Epstein-Barr viruses in their myocardium. Myocarditis is a condition characterized by inflammation of the heart muscle, known as the myocardium. There are several types of myocarditis, each with distinct characteristics and causes:

1. Acute Myocarditis:Acute myocarditis refers to a rapid onset of the condition, often caused by viral infections. Symptoms can develop suddenly and may resolve quickly as well.
2. Chronic Myocarditis: Chronic myocarditis occurs when the disease takes longer to treat or when symptoms reappear after initial improvement. This type can be associated with autoimmune disorders where the immune system attacks healthy cells and tissues.
3. Lymphocytic Myocarditis:Lymphocytic myocarditis is a rare form that can lead to hospitalization for acute care. It is characterized by the infiltration of white blood cells (lymphocytes) into the heart muscle, causing inflammation. This type can occur following a viral infection.
4. Rare Types: Rare types of myocarditis include endocarditis, which is an infection or inflammation of the heart valves, and giant cell myocarditis.

Myocarditis can present with symptoms such as chest pain, fatigue, abnormal heart rhythms, signs of infection, shortness of breath, and leg swelling. Diagnosis involves a thorough medical history review and various tests like blood tests, chest X-rays, electrocardiograms (ECG), echocardiograms, and in some cases, cardiac MRI or biopsy may be necessary. The condition is most commonly caused by infections in the body, with viral infections being a common culprit

Elkattawy S et al. Cocaine induced heart failure: report and literature review. J Community Hosp Intern Med Perspect. 2021 Jun 21;11(4):547-550. PMID: 34211666

8.20 Managing Hypertrophic Cardiomyopathy

Case 141

A 25-year-old male with a family history of hypertrophic cardiomyopathy (HCM) presents to the clinic with exertional dyspnea and occasional palpitations. He denies any syncope or chest pain. He is an amateur soccer player and is concerned about his risk of sudden cardiac death. Physical examination reveals a harsh systolic murmur that increases in intensity with the Valsalva maneuver. An echocardiogram shows asymmetric septal hypertrophy with a maximum wall thickness of 2.3 cm and systolic anterior motion of the mitral valve leaflet causing left ventricular outflow tract (LVOT) obstruction. There is no mitral regurgitation at rest, and the left ventricular ejection fraction is 75%. The patient's blood pressure is 130/85 mmHg, and his heart rate is 70 beats per minute at rest.
Which of the following is the most appropriate next step in the management of this patient?

- A. Initiate treatment with a high-dose beta-blocker to reduce myocardial contractility and relieve LVOT obstruction.
- B. Refer the patient for surgical myectomy due to the high risk of sudden cardiac death associated with his family history and wall thickness.
- C. Advise the patient to discontinue competitive sports and begin a moderate-intensity exercise program to reduce the risk of sudden cardiac death.
- D. Prescribe a calcium channel blocker and recommend genetic counseling and testing for pathogenic variants associated with HCM.

The correct answer is C. Advise the patient to discontinue competitive sports and begin a moderate-intensity exercise program to reduce the risk of sudden cardiac death. In patients with HCM, particularly those with a family history of sudden cardiac death, participation in competitive sports is generally contraindicated due to the increased risk of life-threatening arrhythmias during intense physical activity. Moderate-intensity exercise may be safer and is often recommended to maintain cardiovascular health. This recommendation is in line with the 2020 ACC/AHA guidelines on the diagnosis and treatment of HCM, which emphasize the importance of lifestyle modification in the management of patients with HCM. Option A is incorrect because while beta-blockers are a mainstay of treatment in HCM to reduce myocardial contractility and relieve LVOT obstruction, there is no indication that the patient is symptomatic enough at this point to warrant high-dose beta-blocker therapy. Treatment is typically initiated for symptom control, and the patient's symptoms are mild. Option B is incorrect because surgical myectomy is considered in patients with HCM who are symptomatic despite optimal medical therapy, particularly those with severe LVOT obstruction and symptoms refractory to medical management. This patient has not yet been trialed on medical therapy and does not have symptoms at rest. Option D is incorrect because while calcium channel blockers can be used to manage symptoms in HCM, they are not the first-line treatment in patients with significant LVOT obstruction and symptoms. Genetic counseling and testing may be appropriate for this patient, but it is not the most immediate next step in management regarding his risk of sudden cardiac death and participation in competitive sports. In 2020, the ACC and AHA joint committee on clinical practice guidelines released updated recommendations for the diagnosis and management of hypertrophic cardiomyopathy (HCM). These guidelines offer a comprehensive set of clinically relevant suggestions covering various clinical scenarios. HCM is identified when left ventricular hypertrophy (LVH) is present without pressure or volume overload. The definition of HCM has evolved over time, transitioning from being solely associated with left ventricular outflow obstruction due to septal hypertrophy to encompassing any degree of LV wall involvement, even in the absence of outflow obstruction. This broader definition allows for the recognition of diverse forms of HCM that do not impede LV outflow. Thickening of the LV wall can increase ejection fraction, reduce LV systolic stress, and potentially lead to an "empty ventricle" at the end of systole.

Asymmetric septal hypertrophy denotes uneven thickening of the septum, although hypertrophy can also localize to the mid-ventricle or apex. In HCM, LV obstruction may trap blood just above the apex, elevating LV pressure significantly and potentially causing an aneurysmal apex. The hypertrophied septum often narrows the LV outflow tract during systole, resulting in systolic anterior motion of the mitral valve leaflet into the outflow tract. Factors that enhance myocardial contractility (e.g., sympathetic stimulation, digoxin) or reduce left ventricular filling (e.g., Valsalva maneuver, peripheral vasodilators) can exacerbate obstruction. The degree of obstruction varies daily based on preload and afterload conditions.

HCM is an autosomal dominant trait with variable penetrance inherited within families. It is linked to pathogenic variants in numerous genes, many encoding proteins or heavy chains involved in calcium regulation or myosin function. Prognosis is influenced by the specific pathogenic gene variant, with most patients experiencing symptoms in early adulthood.

While elite athletes may exhibit significant hypertrophy that resembles HCM, they typically lack diastolic dysfunction seen in pathological HCM cases, aiding in differentiation between athletic hypertrophy and disease. The 2020 AHA/ACC guidelines provide essential recommendations for the diagnosis and treatment of patients with Hypertrophic Cardiomyopathy (HCM). Here are some key points based on the guidelines:

1. Surgical Septal Myectomy: For patients with HCM undergoing surgical septal myectomy, it is recommended to use intraoperative transesophageal echocardiogram (TEE) to assess mitral valve anatomy.
2. Assessment Tools: The guidelines emphasize the use of various diagnostic tools such as echocardiography, cardiovascular magnetic resonance, exercise stress testing, and genetic testing for accurate diagnosis and risk stratification.
3. Treatment Options: The guidelines cover a range of treatment options including septal alcohol ablation, septal reduction therapy, implantable cardioverter defibrillator (ICD) placement, and shared decision-making in the management of HCM patients.
4. Risk Stratification: Risk stratification for sudden cardiac death is a crucial aspect addressed in the guidelines, highlighting the importance of identifying high-risk individuals who may benefit from specific interventions like ICD placement.
5. Family Screening: Recommendations include screening family members of HCM patients for early detection and management of the condition due to its genetic nature

Maron BJ et al. Diagnosis and Evaluation of Hypertrophic Cardiomyopathy: JACC State-of-the-Art Review. J Am Coll Cardiol. 2022 Feb 1;79(4):372-389. PMID: 35086660

Case 141B

A 46-year-old male with a known history of hypertension presents to the clinic complaining of shortness of breath and chest pain that occurs during exertion. He mentions that he recently experienced a near-syncopal episode after jogging. His family history is significant for sudden cardiac death in his father at the age of 60. On examination, his blood pressure is 145/90 mm Hg, heart rate is 88 bpm, and respiratory rate is 18 breaths per minute. The cardiac examination reveals a bisferiens carotid pulse and a triple apical impulse. Auscultation of the heart demonstrates a loud S4 and a harsh systolic murmur along the left sternal border that increases with the Valsalva maneuver. An ECG shows left ventricular hypertrophy with deep, narrow Q waves in the lateral leads. An echocardiogram confirms left ventricular hypertrophy, predominantly of the septum, with systolic anterior motion of the mitral valve and a small, hypercontractile left ventricle.
What is the most appropriate next step in the management of this patient?

- A) Initiate high-dose statin therapy
- B) Begin beta-blocker therapy
- C) Perform an immediate coronary angiography
- D) Schedule the patient for septal myectomy surgery

The correct answer is B) Begin beta-blocker therapy. This patient presents with signs and symptoms consistent with hypertrophic cardiomyopathy (HCM), including exertional dyspnea, chest pain, a history of syncope, a bisferiens carotid pulse, a triple apical impulse, and a systolic murmur that increases with Valsalva maneuver. The ECG and echocardiogram findings support the diagnosis of HCM with left ventricular hypertrophy and systolic anterior motion of the mitral valve. Beta-blockers are a mainstay of treatment in HCM as they reduce heart rate, increase diastolic filling time, and decrease the left ventricular outflow tract gradient, which can alleviate symptoms and reduce the risk of arrhythmias. Option A) Initiate high-dose statin therapy is not indicated as the primary treatment for HCM. Statins are used for cholesterol management and the prevention of coronary artery disease, which is not the primary concern in this case. Option C) Perform an immediate coronary angiography is not the first-line investigation for HCM unless there is a suspicion of concomitant coronary artery disease, which is not indicated by the patient's presentation or diagnostic findings. Option D) Schedule the patient for septal myectomy surgery may be considered in patients with HCM who are symptomatic despite optimal medical therapy or who have severe left ventricular outflow tract obstruction. However, this is an invasive option and is not the first step in management before attempting medical therapy with beta-blockers. In conclusion, the most appropriate next step in the management of this patient with hypertrophic cardiomyopathy is to begin beta-blocker therapy to improve symptoms and reduce the risk of arrhythmias and potential sudden cardiac death. Diagnostic features of hypertrophic cardiomyopathy (HCM on echocardiogram include left ventricular hypertrophy (LVH), commonly affecting the septum more than the posterior walls, systolic anterior motion of the mitral valve, early closure followed by reopening of the aortic valve, a small and hypercontractile left ventricle, and delayed relaxation and filling of the left ventricle during diastole. Typically, the septal thickness is 1.3–1.5 times that of the posterior wall, with reduced septal motion. Doppler ultrasound can reveal turbulent flow, a dynamic gradient, and often mitral regurgitation in the left ventricular outflow tract, with 80% of patients showing abnormalities in diastolic filling patterns. Echocardiography aids in distinguishing HCM from ventricular noncompaction, a congenital myocardial disease characterized by trabeculation that incompletely fills the left ventricle cavity. Myocardial perfusion imaging can detect septal ischemia in the presence of normal coronary arteries. Cardiac MRI confirms hypertrophy, while contrast enhancement may reveal scarring where the right ventricle meets the interventricular septum. Cardiac catheterization helps confirm the diagnosis and assess for coronary artery disease (CAD), with coronary arterial bridging often seen in septal arteries during systole. Exercise studies are recommended to detect ventricular arrhythmias and assess blood pressure response, while loop monitoring is a valuable tool for identifying ventricular ectopy. These diagnostic modalities play a crucial role in accurately diagnosing and differentiating HCM from other cardiac conditions, guiding appropriate management strategies for patients with this complex cardiac disorder.

Case 141C

A 43-year-old female with a known diagnosis of hypertrophic cardiomyopathy (HCM) presents to the clinic with worsening exertional dyspnea and intermittent palpitations over the past 6 months. She has a history of paroxysmal atrial fibrillation and is currently on metoprolol 50 mg twice daily. On examination, her blood pressure is 130/80 mmHg, heart rate is 68 beats per minute, and she has a IV/VI systolic murmur best heard at the left sternal border that increases with the Valsalva maneuver. An echocardiogram reveals asymmetric septal hypertrophy with a maximum wall thickness of 2.1 cm, systolic anterior motion of the mitral valve, and a dynamic left ventricular outflow tract (LVOT) gradient of 85 mmHg at rest. There is mild mitral regurgitation and left atrial enlargement. Her LVEF is 70
Which of the following is the most appropriate next step in the management of this patient?

- A. Increase the dose of metoprolol to improve beta-blockade and reduce the LVOT gradient.
- B. Add verapamil to the regimen to improve diastolic filling and reduce the LVOT gradient.
- C. Initiate disopyramide in addition to metoprolol to reduce the LVOT gradient and control atrial arrhythmias.
- D. Start oral diuretics to manage symptoms related to elevated left atrial pressures.

The correct answer is C. Initiate disopyramide in addition to metoprolol to reduce the LVOT gradient and control atrial arrhythmias. This patient with HCM is symptomatic with exertional dyspnea and palpitations, which may be related to her paroxysmal atrial fibrillation and the dynamic LVOT obstruction. Disopyramide is a Class IA antiarrhythmic drug with negative inotropic effects, which can help reduce the LVOT gradient and improve symptoms in patients with HCM. It is particularly useful in patients who remain symptomatic despite beta-blocker therapy and have concomitant atrial arrhythmias, as in this case. Option A is incorrect because the patient is already on a moderate dose of metoprolol, and simply increasing the dose may not adequately control her symptoms or the LVOT gradient. Moreover, the patient's heart rate is well-controlled, suggesting that she is already receiving an adequate beta-blockade. Option B is incorrect because while verapamil can improve diastolic filling, it is contraindicated in patients with significant resting gradients (over 50 mmHg) due to the risk of exacerbating outflow obstruction and causing hypotension. This patient has a resting gradient of 85 mmHg, making verapamil a less suitable option. Option D is incorrect because while diuretics can help manage symptoms related to elevated left atrial pressures, they should be used cautiously in HCM due to the risk of reducing preload and exacerbating LVOT obstruction. The patient's primary issue seems to be the LVOT gradient and atrial arrhythmias, which would be more directly addressed with disopyramide. The initial treatment for symptomatic individuals with hypertrophic cardiomyopathy (HCM), particularly those with dynamic outflow obstruction as detected on echocardiogram, should consist of beta-blockers. Slowing cardiac rates facilitates the diastolic filling of the rigid left ventricle. Symptoms such as angina, dyspnea, and arrhythmias show a response rate of approximately 50% among patients. Calcium channel blockers like verapamil have demonstrated efficacy in managing symptomatic patients. Class I recommendations include verapamil and non-dihydropyridine calcium channel blockers, such as diltiazem. Although enhanced diastolic function is the primary cause of their effect, their vasodilatory mechanisms may also contribute to outflow obstruction and hypotension. Verapamil contraindications include hypotension and a resting gradient greater than 100 mm Hg. Negative inotropic effects contribute to disopyramide's efficacy; however, it is typically employed as a supplementary component to the medical regimen rather than as the sole treatment or to assist in the management of atrial arrhythmias. Due to the high LV diastolic pressure and elevated LA pressures, oral diuretics are often required; however, they must be administered with caution to prevent dehydration, which could worsen obstruction. With rare exceptions, digoxin is contraindicated for rate control in atrial fibrillation. In cases of acute hypotension unresponsive to fluid administration, phenylephrine may be considered. When HCM patients do not have outflow obstruction, comparable treatment should be administered only if they exhibit symptoms; oral diuretics are a safer alternative. A very small subset of these patients may be candidates for apical myomectomy. Patients respond most favorably to sinus rhythm, whereas atrial fibrillation necessitates prompt intervention via radiofrequency ablation or antiarrhythmics. The use of DOACs is preferred over warfarin in the event of atrial fibrillation. Treatment of patients with HCM is recommended irrespective of their CHA2DS2-VASc score.

Case 141D

A 32-year-old male with a diagnosis of hypertrophic cardiomyopathy (HCM) presents to the cardiology clinic for a follow-up visit. He has no personal history of syncope, ventricular arrhythmias, or cardiac arrest. However, his 45-year-old brother recently suffered a sudden cardiac death while playing basketball. On examination, his blood pressure is 125/75 mmHg, heart rate is 60 beats per minute, and he has a II/VI systolic murmur that increases with standing. An echocardiogram shows asymmetric septal hypertrophy with a maximum wall thickness of 28 mm and no left ventricular outflow tract obstruction at rest. His left ventricular ejection fraction is 60%. A cardiac MRI confirms the echocardiographic findings and shows no late gadolinium enhancement. The patient is an active individual who enjoys recreational basketball and inquires about his risk of sudden cardiac death and the need for an implantable cardioverter-defibrillator (ICD). Which of the following is the most appropriate next step in the management of this patient?

- A. Recommend an ICD based on the family history of sudden cardiac death and significant LV wall thickness.
- B. Advise against competitive sports and reassess the need for an ICD if late gadolinium enhancement develops on subsequent cardiac MRI.
- C. Prescribe an angiotensin-converting enzyme inhibitor to reduce myocardial hypertrophy and prevent sudden cardiac death.
- D. Schedule an electrophysiological study to stratify the risk of ventricular arrhythmias before deciding on ICD implantation.

The correct answer is A. Recommend an ICD based on the family history of sudden cardiac death and significant LV wall thickness. According to the 2020 AHA/ACC guidelines, this patient has two major risk factors for sudden cardiac death (SCD) in the context of HCM: a first-degree relative who suffered sudden cardiac death at an age younger than 50 years and significant left ventricular hypertrophy with a wall thickness of 28 mm (just 2 mm shy of the 30 mm threshold). These risk factors place him in a category where an ICD is a class IIa recommendation, meaning it is reasonable to consider ICD implantation to prevent SCD. Option B is incorrect because the patient already has sufficient risk factors for SCD, and waiting for late gadolinium enhancement to develop on cardiac MRI may delay necessary intervention. Additionally, advising against competitive sports is appropriate, but it does not address the immediate risk of SCD. Option C is incorrect because there is no evidence that angiotensin-converting enzyme inhibitors reduce myocardial hypertrophy or prevent SCD in patients with HCM. The primary treatment for HCM is to manage symptoms and prevent SCD with appropriate risk stratification and interventions. Option D is incorrect because electrophysiological studies are not routinely used for risk stratification in HCM. The decision to implant an ICD should be based on clinical risk factors, as outlined in the guidelines, rather than inducibility of ventricular arrhythmias on electrophysiological study. The 2020 AHA/ACC guidelines recommend the use of preventive implantable cardioverter-defibrillators (ICDs) for hypertrophic cardiomyopathy (HCM) patients diagnosed with sustained ventricular tachycardia (class I) or documented cardiac arrest. For class IIa patients, an ICD is advised if they have specific risk factors, including a family history of sudden death at a young age, left ventricular (LV) wall thickness of 30 mm or greater, recent syncope likely due to arrhythmias, LV apical aneurysm, or LV systolic dysfunction with an ejection fraction (EF) below 50%. If substantial late gadolinium enhancement on cardiac MRI is present (greater than 15%), it is a class IIb recommendation for an ICD. To reduce shocks, antitachycardia pacing should be programmed in ICD recipients. However, using an ICD solely to allow participation in competitive athletics is not advisable. Surgical myotomy-myomectomy can be performed by skilled surgeons for symptomatic patients unresponsive to standard medical therapy. Some surgeons advocate mitral valve replacement to eliminate associated gradients and mitral regurgitation. Myomectomy may involve Alfieri stitching on the mitral valve to join the midportion of the leaflets. Patients with severe symptoms or rare progression to left ventricular dilation may be candidates for cardiac transplantation. Septal ablation using alcohol injection into septal branches of the left coronary artery is a nonsurgical option for thick-walled areas with refractory LV outflow tract obstruction exceeding 50 mm Hg when medical or surgical interventions are not feasible. For "burned out" HCM cases resembling dilated cardiomyopathy, similar medical management is recommended. Cardiac transplantation is a viable option for patients with heart failure (HF) or refractory arrhythmias. Pregnant individuals with symptoms or outflow tract gradients over 50 mm Hg are at higher risk and should undergo genetic counseling before planned pregnancy. Pregnant HCM patients should continue beta-blocker therapy for optimal management.

Ommen SR et al.2020 AHA/ACC Guideline for the Diagnosis and Treatment of Patients With Hypertrophic Cardiomyopathy: Executive Summary: A Report of the American College of Cardiology/American Heart Association Joint Committee on Clinical Practice Guidelines. Circulation. 2020 Dec 22;142(25):e533-e557. PMID: 33215938

8.21 A Case of Progressive Dyspnea and Edema in an Elderly Woman

Case 142

A 65-year-old woman presents with progressive dyspnea on exertion and bilateral lower extremity edema over the past six months. She has a past medical history of hypertension and type 2 diabetes mellitus. On physical examination, her blood pressure is 130/80 mmHg, heart rate is 88 beats per minute, and jugular venous pressure is elevated. A pericardial knock is not appreciated. Cardiac auscultation reveals a low-pitched, rumbling diastolic murmur at the apex. There is no pulsus paradoxus. The liver is palpable 3 cm below the right costal margin, and there is pitting edema up to the shins. An electrocardiogram shows low voltage QRS complexes and nonspecific ST-T wave abnormalities. An echocardiogram demonstrates normal left ventricular size with increased ventricular wall thickness, biatrial enlargement, and normal systolic function but impaired diastolic filling. Doppler imaging shows a restrictive filling pattern. The pulmonary artery systolic pressure is estimated at 45 mmHg. Serum brain natriuretic peptide (BNP) is elevated.
What is the most appropriate next step in the diagnosis of this patient's condition?

- A. Cardiac magnetic resonance imaging (MRI)
- B. Right heart catheterization
- C. Endomyocardial biopsy
- D. Serum and urine protein electrophoresis with immunofixation

Correct Answer: D. Serum and urine protein electrophoresis with immunofixation The patient's clinical presentation and echocardiographic findings are suggestive of restrictive cardiomyopathy, which can be caused by infiltrative diseases such as amyloidosis. The absence of a pericardial knock and pulsus paradoxus makes constrictive pericarditis less likely. The presence of a restrictive filling pattern on Doppler imaging, along with increased ventricular wall thickness and biatrial enlargement, further supports the diagnosis of restrictive cardiomyopathy.

The elevated pulmonary artery pressure is consistent with the increased left ventricular filling pressures often seen in restrictive cardiomyopathy, which can lead to pulmonary hypertension. The nonspecific ST-T wave abnormalities and low voltage on the ECG are also common in amyloidosis due to the infiltration of the myocardium.

Given the suspicion of amyloidosis, the most appropriate next step is to perform serum and urine protein electrophoresis with immunofixation. This test can detect monoclonal proteins, which are present in the majority of patients with AL (primary) amyloidosis. The identification of a monoclonal protein spike is crucial for the diagnosis and will guide further management, including potential chemotherapy for AL amyloidosis.

While cardiac MRI (Option A) can offer additional insights into tissue characteristics and potentially indicate amyloidosis, it is not definitive for diagnosis. Right heart catheterization (Option B) can aid in distinguishing between restrictive cardiomyopathy and constrictive pericarditis by assessing hemodynamics, but its invasive nature makes it unnecessary at this stage. Endomyocardial biopsy (Option C) is considered the gold standard for diagnosing restrictive cardiomyopathy; however, it is typically reserved for situations where the diagnosis remains uncertain after noninvasive tests or when treatment decisions hinge on biopsy results. Given the high clinical suspicion of amyloidosis in this case, initial noninvasive serum and urine tests for monoclonal proteins should be conducted.

Frequent conduction abnormalities are commonly observed. The presence of both low ECG voltage and echocardiographic ventricular hypertrophy is indicative of disease. Technetium pyrophosphate imaging (bone scan imaging) has emerged as the preferred noninvasive imaging method for detecting amyloid deposition in the myocardium, particularly in transthyretin amyloidosis cases where typical scintigraphic findings obviate the need for biopsy in the absence of monoclonal gammopathy.

Cardiac MRI serves as a valuable screening tool, revealing a distinct pattern of diffuse gadolinium hyperenhancement in amyloidosis. Extensive late gadolinium hyperenhancement signifies more extensive cardiac involvement. Echocardiography may show biatrial enlargement, rapid early diastolic filling (via mitral inflow Doppler), and a small, thickened left ventricle with speckled myocardium. Unique longitudinal strain patterns in cardiac amyloidosis can aid in diagnosis. Atrial septal hypertrophy may be evident, with a variant affecting primarily the atria identified. While extracardiac biopsies can confirm systemic involvement, a negative result does not exclude myocardial participation; thus, endomyocardial biopsy remains crucial for confirming cardiac amyloid presence. Immunohistochemical analyses and genetic testing are essential post-biopsy to identify the specific protein involved. Patients suspected of TTR wild type or variant should undergo TTR gene sequencing and mass spectroscopy on relevant tissues. Elevated BNP and NT-proBNP levels have historically aided in distinguishing constrictive pericarditis from restrictive cardiomyopathy.

Rapezzi C et al. Restrictive cardiomyopathy: definition and diagnosis. Eur Heart J. 2022 Dec 1;43(45):4679-4693. PMID: 36269634

8.22 Management of Heart Failure in a Patient with AL Amyloidosis

Case 143

A 58-year-old man with a history of chronic heart failure presents with worsening dyspnea, fatigue, and bilateral lower extremity edema. He was recently hospitalized for a heart failure exacerbation and was discharged on a regimen of furosemide, spironolactone, and carvedilol. Despite adherence to his medications and dietary restrictions, he reports a weight gain of 5 kg over the past month. His blood pressure is 105/70 mmHg, heart rate is 88 bpm, and he has an irregularly irregular pulse. Physical examination reveals jugular venous distension, bibasilar crackles, an S3 gallop, and 3+ pitting edema up to the mid-shins. Laboratory tests show a serum creatinine of 1.8 mg/dL (baseline 1.2 mg/dL), BNP of 900 pg/mL, and an INR of 1.0. An echocardiogram shows increased ventricular wall thickness with a speckled appearance, biatrial enlargement, and a small pericardial effusion. The ejection fraction is preserved. An electrocardiogram demonstrates atrial fibrillation with a ventricular rate of 110 bpm and low QRS voltages. A fat pad biopsy confirms the diagnosis of AL amyloidosis.
What is the most appropriate next step in the management of this patient's heart failure?

- A. Increase the dose of furosemide.
- B. Initiate anticoagulation with warfarin.
- C. Start treatment with tafamidis.
- D. Discontinue carvedilol and start verapamil.

Correct Answer: B. Initiate anticoagulation with warfarin. This patient with AL amyloidosis presents with signs and symptoms of worsening heart failure and atrial fibrillation. In amyloidosis, the deposition of amyloid fibrils in the myocardium leads to diastolic dysfunction and heart failure with preserved ejection fraction (HFpEF). Atrial fibrillation is common in amyloidosis due to atrial infiltration and dysfunction, which increases the risk of thromboembolic events, including stroke. Given the presence of atrial fibrillation and heart failure, which are both risk factors for thrombus formation, anticoagulation is indicated to reduce the risk of stroke.

Option A, increasing the dose of furosemide, may seem appropriate given the signs of volume overload. However, excessive diuresis in amyloidosis can lead to worsening renal function and hypotension due to the restrictive physiology and limited cardiac output. The patient's current blood pressure is on the lower side, and his renal function has worsened, suggesting that he may already be experiencing the adverse effects of aggressive diuresis.

Option C, starting treatment with tafamidis, is a treatment for transthyretin amyloidosis (ATTR), not AL amyloidosis. This patient has AL amyloidosis, as confirmed by the fat pad biopsy, so tafamidis would not be appropriate.

Option D, discontinuing carvedilol and starting verapamil, is not recommended. Beta-blockers are generally beneficial in heart failure for rate control, especially in the presence of atrial fibrillation. Verapamil is a non-dihydropyridine calcium channel blocker that can negatively affect systolic function and is generally avoided in patients with heart failure. Additionally, verapamil can increase the risk of bradycardia and exacerbate heart failure symptoms. Therefore, the most appropriate next step in the management of this patient's heart failure, given the new onset of atrial fibrillation and the increased risk of thromboembolism, is to initiate anticoagulation with warfarin. This decision should be made after careful consideration of the patient's bleeding risk and potential need for close monitoring of renal function and anticoagulation levels. Alkylator-based chemotherapy or high-dose melphalan, followed by autologous stem cell transplantation, are viable treatment options for AL amyloidosis. Stem cell rescue combined with standard or high-dose chemotherapy is commonly used in the management of immunoglobulin light-chain amyloidosis. The treatment landscape for ATTR amyloidosis is evolving. Tafamidis is currently approved to prevent the misfolding of the TTR tetramer, while Patisiran offers an alternative by inhibiting the synthesis of both variant and wild-type TTR. Inotersen, administered subcutaneously, can address variant TTR polyneuropathy by binding to TTR mRNA and inhibiting its transcription. In cases of acute heart failure, diuretics can be effective; however, caution is advised as excessive diuresis may worsen kidney function. Aldosterone antagonists, loop diuretics, and thiazides are beneficial for most patients with severe right heart failure. While atrial thrombi are common, the role of anticoagulation in amyloidosis remains uncertain. Digoxin should be avoided due to the risk of precipitating arrhythmias. Beta-blockers can help prolong diastolic time, slowing heart rate and improving filling. Verapamil likely promotes myocardial relaxation and delays diastolic filling time. The goal of maintaining a lower heart rate is to allow for extended diastolic filling time. Inhibiting ACE or blocking angiotensin II receptors may enhance diastolic relaxation and filling; these approaches can be considered cautiously if systemic blood pressure is stable. Corticosteroids have shown greater efficacy in managing conduction abnormalities associated with sarcoidosis compared to heart failure.

Rapezzi C et al. Restrictive cardiomyopathy: definition and diagnosis. Eur Heart J. 2022 Dec 1;43(45):4679-4693. PMID: 36269634

Case 143B

A 68-year-old man presents with progressive shortness of breath, lower extremity edema, and fatigue over the past 6 months. His medical history is significant for hypertension and chronic kidney disease stage 3. Physical examination reveals jugular venous distension, bibasilar crackles, and 2+ pitting edema in the lower extremities. Echocardiography shows concentric left ventricular hypertrophy, biatrial enlargement, and a restrictive filling pattern consistent with cardiac amyloidosis. Serum and urine protein electrophoresis reveal a monoclonal spike, and a fat pad biopsy confirms AL (light chain) amyloidosis. Which of the following is the most appropriate next step in management?

- A. Initiate high-dose melphalan followed by autologous stem cell transplantation
- B. Start tafamidis to prevent transthyretin misfolding
- C. Prescribe patisiran to inhibit transthyretin production
- D. Administer inotersen subcutaneously to bind transthyretin mRNA

The best answer is A. Initiate high-dose melphalan followed by autologous stem cell transplantation. This is the most appropriate next step in management for this patient with AL (immunoglobulin light chain) amyloidosis based on the clinical presentation and diagnostic findings. Rationale: AL amyloidosis is caused by misfolded immunoglobulin light chains produced by an underlying plasma cell dyscrasia. The treatment aims to reduce or eliminate the pathogenic light chain production by targeting the underlying clonal plasma cell disorder. High-dose melphalan followed by autologous stem cell transplantation (HDM/ASCT) is considered the standard of care for newly diagnosed AL amyloidosis patients who are eligible candidates. HDM/ASCT leads to deeper hematologic responses and improved survival compared to conventional chemotherapy regimens. The other options are not appropriate for this patient with AL amyloidosis: B) Tafamidis is indicated for the treatment of transthyretin amyloid cardiomyopathy (ATTR), not AL amyloidosis. It stabilizes the tetrameric structure of transthyretin and prevents dissociation into monomers that can misfold and form amyloid fibrils. C) Patisiran is an RNA interference therapeutic that inhibits the production of both wild-type and mutant transthyretin. It is approved for the treatment of hereditary ATTR amyloidosis with polyneuropathy, not AL amyloidosis. D) Inotersen is a antisense oligonucleotide that binds to transthyretin mRNA, preventing its translation. It is used for the treatment of hereditary transthyretin amyloidosis with polyneuropathy, not AL amyloidosis caused by light chain deposition. In summary, for a patient with newly diagnosed AL amyloidosis who is an eligible candidate, high-dose melphalan followed by autologous stem cell transplantation is the preferred treatment approach to target the underlying clonal plasma cell disorder and reduce light chain production, thereby preventing further amyloid deposition and potentially improving outcomes. The treatment of AL amyloidosis, a rare and serious condition characterized by the abnormal deposition of amyloid proteins in various organs, can be associated with several potential side effects. These side effects can vary depending on the specific treatment regimen employed, which may include chemotherapy drugs, immunomodulatory agents, steroids, and stem cell transplantation. Careful monitoring and supportive care are crucial in managing these potential toxicities.

Gastrointestinal Side Effects

- Nausea and vomiting
- Diarrhea or constipation
- Loss of appetite
- Taste changes

Hematologic Side Effects

Low blood counts (anemia, neutropenia, thrombocytopenia) leading to fatigue, increased infection risk, and bleeding/bruising

Peripheral Neuropathy

- Numbness, tingling, and pain in the hands and feet
- Caused by certain chemotherapies like bortezomib

Kidney Problems

- Worsening kidney function
- Protein in the urine

Steroid Side Effects (from dexamethasone, prednisone)

- Increased appetite and weight gain
- Insomnia and restlessness
- High blood sugar
- Mood changes
- Increased infection risk

Fertility Issues

- Early menopause in women
- Low sperm count in men

General Side Effects

- Fatigue and weakness
- Hair loss
- Skin changes like rash and bruising
- Increased infection risk

The severity of these side effects can vary based on the specific treatment regimen used, which may include chemotherapy drugs like melphalan, cyclophosphamide, bortezomib, immunomodulatory drugs like lenalidomide, steroids, and stem cell transplantation. Careful monitoring and supportive care are essential to manage these potential toxicities effectively.

9

VASCULAR DISEASES

9.1 Progressing Intermittent Claudication: Evaluating Treatment Options

Case 144

A 72-year-old man with a history of smoking and controlled hypertension presents with a 6-month history of intermittent claudication. His symptoms have progressively worsened, and he now experiences pain in his calves after walking less than two blocks, which was previously not the case. He denies any rest pain or non-healing wounds on his feet. His physical examination reveals diminished femoral pulses bilaterally and absent popliteal and pedal pulses. Ankle-brachial index (ABI) is 0.55 on the right and 0.58 on the left. A computed tomography angiogram (CTA) of the abdomen and pelvis shows extensive calcified plaques and bilateral severe stenosis of the common iliac arteries. The patient has tried supervised exercise therapy for the past 3 months without significant improvement in his symptoms.
What is the most appropriate next step in the management of this patient's peripheral arterial disease (PAD)?

- A. Continue supervised exercise therapy and add cilostazol.
- B. Schedule for aorto-femoral bypass surgery.
- C. Perform percutaneous transluminal angioplasty (PTA) with stenting of the iliac arteries.
- D. Initiate a trial of high-dose statin therapy and reassess in 6 months.

Correct Answer: B. Schedule for aorto-femoral bypass surgery. This patient presents with lifestyle-limiting intermittent claudication due to severe bilateral common iliac artery stenosis, as evidenced by a low ABI and confirmed by CTA. Given the extensive nature of the disease and the failure of supervised exercise therapy, which is a first-line treatment for claudication, more invasive options should be considered.

Option A, continuing supervised exercise therapy and adding cilostazol, is a reasonable non-invasive approach for PAD with intermittent claudication. However, this patient has already failed to improve with exercise therapy, and while cilostazol can improve symptoms, it is unlikely to provide significant relief given the severity of the stenosis.

Option C, performing PTA with stenting, is less invasive than surgery and may be considered for patients with focal stenosis. However, the scenario describes extensive disease, and endovascular approaches are less durable in such cases, with higher recurrence rates.

Option D, initiating high-dose statin therapy, is an important part of medical management for PAD to reduce cardiovascular risk, but it is unlikely to provide immediate or significant symptomatic relief for severe bilateral stenosis and would not be the most appropriate next step for someone with lifestyle-limiting claudication.

Therefore, the most appropriate next step is Option B, scheduling for aorto-femoral bypass surgery. This procedure is highly effective and durable, particularly in patients with extensive aortoiliac disease, and can provide excellent symptomatic relief. The patient's symptoms have progressed to the point where they significantly limit his lifestyle, and surgical intervention is warranted to improve his quality of life and walking distance. While there is a risk of complications, the mortality rate is relatively low, and the long-term patency rate is high.

The ankle-brachial index (ABI), a measure of the ratio between systolic blood pressure at the ankle and the brachial artery, typically falls below 0.9 during Doppler examination (with the normal range being 0.9–1.2). This discrepancy is often exacerbated by physical activity. When assessing ABI, pressures from both the dorsalis pedis and posterior tibial arteries are taken into account, with the calculation based on the higher of the two values. Utilizing segmental waveforms or pulse volume recordings through blood pressure monitors and strain gauge technology can reveal reduced arterial inflow to the lower extremities.

Magnetic resonance angiography (MRA) and CT angiography (CTA) are valuable tools for pinpointing the specific anatomical location of arterial disease. Duplex ultrasound imaging of the aortoiliac segment may be limited by bowel interference. Imaging is typically reserved for cases where symptoms necessitate intervention; otherwise, a combination of medical history, physical examination, and vascular testing can accurately identify affected areas within the arterial tree. Focal atherosclerotic lesions in the aortic or iliac regions can often be effectively treated with angioplasty and stenting. While this approach yields favorable surgical outcomes for single stenoses, its effectiveness may diminish with prolonged or multiple stenoses. For cases requiring bypass surgery, a prosthetic aorto-femoral graft is a highly successful and durable option, bypassing diseased segments in the iliac or aorta. In instances of unilateral iliac disease, patients may benefit from grafts originating from femoral arteries or contralateral femoral arteries (such as axillo-femoral or femoral-femoral bypass grafts). These procedures carry reduced operative risks compared to those involving abdominal entry and aortic clamping; however, they may result in grafts with slightly inferior durability.

Shi R et al.Modern approaches and innovations in the diagnosis and treatment of peripheral vascular diseases. Front Biosci (Schol Ed). 2021 Dec 3;13(2):173-180. PMID: 34879469.

Case 144B

A 68-year-old male with a history of diabetes mellitus and chronic kidney disease presents with a 1-year history of intermittent claudication. He reports calf pain after walking approximately one block, which resolves with rest. He has tried a supervised exercise program for the past 6 months with minimal improvement. His medications include aspirin, metformin, and atorvastatin. On physical examination, his blood pressure is 142/86 mmHg, heart rate is 78 bpm, and he has diminished hair growth on his lower extremities. The skin on his feet is shiny and atrophic. His right foot appears dusky when elevated and becomes ruborous when dependent. Palpation reveals a normal right common femoral pulse, but his right popliteal and pedal pulses are not palpable. Ankle-brachial index (ABI) on the right is 0.35. Duplex ultrasonography of the right leg shows occlusion of the superficial femoral artery with reconstitution at the popliteal artery.
What is the most appropriate next step in the management of this patient's peripheral arterial disease (PAD)?

- A. Increase the dose of atorvastatin and continue the exercise program.
- B. Add cilostazol to the current regimen.
- C. Refer for percutaneous transluminal angioplasty (PTA) with possible stenting of the superficial femoral artery.
- D. Begin dual antiplatelet therapy with clopidogrel and continue the exercise program.

Correct Answer: C. Refer for percutaneous transluminal angioplasty (PTA) with possible stenting of the superficial femoral artery. This patient has chronic limb-threatening ischemia (CLTI) as evidenced by an ABI of 0.35 and symptoms of intermittent claudication after walking one block, which indicates severe ischemia. The duplex ultrasonography findings of occlusion of the superficial femoral artery with reconstitution at the popliteal artery further support the diagnosis of CLTI. Option A, increasing the dose of atorvastatin and continuing the exercise program, is part of the standard medical therapy for PAD. However, this patient has already been on high-dose statin therapy and has not had significant improvement with exercise therapy alone. Option B, adding cilostazol, may improve symptoms of intermittent claudication, but given the severity of the patient's symptoms and the low ABI, medical therapy alone is unlikely to be sufficient. Cilostazol is also contraindicated in patients with heart failure, which needs to be considered in patients with PAD due to the common risk factors. Option D, beginning dual antiplatelet therapy with clopidogrel, is not indicated in this scenario. While dual antiplatelet therapy may be used in certain settings, such as after revascularization, there is no evidence to suggest that it would be beneficial in this patient who has not yet undergone revascularization. Therefore, the most appropriate next step is Option C, referring the patient for PTA with possible stenting. This patient's lifestyle-limiting claudication and evidence of severe ischemia on ABI and duplex ultrasonography indicate that he is likely to benefit from revascularization. PTA with or without stenting is a less invasive option compared to surgical bypass and can provide significant symptom relief and improve quality of life in patients with CLTI. Mitigating risk factors is crucial in the management of peripheral artery disease (PAD). This includes quitting smoking, using antiplatelet therapy, controlling lipids and blood pressure, and achieving weight loss. While primary prevention of cardiovascular disease is no longer recommended, antiplatelet agents like clopidogrel or low-dose aspirin (81 mg orally daily) remain vital for reducing peripheral vascular morbidity and preventing cardiovascular events in PAD patients. Symptomatic individuals may benefit from combining low-dose rivaroxaban (2.5 mg orally twice daily) with aspirin to reduce cardiovascular and limb-related adverse events. All PAD patients should receive a high-dose statin such as atorvastatin 80 mg daily (if tolerated) to manage hypercholesterolemia and arterial inflammation. Cilostazol (100 mg twice daily orally) may improve walking distance in about two-thirds of patients, with full effects potentially taking up to 12 weeks to manifest. Supervised exercise programs have shown to be more effective than endovascular treatments alone in alleviating pain, increasing walking distance, and improving quality of life for PAD patients. A structured regimen involving 30–45 minutes of walking three days a week for at least 12 weeks is recommended. Alternative exercises like upper-body ergometry and cycling can also be beneficial. A patient-facing mobile application, the Society for Vascular Surgery Supervised Exercise Therapy App, may prove beneficial.

Sontheimer DL. Peripheral vascular disease: diagnosis and treatment. Am Fam Physician. 2006 Jun 1;73(11):1971-6. PMID: 16770929

9.2 Acute Limb Ischemia in a Patient with Chronic Atrial Fibrillation

Case 145

A 73-year-old woman with a history of chronic atrial fibrillation, for which she is not on anticoagulation due to a prior intracranial hemorrhage, presents to the emergency department with a 3-hour history of severe right leg pain. She reports no recent trauma or injury. On examination, her right leg is pale, cold to the touch, and mottled with absent pulses distal to the femoral artery. She is unable to move her toes or feel light touch. Her left leg is normal. Her vital signs are stable, and she is afebrile. Doppler ultrasound of the right leg shows no flow in the popliteal, anterior tibial, or posterior tibial arteries. Laboratory tests reveal a serum creatinine of 1.9 mg/dL (elevated from a baseline of 1.2 mg/dL), a potassium of 5.8 mEq/L, and an arterial blood gas showing metabolic acidosis with a pH of 7.28.
What is the most appropriate next step in the management of this patient's condition?

- A. Immediate heparinization and vascular surgery consultation for possible embolectomy.
- B. Intravenous administration of tissue plasminogen activator (tPA).
- C. Obtain a computed tomography angiogram (CTA) to confirm the diagnosis of arterial occlusion.
- D. Start broad-spectrum antibiotics and admit to the hospital for observation.

Correct Answer: A. Immediate heparinization and vascular surgery consultation for possible embolectomy. This patient presents with signs and symptoms consistent with acute limb ischemia (ALI), likely secondary to an embolic event given her history of atrial fibrillation and the absence of anticoagulation. The clinical findings of a pale, cold, mottled leg with absent pulses and impaired neurologic function are indicative of severe ischemia and the need for urgent intervention to prevent irreversible damage and potential limb loss.

Option A is the correct answer because immediate heparinization will help to prevent propagation of the thrombus and reduce the risk of further embolic events. An urgent vascular surgery consultation is necessary for possible embolectomy, which is the treatment of choice for acute embolic occlusion of a major artery.

Option B, intravenous administration of tPA, is a thrombolytic therapy that could be considered in certain cases of ALI. However, given the severity of the patient's presentation and the high risk of limb loss, immediate surgical intervention is preferred over thrombolytic therapy, which can take time to work and has a risk of bleeding, especially in a patient with a history of intracranial hemorrhage.

Option C, obtaining a CTA, is not appropriate as the first step because it may delay definitive treatment. While CTA can confirm the diagnosis and define the anatomy, the clinical presentation is already highly suggestive of ALI, and immediate treatment should not be delayed for imaging.

Option D, starting broad-spectrum antibiotics, is not indicated at this time as there is no evidence of infection. The patient's presentation is consistent with ALI, not an infectious process, and antibiotics would not address the underlying issue. Therefore, the most appropriate next step is immediate heparinization and vascular surgery consultation for possible embolectomy to restore perfusion and minimize the risk of limb loss. Due to the presence of an embolus or thrombosis within a diseased atherosclerotic segment, there is a risk of acute occlusion. When emboli are large enough to block proximal arteries in the lower extremities, they typically originate from the heart, with atrial fibrillation being a primary cause of cardiac thrombus formation. Valvular disease and thrombus formation on the ventricular surface following a significant anterior myocardial infarction also contribute to this condition. Smaller emboli from arterial sources, such as calcified excrescences or arterial ulcerations, tend to travel to the distal arterial tree (toes). Patients experiencing primary thrombosis often report a sudden worsening of symptoms and a history of claudication. In cases of chronic stenosis, collateral blood vessels develop, leading to a gradual occlusion that may cause only mild symptom exacerbation. Doppler examination of distal vessels may show minimal or negligible blood flow. Imaging studies can reveal a sudden lack of contrast in the presence of embolic occlusion. Blood tests may detect metabolic acidosis and myoglobinemia. Immediate revascularization is crucial in all cases of symptomatic acute arterial thrombosis. If neurologic injury symptoms like loss of light touch sensation are present, indicating inadequate collateral flow to sustain limb viability, revascularization should be performed within three hours to prevent irreversible tissue damage, which can approach 100% after six hours. An initial intravenous bolus of unfractionated heparin (80 U/kg) should be administered immediately following the diagnosis. Subsequently, a continuous heparin infusion should be maintained to ensure that the activated partial thromboplastin time (aPTT) remains within the therapeutic range of 60–85 seconds (12–18 units/kg/hour). This prevents the spread of clots and may also alleviate vessel spasms that are associated with them. Although anticoagulation may alleviate symptoms, revascularization will ultimately be necessary.

Ferrer C et al. Acute ischemia of the upper and lower limbs: Tailoring the treatment to the underlying etiology. Semin Vasc Surg. 2023 Jun;36(2):211-223. PMID: 37330235

9.3 Management of Asymptomatic Carotid Stenosis

Case 146

A 67-year-old man with a history of hypertension and hyperlipidemia presents to the clinic for a routine follow-up. He has no history of cerebrovascular symptoms. His medications include lisinopril and atorvastatin. On physical examination, a bruit is auscultated over the right carotid artery. His neurological examination is normal. Duplex ultrasonography of the carotid arteries reveals 70% stenosis of the right internal carotid artery. The patient is asymptomatic with no history of transient ischemic attacks (TIAs) or stroke. His life expectancy is greater than 5 years, and he is interested in any interventions that may reduce his risk of future stroke.
What is the most appropriate next step in the management of this patient's carotid stenosis?

- A. Initiate antiplatelet therapy with aspirin and schedule for carotid endarterectomy (CEA).
- B. Obtain a confirmatory computed tomography angiogram (CTA) or magnetic resonance angiography (MRA) of the carotid arteries.
- C. Increase the dose of atorvastatin to achieve LDL cholesterol ¡70 mg/dL and continue to monitor with duplex ultrasonography.
- D. Refer for carotid artery stenting given the patient's preference for less invasive procedures.

Correct Answer: B. Obtain a confirmatory computed tomography angiogram (CTA) or magnetic resonance angiography (MRA) of the carotid arteries. This patient has asymptomatic carotid stenosis of 70% as detected by duplex ultrasonography. While large studies have shown a reduction in the 5-year stroke rate with surgical treatment of asymptomatic carotid stenosis greater than 60%, the decision to intervene depends on an accurate assessment of the degree of stenosis. Given the potential risks associated with carotid intervention, it is crucial to confirm the degree of stenosis with a second imaging modality before proceeding with invasive procedures.

Option A, initiating antiplatelet therapy with aspirin and scheduling for CEA, is premature without confirmation of the degree of stenosis by another imaging modality. While CEA may be beneficial for patients with significant asymptomatic carotid stenosis, the indication is based on accurate measurement of the degree of stenosis.

Option C, increasing the dose of atorvastatin to achieve LDL cholesterol ¡70 mg/dL, is part of aggressive risk factor modification and is recommended for patients with carotid stenosis. However, this does not address the immediate need to confirm the degree of stenosis before considering an intervention.

Option D, referring for carotid artery stenting, may be considered in certain patients, particularly those who are not good candidates for surgery. However, as with CEA, the degree of stenosis should be confirmed with another imaging modality before proceeding with this less invasive procedure.

Therefore, the most appropriate next step is Option B, obtaining a confirmatory CTA or MRA. This will provide a more comprehensive assessment of the cerebrovascular anatomy and confirm the degree of stenosis. If the stenosis is confirmed to be greater than 60%, and the patient's surgical risk is low, he may benefit from carotid intervention, considering his life expectancy is greater than 5 years.

Stroke rates have shown a significant decrease from 11.5% to 5% over a five-year period when surgical treatment for asymptomatic carotid stenosis surpasses 60%, as indicated by extensive studies. Patients with a life expectancy exceeding five years and a low risk of complications related to intervention may derive benefits from carotid intervention. For such individuals, aggressive management of risk factors, including the use of high-potency statins, could be equally advantageous compared to surgical procedures. The CREST2 study, strongly endorsed by the NIH, is actively investigating this aspect. In cases of mild to moderate disease (30–50% stenosis), ongoing monitoring and proactive adjustment of risk factors are essential. The presence of acutely worsening carotid stenosis suggests an unstable plaque, significantly elevating the risk of embolic stroke for the patient. For symptomatic individuals: Patients who have experienced TIAs or strokes and have fully or nearly fully recovered may benefit from carotid intervention if the ipsilateral carotid artery exhibits a stenosis of at least 70%. They are also likely to benefit if the stenosis ranges from 50% to 69%, based on findings from large randomized trials. Evidence supports that carotid endarterectomy (CEA) and, in specific cases, carotid artery stenting can effectively and durably prevent subsequent events in these scenarios. Planning interventions for symptomatic patients should ideally occur within two weeks, as delaying increases the risk of recurrence.

Ismail A et al. Carotid Artery Stenosis: A Look Into the Diagnostic and Management Strategies, and Related Complications. Cureus. 2023 May 9;15(5):e38794. PMID: 37303351

9.4 Management of Acute Abdominal Pain in a Patient with Atrial Fibrillation

Case 147

A 72-year-old woman with a history of atrial fibrillation and previous myocardial infarction presents to the emergency department with sudden onset of severe, diffuse abdominal pain that began 6 hours ago. She describes the pain as steady and unrelenting. She has a history of chronic, postprandial abdominal pain for which she did not seek medical attention. Her current medications include aspirin and metoprolol. On examination, her abdomen is soft with minimal tenderness to palpation, but she appears to be in significant distress. Her vital signs reveal a blood pressure of 100/60 mmHg, heart rate of 110 bpm, and a respiratory rate of 22 breaths per minute. Laboratory tests show a white blood cell count of 16,000/uL, serum lactate of 5 mmol/L, and a normal lipase. An electrocardiogram shows atrial fibrillation with a rapid ventricular response. What is the most appropriate next step in the management of this patient's condition?

- A. Immediate surgical consultation and consideration for exploratory laparotomy.
- B. Administration of broad-spectrum antibiotics and fluid resuscitation.
- C. Computed tomography angiography (CTA) of the abdomen to assess for mesenteric ischemia.
- D. Upper endoscopy to evaluate for possible peptic ulcer disease.

Correct Answer: C. Computed tomography angiography (CTA) of the abdomen to assess for mesenteric ischemia. This patient presents with symptoms suggestive of acute mesenteric ischemia (AMI), which is a vascular emergency. The clinical picture of severe, diffuse abdominal pain with minimal physical findings ("pain out of proportion"), a high white blood cell count, and elevated lactate levels is classic for AMI. Given her history of atrial fibrillation, she is at risk for embolic phenomena, which could include an embolism to the mesenteric vessels.

Option A, immediate surgical consultation and consideration for exploratory laparotomy, may be necessary if the patient were hemodynamically unstable or if there were signs of peritonitis, which would suggest bowel infarction. However, without imaging to confirm the diagnosis, exploratory surgery may not be the most appropriate initial step.

Option B, administration of broad-spectrum antibiotics and fluid resuscitation, is part of the management of sepsis and may be part of the supportive care for AMI, but it does not address the need for a definitive diagnosis.

Option D, upper endoscopy, is not indicated at this time as the patient's presentation is not consistent with peptic ulcer disease, and it would not be the appropriate modality to diagnose AMI. Therefore, the most appropriate next step is Option C, a CTA of the abdomen. This imaging modality can rapidly provide detailed information about the mesenteric vasculature and can help confirm the diagnosis of AMI, differentiate between embolic and thrombotic causes, and guide further management, which may include surgical intervention or endovascular therapy. Prompt diagnosis and treatment are critical to improve outcomes in AMI due to the high risk of bowel infarction and mortality associated with delayed treatment.

- Acute mesenteric ischemia presents with visceral arterial embolism, where severe abdominal pain is the primary symptom. Conversely, individuals with primary visceral arterial thrombosis often have a medical history indicative of chronic mesenteric ischemia. The acute form is characterized by diffuse, persistent, and intense abdominal pain without focal tenderness or distention. The concept of "pain out of proportion" to physical exam findings occurs because initial ischemia affects the mucosa before involving the peritoneum, leading to inflammation.

Diagnosis may involve lactic acidosis, abdominal distention, elevated WBC count, or hypotension.

- Chronic mesenteric ischemia typically affects individuals over 45 years old, often showing signs of atherosclerosis in other arteries. Symptoms include postprandial epigastric or periumbilical discomfort lasting one to three hours. Patients may reduce food intake to ease pain and may develop an aversion to eating, leading to weight loss. Severe cases can lead to dehydration, potentially causing hypotension and acute thrombosis.
- Ischemic colitis manifests as intestinal cramping, tenderness, and discomfort in the left lower quadrant, along with mild diarrhea (bloody or non-bloody) and abdominal cramping. Rectal discharge may appear viscous or bloody in nature.

1. Acute mesenteric ischemia—Immediate exploration to evaluate bowel viability is required in the presence of a strong suspicion of acute mesenteric ischemia. In the event that the bowel retains its viability, arterial bypass can be performed via a prosthetic conduit connecting the celiac and superior mesentery arteries via the supra-celiac aorta or common iliac artery. Although angioplasty and stenting of the arteries may be utilized, a surgical evaluation of bowel viability is still required.
2. Chronic mesenteric ischemia—Depending on the anatomical characteristics of the stenosis, angioplasty and stenting of the proximal vessel might be advantageous. When an endovascular solution is unavailable, the most preferable course of treatment is an aorto-visceral artery bypass. Extremely durable long-term results are observed.
3. Management of ischemic colitis—Until collateral circulation becomes well-established, blood pressure and perfusion maintenance are the cornerstones of treatment. It is critical to closely monitor the patient for any indications of perforation that could require resection.

Bala M et al. Acute mesenteric ischemia: updated guidelines of the World Society of Emergency Surgery. World J Emerg Surg. 2022 Oct 19;17(1):54. PMID: 36261857;

9.5 Management of Infrarenal Abdominal Aortic Aneurysm

Case 148

A 65-year-old man with a history of hypertension and smoking presents to his primary care physician for a routine health maintenance visit. He has no complaints and is asymptomatic. His blood pressure is well controlled on lisinopril, and he has a 30-pack-year smoking history. On examination, a pulsatile mass is palpable in the mid-abdomen. There is no tenderness, and the mass is not associated with any bruit on auscultation. The remainder of the physical examination is unremarkable. Given the clinical findings, an abdominal ultrasound is performed, which reveals an infrarenal abdominal aortic aneurysm (AAA) measuring 4.5 cm in maximum diameter.

What is the most appropriate next step in the management of this patient's AAA?

- A. Schedule an immediate open surgical repair of the AAA.
- B. Initiate a beta-blocker to reduce the rate of aneurysm expansion.
- C. Refer the patient for endovascular aneurysm repair (EVAR).
- D. Arrange for regular surveillance with abdominal ultrasound in 6 months.

Correct Answer: D. Arrange for regular surveillance with abdominal ultrasound in 6 months. This patient has an asymptomatic infrarenal AAA that is less than 5 cm in diameter. The risk of rupture for aneurysms of this size is relatively low, and immediate surgical intervention is not typically indicated. The current guidelines recommend regular surveillance for aneurysms that are between 4.0 and 5.4 cm in diameter.

Option A, scheduling an immediate open surgical repair, is not indicated at this time because the aneurysm is below the threshold size (5.5 cm for men, 5.0 cm for women) at which elective repair is recommended to prevent rupture, provided the patient has a reasonable operative risk profile.

Option B, initiating a beta-blocker, is a strategy that has been investigated to potentially reduce the rate of aneurysm expansion by lowering arterial pressure and the force of the arterial pulse wave. However, beta-blockers are not currently recommended solely for the purpose of limiting aneurysm expansion, as the evidence supporting their use for this indication is not strong.

Option C, referring the patient for EVAR, is not indicated at this time for the same reasons as Option A. EVAR is typically reserved for aneurysms that have reached a size where the risk of rupture outweighs the risk of the procedure, or for patients who have symptoms attributable to the aneurysm.

Therefore, the most appropriate next step is Option D, to arrange for regular surveillance with abdominal ultrasound in 6 months. Surveillance intervals for AAA are typically based on the size of the aneurysm; smaller aneurysms (3.0-3.9 cm) may be monitored every 2-3 years, while those approaching the threshold for repair (4.0-5.4 cm) are generally monitored more frequently, such as every 6-12 months. This strategy allows for the timely detection of significant growth that may necessitate intervention while avoiding unnecessary procedures in the interim. Age-related dilation of the infrarenal aorta is a common consequence. The aorta of a young, healthy male typically measures around 2 centimeters in length. Although aneurysm rupture is rare until their diameter exceeds 5 cm, aneurysm presence is confirmed when the aortic diameter rises above 3 cm. Abdominal aortic aneurysms (AAAs) are detected in 2% of men aged 55 and older, with a 4:1 male-to-female ratio. The origin of 90% of abdominal atherosclerotic aneurysms is inferior to the renal arteries. Aneurysms frequently affect the common iliac arteries and often manifest at the aortic bifurcation. Initial abdominal ultrasound screening is the preferred diagnostic procedure for identifying the presence of an aneurysm. Plain radiographs of the abdomen or back may reveal curvilinear calcifications delineating segments of the aneurysm wall in around 75% of patients diagnosed with aneurysms. For a more reliable evaluation of aneurysm diameter, computed tomography (CT) imaging should be performed when the aneurysm approaches the treatment threshold of 5.5 cm in diameter. CT scans with contrast reveal the arteries both above and below the aneurysm. Frequently, mural thrombus within the aneurysm can be detected via CT imaging; therefore, anticoagulation is not warranted. Routine follow-up with ultrasound will determine the size and growth rate of an identified aneurysm. Imaging is performed at regular intervals of three years for aneurysms measuring 3-3.9 cm, every twelve months for aneurysms measuring 4-4.9 cm, and every six months for aneurysms measuring 5 cm or more in diameter. A CTA with contrast should be performed when an aneurysm measures approximately 5 cm in order to define arterial anatomy and assess aneurysm size more precisely. Although abdominal ultrasound screening is recommended for men aged 65-75 who have smoked 100 or more cigarettes in their lifetime, there is disagreement among guidelines regarding whether or not women with the same level of lifetime cigarette exposure should also undergo screening. When the aortic diameter is between 2 and 2.9 centimeters, recommendations call for a subsequent imaging procedure to be conducted in 10 years. Patients are advised to cease smoking and receive treatment for any pre-existing hypertension, hyperlipidemia, or diabetes while under observation. As aneurysm diameter increases, so does the risk of rupture. Elective repair is generally recommended for abdominal aortic aneurysms measuring at least 5.5 cm in diameter in males and 5 cm in diameter in females. An additional indication that necessitates repair is aneurysm growth that surpasses 0.5 cm within a six-month period. Symptoms such as pain or tenderness, irrespective of the aneurysm's diameter, may indicate an imminent rupture and necessitate immediate repair.

Sakalihasan et al. Abdominal aortic aneurysms. Nat Rev Dis Primers. 2018 Oct 18;4(1):34.PMID: 30337540

9.6 Management of Suspected Aortic Dissection

Case 149

A 55-year-old woman with a history of hypertension and smoking presents to the emergency department with sudden onset of severe, sharp chest pain radiating to her back. She describes the pain as "tearing" in nature. Her blood pressure is 180/95 mmHg in the right arm and 170/90 mmHg in the left arm. Physical examination reveals a diastolic murmur heard best at the right sternal border, mild dysphagia, and hoarseness. She has a history suggestive of Marfan syndrome but has never been formally diagnosed. A chest X-ray shows a widened mediastinum. An electrocardiogram (ECG) shows left ventricular hypertrophy with no signs of ischemia. What is the most appropriate next step in the management of this patient's condition?

- A. Immediate transthoracic echocardiogram (TTE) to assess for aortic regurgitation.
- B. Computed tomography angiography (CTA) of the chest to evaluate for thoracic aortic aneurysm.
- C. Magnetic resonance angiography (MRA) of the chest to evaluate for thoracic aortic aneurysm.
- D. Initiate antihypertensive therapy with intravenous beta-blockers and arrange for urgent cardiac surgery consultation.

Correct Answer: B. Computed tomography angiography (CTA) of the chest to evaluate for thoracic aortic aneurysm. This patient presents with symptoms and signs suggestive of an acute thoracic aortic aneurysm, possibly an aortic dissection, given the severe, sharp, "tearing" chest pain radiating to the back, a diastolic murmur that could indicate aortic regurgitation, and hoarseness which may be due to stretching of the left recurrent laryngeal nerve. The widened mediastinum on chest X-ray further supports this diagnosis. In the setting of suspected acute aortic dissection, rapid imaging to confirm the diagnosis is critical. Option A, an immediate TTE, can be useful in assessing for aortic regurgitation and can sometimes visualize the ascending aorta, but it is not the diagnostic test of choice for suspected aortic dissection because it may not adequately visualize the entire thoracic aorta, especially in the acute setting where time is of the essence. Option C, an MRA of the chest, is a good imaging modality for thoracic aortic aneurysms, but it is less practical in the acute setting due to longer imaging times and less availability in emergency situations. Option D, initiating antihypertensive therapy with intravenous beta-blockers, is part of the management of aortic dissection after the diagnosis has been confirmed, as it helps to reduce the shear stress on the aortic wall. However, it should not precede the confirmation of the diagnosis, as there are other potential causes of chest pain that need to be ruled out. Therefore, the most appropriate next step is Option B, a CTA of the chest. CTA is the diagnostic test of choice for suspected aortic dissection because it is rapid, widely available, and highly sensitive and specific for diagnosing aortic dissection. It can provide detailed images of the aorta and can help identify the extent of the dissection, involvement of branch vessels, and any complications such as impending rupture. Once the diagnosis is confirmed, immediate management including blood pressure control with IV beta-blockers and urgent surgical consultation is indicated. Syphilis is a rare cause of thoracic aortic aneurysms, with atherosclerosis being the predominant etiology. Connective tissue disorders like Ehlers-Danlos syndromes and Marfan syndromes, although uncommon, have significant therapeutic implications. Traumatic false aneurysms beyond the left subclavian artery's origin can result from deceleration-induced partial rupture of the aortic wall. Thoracic aortic aneurysms represent only 10% of all aortic aneurysms. A chest radiograph can aid in diagnosing aneurysms based on the calcified outline of the dilated aorta, while CT scanning with contrast enhancement is the preferred imaging modality. MRA can be used to differentiate aneurysm-like lesions from actual aneurysms and assess their anatomy and extent.

Coronary catheterization and echocardiography may be necessary to understand the relationship between ascending aortic aneurysms and coronary vessels. Repair decisions depend on factors such as location of dilation, progression rate, symptoms, and overall health status. Aneurysms involving the ascending aorta or proximal aortic arch are challenging to manage and may require repair at 5.5 cm. Open surgery is often needed for these cases, carrying risks like stroke and neurologic complications.

Descending thoracic aneurysms measuring 5.5 cm or more should be considered for reconstructive treatment due to a 5-year survival rate of 54% without intervention. Endovascular grafting is the standard approach for descending thoracic aortic aneurysms. Repair of aortic arch aneurysms should be performed by experienced surgical teams with a successful history in complex procedures. Despite advancements in endovascular techniques, repair indications for thoracic aortic aneurysms remain consistent, emphasizing the need for careful evaluation and appropriate management strategies.

Senser EM et al. Thoracic Aortic Aneurysm: A Clinical Review. Cardiol Clin. 2021 Nov;39(4):505-515.PMID: 34686263

9.7 Acute Management of Aortic Dissection

Case 150

A 57-year-old male with a 10-year history of uncontrolled hypertension and a 20-pack year smoking history presents to the emergency department with sudden onset severe chest pain. The pain started an hour ago while he was at rest, and he describes it as a tearing sensation that radiates to his back. He also reports feeling lightheaded and sweaty. He denies any shortness of breath, nausea, or vomiting. His blood pressure is 180/110 mm Hg in the right arm and 160/100 mm Hg in the left arm. His heart rate is 110 beats/min, and his respiratory rate is 22 breaths/min. On physical examination, he appears diaphoretic and in distress. His heart sounds are regular without any murmurs, rubs, or gallops. His lungs are clear to auscultation bilaterally. An EKG shows no signs of myocardial infarction or ischemia.
Question: What is the most appropriate next step in the management of this patient?

- A. Administer morphine sulfate for pain relief
- B. Start intravenous infusion of labetalol
- C. Start intravenous infusion of nicardipine
- D. Administer a loading dose of esmolol

Correct Answer: B. Start intravenous infusion of labetalol The patient's presentation is highly suggestive of aortic dissection, a life-threatening condition that requires immediate management. The goal in aortic dissection is to reduce the shear stress on the aortic wall by lowering the blood pressure and heart rate. Beta-blockers are the first-line therapy as they reduce the left ventricular ejection force that weakens the arterial wall. Labetalol, both an alpha- and beta-blocker, can lower heart rate and achieve rapid blood pressure control. It can be given as 20 mg over 2 minutes by intravenous injection, with additional doses of 40–80 mg intravenously every 10 minutes (maximum dose 300 mg) until the desired blood pressure has been reached. Alternatively, 2 mg/min may be given by intravenous infusion, titrated to the desired effect.

A. Administer morphine sulfate for pain relief While morphine sulfate is an important component of managing the pain associated with aortic dissection, it is not the most appropriate next step in this scenario. Morphine sulfate is an opioid analgesic that reduces the emotional response to pain and changes the perception of the pain experience. However, it does not address the underlying cause of the pain, which in this case is the dissection of the aorta. Moreover, it doesn't have any effect on the blood pressure or heart rate, which are critical parameters that need immediate control in aortic dissection to prevent rupture and other complications. Therefore, while morphine sulfate may be used as an adjunct therapy to relieve the patient's pain, it is not the primary treatment in the management of aortic dissection.

B. Start intravenous infusion of labetalol This is the correct answer. The immediate priority in the management of aortic dissection is to control blood pressure and heart rate to minimize the risk of aortic rupture, which is a life-threatening complication. Beta-blockers, such as labetalol, are the first-line therapy for achieving this goal. Labetalol is a non-selective beta-blocker and alpha-1 blocker. It reduces the force of the heart's contractions, which decreases the blood pressure and the heart rate. This slows the progression of the aortic dissection. Labetalol can be given by intravenous injection or infusion and can be titrated to achieve the desired blood pressure and heart rate.

C. Start intravenous infusion of nicardipine Nicardipine is a calcium channel blocker that can be used to control blood pressure. It works by relaxing the muscles of your heart and blood vessels. However, it should be used as a second-line treatment or in patients who cannot tolerate beta-blockers. It does not decrease the heart rate or the force of ventricular ejection as effectively as beta-blockers, which is crucial in aortic dissection management. Therefore, while nicardipine is a treatment option, it is not the most appropriate next step in this scenario.

D. Administer a loading dose of esmolol Esmolol is a short-acting beta-1 selective blocker that can be used to rapidly control heart rate and blood pressure. Its short half-life allows for rapid titration and for testing a patient's reaction to a beta-blocker if there are concerns about asthma or bradycardia. However, given its short half-life and the need for continuous monitoring and titration, it is typically reserved for use in the critical care or operating room settings. While esmolol can be used in the management of aortic dissection, it is not typically the first-line therapy and therefore is not the most appropriate next step in this patient's management.

Surgery options:

1. Type A dissection—Immediate surgical intervention is necessary for all type A dissections. If a proficient cardiovascular team is not accessible, the patient should be transferred to a suitable facility. The process includes replacing the affected part of the arch with a graft and performing a brachiocephalic vessel bypass if needed. Replacing the aortic valve may be necessary along with reattaching the coronary arteries.
2. Type B dissection with malperfusion—Immediate surgery is necessary for type B dissections if there is aortic branch compromise leading to malperfusion of the renal, visceral, or extremity vessels. The primary aim of surgery is to reestablish blood flow to the ischemic tissue. Stenting the entry tear at the subclavian artery level can close the false lumen and improve flow into the branch vessel from the true lumen. The outcomes can be unpredictable and should only be pursued by a skilled team.
3. For acute type B dissections without malperfusion, blood pressure control is the primary treatment. Survival and aneurysm rates are better with early repair using thoracic stent grafts, particularly in healthy patients with high-risk anatomic features.

Kaji S. Acute medical management of aortic dissection. Gen Thorac Cardiovasc Surg. 2019 Feb;67(2):203-207. PMID: 30456591

9.8 Progressive swelling of the neck, face

Case 151

A 62-year-old male patient presents with progressive swelling of the neck, face, and upper extremities over the past 2 weeks. He also reports headaches, dizziness, and occasional episodes of syncope. Physical examination reveals dilated cutaneous veins on the upper chest and lower neck, flushing of the face and neck, and brawny edema of the face, neck, and arms. The patient's symptoms worsen when bending over or lying down. Relevant Patient History:Former smoker (quit 5 years ago, 30 pack-year history) No significant medical history Physical Examination Findings Vital signs: BP 140/90 mmHg, HR 92 bpm, RR 18 breaths/min, SpO2 96% on room air Dilated cutaneous veins on the upper chest and lower neck. Flushing of the face and neck Brawny edema of the face, neck, and arms No palpable lymphadenopathy Diagnostic Test Results: Chest X-ray: Widened mediastinum with a right hilar mass CT scan of the chest: 4 cm right hilar mass encasing and obstructing the superior vena cava
What is the most appropriate next step in the management of this patient?

- A. Initiate anticoagulation therapy
- B. Perform a percutaneous stent placement
- C. Initiate chemotherapy
- D. Initiate radiation therapy

The correct answer is B. Perform a percutaneous stent placement. In this clinical scenario, the patient presents with signs and symptoms suggestive of superior vena cava syndrome (SVCS), which is a relatively rare condition caused by obstruction of the superior vena cava. The diagnostic test results indicate the presence of a right hilar mass encasing and obstructing the superior vena cava, which is likely the underlying cause of the patient's symptoms. Percutaneous stent placement is the most appropriate next step in the management of this patient. Stent placement is a minimally invasive procedure that can rapidly relieve the obstruction and alleviate the symptoms of SVCS. It is the preferred initial treatment for SVCS caused by malignant obstruction, as it provides prompt symptom relief and allows for subsequent treatment of the underlying malignancy. Anticoagulation therapy (option A) is not the most appropriate next step, as it does not address the underlying obstruction and may increase the risk of bleeding complications. Initiating chemotherapy (option C) or radiation therapy (option D) may be appropriate subsequent steps after relieving the obstruction, depending on the underlying malignancy and its staging. However, these options do not provide immediate relief of the SVCS symptoms and should not be the initial management approach in this acute setting. The main treatment options for partial or complete obstruction of the superior vena cava (superior vena cava syndrome or SVCS) are:

1. Percutaneous stent placement: This is considered the first-line treatment and preferred initial approach for relieving the obstruction and alleviating symptoms rapidly. A stent is placed via a minimally invasive procedure to open up the blocked superior vena cava.
2. Percutaneous transluminal angioplasty (PTA): This involves using a balloon catheter to dilate and open up the obstructed vein.
3. Thrombolysis: For cases where a thrombus (blood clot) is causing the obstruction, thrombolytic medications can be used to dissolve the clot.
4. Anticoagulation therapy: Anticoagulants like heparin may be used, especially when the obstruction is caused by a thrombus around a central venous catheter.
5. Radiation therapy: Radiotherapy can be used to shrink the tumor mass that is compressing and obstructing the superior vena cava, especially in cases of malignancy like lung cancer or lymphoma.
6. Chemotherapy: For chemosensitive tumors causing SVCS, chemotherapy may be preferred over radiation therapy.
7. Surgical bypass: In carefully selected cases, surgical bypass procedures can be performed to create an alternative route for venous drainage and palliate symptoms.
8. Corticosteroids or diuretics: These may be used as emergency treatments when brain edema, decreased cardiac output, or upper airway edema is present due to severe SVCS.

10

INFECTIVE ENDOCARDITIS

10.1 Suspected Infective Endocarditis in a Patient with Mitral Valve Prolapse

Case 152

A 60-year-old male with a history of mitral valve prolapse presents to the hospital with a two-week history of intermittent fever, fatigue, and a new-onset regurgitant murmur. He recently underwent a dental extraction. His temperature is 38.5C, blood pressure is 130/85 mmHg, and heart rate is 95 bpm. Physical examination reveals Osler's nodes on his fingers and Janeway lesions on his palms. Blood cultures have been obtained , and an echocardiogram has revealed vegetations on the mitral valve .
Given the patient's history, physical examination findings, and diagnostic test results, what is the most appropriate next step in the management of this patient?

- A) Initiate empirical antibiotic therapy targeting viridans streptococci and staphylococci
- B) Await final blood culture results before starting antibiotic therapy
- C) Perform a colonoscopy to evaluate for polyps or colon cancer
- D) Treat for Clostridium difficile infection

Correct Answer: A) Initiate empirical antibiotic therapy targeting viridans streptococci and staphylococci The patient presents with clinical features suggestive of infective endocarditis, including fever, a new regurgitant murmur, Osler's nodes, Janeway lesions, and echocardiographic evidence of mitral valve vegetations. The recent dental extraction is a significant risk factor for bacteremia caused by oral flora, particularly viridans streptococci, which are common causes of native-valve endocarditis (NVE). Staphylococci are also important pathogens in NVE, especially in patients with pre-existing valvular heart disease. The presence of gram-positive rods in the blood culture could suggest a variety of organisms, including streptococci. While the final identification and susceptibility results of the blood cultures are pending, it is critical to initiate empirical antibiotic therapy promptly in a patient with suspected infective endocarditis to prevent further complications such as heart failure, systemic emboli, or abscess formation.

A colonoscopy may be indicated if Streptococcus gallolyticus (formerly S. bovis) is identified, given its association with colonic neoplasia. However, this is not the immediate next step in the management of a patient with suspected NVE and evidence of systemic infection.

Treatment for Clostridium difficile infection should be considered if the patient has symptoms of colitis and a positive stool test. However, in the context of suspected NVE, the priority is to address the endocarditis, which is a life-threatening condition.

Therefore, the most appropriate next step is to initiate empirical antibiotic therapy targeting the most likely pathogens, viridans streptococci and staphylococci, while awaiting the final blood culture results. Antibiotic therapy can be adjusted later based on culture results and antibiotic susceptibility testing.

Infective endocarditis is definitively diagnosed when microorganisms are seen histologically in or cultured from endocardial vegetations obtained during cardiac surgery, embolectomy, or autopsy. Echocardiography is a key diagnostic tool, with transesophageal echocardiography (TEE) being more sensitive than transthoracic echocardiography (TTE). Treatment consists of a prolonged course of antimicrobial therapy, and surgery may be required in some cases. The duration of therapy depends on the pathogen and site of valvular infection, typically lasting up to 6 weeks from the first day of negative blood cultures.

Empiric antibiotic therapy should cover Staphylococcus (methicillin-susceptible and resistant), Streptococcus, and Enterococcus. Valve replacement may be considered for patients with persistent infection or complications such as heart failure. Anticoagulation therapy in patients with NVE is controversial and requires careful consideration, especially in those with mechanical valve endocarditis. The potential complications of infective endocarditis include congestive heart failure, systemic emboli, abscess formation, myocardial abscesses, infected and sterile emboli, a variety of immunological processes, severe valvular insufficiency, intractable congestive heart failure, and neurological complications such as meningitis-encephalopathy, ischemic complications, and cerebral hemorrhage. e treatment of bacterial endocarditis can differ between native valve endocarditis (NVE) and prosthetic valve endocarditis (PVE) due to variations in the pathogens involved, the presence of prosthetic material, and the risk of complications. Here are some key differences :

1. Pathogens: NVE is often caused by viridans streptococci, especially in patients with a history of dental procedures, while PVE may be more frequently associated with staphylococci, particularly Staphylococcus epidermidis, due to its ability to adhere to prosthetic materials.
2. Antibiotic Therapy: The choice of antibiotics may differ between NVE and PVE. For example, treatment for Staphylococcus aureus (MSSA) in NVE may involve oxacillin or cefazolin, while PVE treatment may require the addition of rifampin and gentamicin due to the biofilm associated with prosthetic valves.
3. Duration of Treatment: The duration of antibiotic therapy can be longer for PVE compared to NVE. For instance, MSSA NVE may be treated for 4-6 weeks, while MSSA PVE may require 6 weeks of treatment due to the challenges of eradicating infection from prosthetic material.
4. Surgical Intervention: Patients with PVE may have a higher mortality rate and may be more likely to require surgical intervention compared to those with NVE. Surgical indications for PVE include valvular dehiscence, early PVE, and infection with multiresistant organisms.
5. Complications: PVE is associated with a higher risk of complications, including a higher incidence of atrial fibrillation and a much higher mortality rate when compared to NVE. Staphylococcal endocarditis, for example, results in a higher mortality rate in PVE than in NVE/
6. Surgical Timing: The timing of surgery may differ, with PVE often requiring earlier intervention due to the risk of biofilm-associated infection and the potential for rapid deterioration.
7. Anticoagulation: The use of anticoagulation therapy in patients with NVE is controversial and requires careful consideration, especially in those with mechanical valve endocarditis, which is a concern in PVE.

Pathogen	Condition	Treatment	Duration
Staphylococcus (MSSA)	NVE	Oxacillin or Cefazolin/Cefotaxime	4-6 weeks
Staphylococcus (MSSA)	PVE	Oxacillin + Rifampin + Gentamicin	6 weeks
Staphylococcus (MRSA)	NVE/PVE	Vancomycin or Daptomycin	4-6 weeks
Streptococcus (PCN sensitive)	NVE	Penicillin G/Ceftriaxone and Gentamicin	2 weeks
Streptococcus (PCN sensitive)	PVE	Penicillin G/Ceftriaxone/Amoxicillin	6 weeks
Streptococcus (PCN resistant)	NVE	Penicillin G/Ceftriaxone + Gentamicin	4 weeks
Streptococcus (PCN resistant)	PVE	Penicillin G/Ceftriaxone + Gentamicin	6 weeks
Enterococcus	NVE/PVE	Ampicillin + Ceftriaxone	6 weeks

10.2 Postoperative Complications: Evaluating Aortic Valve Replacement

Case 153

A 67-year-old female with a history of aortic valve replacement 8 weeks ago presents with a 1-week history of intermittent fever, chills, and malaise. She reports no recent dental procedures or other invasive interventions. On examination, her temperature is 38.7C, blood pressure is 110/70 mmHg, and heart rate is 102 bpm. A new diastolic murmur is noted. Laboratory findings show elevated inflammatory markers. Three sets of blood cultures have been drawn and are pending. A transthoracic echocardiogram is inconclusive due to the presence of the prosthetic valve.
Diagnostic Test Results:

1. Blood cultures: Pending
2. Transthoracic echocardiogram: Inconclusive
3. Inflammatory markers: Elevated

What is the most appropriate next step in the management of this patient?

- A) Initiate empirical antibiotic therapy targeting common skin flora
- B) Perform a transesophageal echocardiogram (TEE) to assess for valve vegetations
- C) Await blood culture results before initiating any treatment
- D) Schedule immediate valve replacement surgery

Correct Answer: B) Perform a transesophageal echocardiogram (TEE) to assess for valve vegetations The patient presents with signs and symptoms suggestive of prosthetic valve endocarditis (PVE), which is a serious complication following valve replacement surgery. Given the recent surgery (within 2 months), the patient is at risk for early PVE, which is often due to intraoperative contamination or a bacteremic postoperative complication. The most common pathogens associated with early PVE include coagulase-negative staphylococci (CoNS), Staphylococcus aureus, facultative gram-negative bacilli, diphtheroids, or fungi.

While empirical antibiotic therapy is an important consideration in the management of suspected PVE, it is crucial to first establish the diagnosis. A transthoracic echocardiogram (TTE) often has limited sensitivity in the presence of a prosthetic valve due to shadowing and reverberation artifacts. Therefore, a transesophageal echocardiogram (TEE) is the next best step as it provides superior sensitivity and specificity for the detection of vegetations, abscesses, and other complications associated with PVE.

Awaiting blood culture results (Option C) before initiating any treatment may delay necessary therapy in a potentially life-threatening infection. However, it is important to obtain blood cultures before starting antibiotics when possible to ensure the causative organism is identified.

Immediate valve replacement surgery (Option D) is not indicated without first confirming the diagnosis of PVE and assessing the extent of infection and valve function. Surgery is typically reserved for patients who fail medical management or develop complications such as heart failure, uncontrolled infection, or recurrent emboli.

Therefore, the most appropriate next step is to perform a TEE to confirm the diagnosis of PVE and guide further management, including the selection of appropriate empirical antibiotic therapy. The recommended next step after obtaining blood culture results in the management of suspected prosthetic valve endocarditis (PVE) is to initiate empirical antibiotic therapy promptly while awaiting the final blood culture results. This approach is critical to prevent further complications such as heart failure, systemic emboli, or abscess formation associated with infective endocarditis. The choice of empirical antibiotics should target the most likely pathogens, which commonly include coagulase-negative staphylococci (CoNS), Staphylococcus aureus, and other organisms that may be associated with PVE. The antibiotic therapy can be adjusted later based on the culture results and antibiotic susceptibility testing to ensure the most effective treatment. Blood cultures should be taken after 3 to 4 days of treatment to document eradication of the bacteremia in the treatment of prosthetic valve endocarditis (PVE).

The criteria for documenting eradication of bacteremia during the treatment of prosthetic valve endocarditis (PVE) involve obtaining serial blood cultures after 3 to 4 days of antibiotic therapy to ensure that the bacteremia has been cleared.

Table 10.1: Etiology and Microbiology of Different Types of Endocarditis

Type of Endocarditis	Causative Microorganisms	Portal of Entry or Associated Conditions
Native-valve endocarditis (NVE)	Viridans streptococci, staphylococci, HACEK organisms, Streptococcus gallolyticus	Oral, skin, upper respiratory tract, gut (S. gallolyticus)
Health care–associated NVE	Staphylococcus aureus, CoNS, enterococci	Nosocomial or community onset in healthcare-exposed patients
Prosthetic-valve endocarditis (PVE)	CoNS, S. aureus, facultative gram-negative bacilli, diphtheroids, fungi	Intraoperative contamination or bacteremic postoperative complication
CIED-related endocarditis	S. aureus, CoNS (often methicillin-resistant strains)	Device itself or the endothelium at points of device contact
Endocarditis among IV drug users	S. aureus, Pseudomonas aeruginosa, Candida, Bacillus, Lactobacillus, Corynebacterium spp.	Tricuspid valve (common), left-sided valve infections
Culture-negative endocarditis	Granulicatella, Abiotrophia spp., HACEK organisms, Coxiella burnetii, Bartonella spp., Brucella spp., Tropheryma whipplei	Prior antibiotic exposure or infection by fastidious organisms

10.3 Intravenous Drug Use and Infectious Complications

Case 154

A 48-year-old male with a history of intravenous drug use presents to the emergency department with a 2-week history of fever, night sweats, and weight loss. He denies any recent dental work or other invasive procedures. On examination, his temperature is 39.2C, blood pressure is 100/60 mmHg, and heart rate is 120 bpm. A faint diastolic murmur is auscultated. There are no visible skin lesions or Roth's spots, and neurological examination is normal. Laboratory findings reveal elevated white blood cell count and erythrocyte sedimentation rate. Blood cultures have been drawn. A chest X-ray shows multiple nodular pulmonary infiltrates.
Diagnostic Test Results:

1. White blood cell count: Elevated
2. Erythrocyte sedimentation rate: Elevated
3. Blood cultures: Pending
4. Chest X-ray: Multiple nodular pulmonary infiltrates

What is the most appropriate next step in the diagnosis of this patient?

- A) Await blood culture results before initiating any treatment
- B) Perform a transthoracic echocardiogram (TTE) to assess for valvular vegetations
- C) Initiate empirical antibiotic therapy targeting S. aureus and gram-negative bacilli
- D) Schedule a CT scan of the chest to further evaluate pulmonary infiltrates

Correct Answer: B) Perform a transthoracic echocardiogram (TTE) to assess for valvular vegetations The patient's history of intravenous drug use, febrile presentation, and a new diastolic murmur are highly suggestive of infective endocarditis (IE), possibly involving the tricuspid valve, which is common in intravenous drug users. The presence of multiple nodular pulmonary infiltrates on chest X-ray is consistent with septic pulmonary emboli, a complication often seen in tricuspid valve endocarditis.

While awaiting blood culture results (Option A) is important for definitive diagnosis and targeted antibiotic therapy, it is not the most immediate next step given the patient's symptoms and risk factors for IE. Empirical antibiotic therapy (Option C) is also critical in the management of suspected IE, especially in a patient with a high risk of S. aureus infection. However, before initiating antibiotics, it is essential to obtain imaging to support the diagnosis and guide treatment.

A transthoracic echocardiogram (TTE) is the initial imaging modality of choice to assess for valvular vegetations, which are a hallmark of IE. Although TTE has lower sensitivity for detecting vegetations on the tricuspid valve compared to the left-sided heart valves, it is still a necessary diagnostic step and can be performed rapidly to confirm the diagnosis.

A CT scan of the chest (Option D) may provide additional information about the extent of septic emboli but does not replace the need for echocardiographic evaluation of the heart valves in the context of suspected IE. Therefore, the most appropriate next step is to perform a TTE to assess for valvular vegetations, which will help confirm the diagnosis of IE and facilitate the initiation of appropriate empirical antibiotic therapy. Once IE is confirmed and empirical antibiotics are started, further imaging such as a transesophageal echocardiogram (TEE) may be indicated if the TTE is inconclusive or if there is a high clinical suspicion of IE with a negative TTE. Endothelial injury enables direct infection by highly virulent pathogens (e.g., S. aureus) or the formation of a platelet–fibrin thrombus (known as nonbacterial thrombotic endocarditis [NBTE]) that can get infected during temporary bacteremia. There is no text to rewrite. NBTE can result from cardiac conditions like mitral regurgitation, aortic stenosis, and aortic regurgitation, hypercoagulable states leading to marantic endocarditis, and the antiphospholipid antibody syndrome. No text provided. Once in the bloodstream, organisms stick to the endothelium or sites of NBTE using surface adhesin molecules. There is no text to rewrite. The symptoms of endocarditis result from cytokine production, damage to intracardiac structures, embolization of vegetation fragments, hematogenous infection of sites during bacteremia, and tissue injury due to the deposition of immune complexes. Clinical manifestations: The clinical syndrome varies and ranges from acute to subacute presentations. The progression of disease is influenced by the specific causative organisms. S. aureus, -hemolytic streptococci, pneumococci, and Staphylococcus lugdunensis usually manifest acutely, while viridans streptococci, enterococci, CoNS (excluding S. lugdunensis), and the HACEK group typically present subacutely. Constitutional symptoms may include fever, chills, weight loss, myalgias, or arthralgias. **Cardiac manifestations** include heart murmurs, especially new or worsened regurgitant murmurs, which are eventually heard in 85% of patients with acute native valve endocarditis. CHF occurs in 30–40% of patients and is typically caused by valvular dysfunction. Infection extension can lead to perivalvular abscesses, potentially causing intracardiac fistulae. Abscesses can extend from the aortic root into the ventricular septum, disrupting the conduction system, or penetrate through the epicardium, leading to pericarditis. **Noncardiac symptoms**: Arterial emboli, half of which occur before the diagnosis of endocarditis, are found in 50% of patients, with hematogenously seeded focal infection most commonly seen in the skin, spleen, kidneys, bones, and meninges. The risk of embolization is higher with endocarditis from S. aureus, mobile vegetations larger than 10 mm, and infection of the mitral valve (especially the anterior leaflet). **Cerebrovascular emboli** can present as stroke or encephalopathy in 15–35% of cases, with half of these cases occurring before the diagnosis of endocarditis. Evidence of clinically asymptomatic emboli is detected on MRI in 30–65% of patients with left-sided endocarditis. Stroke incidence decreases significantly with antibiotic therapy and is not related to changes in vegetation size. About 3% of strokes occur after 1 week of effective therapy, but these late-occurring embolic events do not necessarily indicate failed antimicrobial therapy. Other neurologic complications may include aseptic or purulent meningitis, intracranial hemorrhage from ruptured mycotic aneurysms, seizures, and microabscesses, particularly with S. aureus. **Immune complex** deposition on the glomerular basement membrane leads to glomerulonephritis and renal dysfunction, which can be treated with antibiotic therapy. **Peripheral manifestations** of subacute endocarditis (e.g., Janeway lesions, Roth's spots) are now rare due to early diagnosis and treatment. Signs of certain underlying conditions: Underlying conditions can impact the signs and symptoms that are presented. **IV drug use**: In cases linked to IV drug use, around half are confined to the tricuspid valve and manifest as fever, faint, or no murmur. **Septic**

pulmonary emboli are indicated by symptoms such as cough, pleuritic chest pain, nodular pulmonary infiltrates, and sometimes empyema or pyopneumothorax, with no peripheral manifestations present. Patients with left-sided cardiac infections typically present with the clinical features of endocarditis. Health care–associated endocarditis: Symptoms are common when there is no intracardiac device present. Endocarditis linked to a transvenous pacemaker or implanted defibrillator can lead to a generator pocket infection, causing fever, minimal murmur, and pulmonary symptoms from septic emboli. **PVE**: In situations where endocarditis develops within 60 days of valve surgery, common symptoms might be hidden by other health issues linked to recent surgery. Paravalvular infection is frequently seen in PVE, leading to partial valve dehiscence, regurgitant murmurs, CHF, or disruption of the conduction system.

Table 10.2: Diagnostic Criteria for Infective Endocarditis

Diagnostic Criteria	Description
Histological and Microbiological Examination	Definitive diagnosis established when vegetations are examined histologically and microbiologically.
Modified Duke Criteria	Emphasizes roles of bacteremia and echocardiographic findings. Definite endocarditis requires two major, or one major and three minor, or five minor criteria. Possible endocarditis requires one major and one minor, or three minor criteria.
Blood Culture Samples	For antibiotic-naïve patients, three sets of blood culture samples from different sites within the first 24 h. If negative after 48–72 h, two or three additional sets should be cultured.
Serology	Useful for implicating Brucella, Bartonella, Legionella, Chlamydia psittaci, or C. burnetii. Histology, culture, direct fluorescent antibody techniques, and/or PCR may identify causative organism in absence of positive blood culture.
Echocardiography	Confirms diagnosis, verifies size of vegetations, detects complications, assesses cardiac function. TTE may suffice for low likelihood of endocarditis. TEE detects vegetations in above 90% of cases, optimal for prosthetic valves and detection of complications.

10.4 A 60-year-old Male with Bioprosthetic Aortic Valve and Persistent Fevers

Case 155

A 60-year-old male with a history of bioprosthetic aortic valve replacement 5 years ago presents with a 1-month history of low-grade fevers, fatigue, and a 5-pound weight loss. He has no known drug allergies and no recent healthcare exposures. On examination, his temperature is 38.3C, blood pressure is 130/80 mmHg, and heart rate is 88 bpm. A grade 3/6 diastolic murmur is heard at the right sternal border. There are no Janeway lesions, Osler nodes, or Roth spots. Laboratory findings show an elevated erythrocyte sedimentation rate and C-reactive protein. Blood cultures grow Enterococcus faecalis, which is sensitive to ampicillin but exhibits high-level resistance to gentamicin and streptomycin.
Diagnostic Test Results:

1. Erythrocyte sedimentation rate: Elevated
2. C-reactive protein: Elevated
3. Blood cultures: Enterococcus faecalis (sensitive to ampicillin, high-level resistance to gentamicin and streptomycin)

What is the most appropriate next step in the management of this patient?

- A) Initiate monotherapy with high-dose intravenous ampicillin for 6 weeks
- B) Initiate combination therapy with intravenous ampicillin and gentamicin
- C) Initiate combination therapy with high-dose intravenous ampicillin and ceftriaxone
- D) Refer the patient for immediate surgical valve replacement

Correct Answer: C) Initiate combination therapy with high-dose intravenous ampicillin and ceftriaxone The patient presents with clinical and laboratory findings consistent with prosthetic valve endocarditis (PVE) caused by Enterococcus faecalis. The standard treatment for enterococcal endocarditis typically includes a synergistic combination of a cell wall–active agent (such as ampicillin) and an aminoglycoside (such as gentamicin or streptomycin). However, in this case, the isolate exhibits high-level resistance to both gentamicin and streptomycin, which precludes the use of these aminoglycosides for synergistic therapy.

Monotherapy with high-dose intravenous ampicillin (Option A) is less effective than combination therapy for enterococcal endocarditis and is not recommended in this scenario. Combination therapy with intravenous ampicillin and gentamicin (Option B) is not appropriate due to the high-level aminoglycoside resistance exhibited by the organism.

Combination therapy with high-dose intravenous ampicillin and ceftriaxone (Option C) is an alternative regimen for Enterococcus faecalis endocarditis with high-level aminoglycoside resistance. This regimen has been shown to be effective and is recommended as an alternative to aminoglycoside-containing regimens in patients with aminoglycoside-resistant enterococcal endocarditis.

Immediate surgical valve replacement (Option D) is considered in patients with PVE who are not responding to medical therapy, who have heart failure due to valvular dysfunction, who have evidence of perivalvular extension of infection, or who have other complications that are not amenable to medical therapy alone. In this clinical scenario, there is no indication provided that the patient has failed medical therapy or has complications necessitating immediate surgery.

Therefore, the most appropriate next step in the management of this patient is to initiate combination therapy with high-dose intravenous ampicillin and ceftriaxone, which provides effective treatment against Enterococcus faecalis with high-level aminoglycoside resistance. The recommended treatment for enterococcal endocarditis with high-level aminoglycoside resistance, specifically caused by Enterococcus faecalis, includes combination therapy with high-dose intravenous ampicillin and ceftriaxone. This regimen is an alternative to aminoglycoside-containing regimens and has been shown to be effective for Enterococcus faecalis endocarditis with high-level aminoglycoside resistance

10.5 Mechanical Mitral Valve Endocarditis

Case 156

A 56-year-old male with a history of mechanical mitral valve replacement 3 years ago presents with a 2-week history of intermittent fever, night sweats, and malaise. He has no known drug allergies and reports no recent invasive procedures. On examination, his temperature is 38.9C, blood pressure is 125/75 mmHg, and heart rate is 110 bpm. A new regurgitant murmur is heard over the mitral area. Laboratory findings reveal an elevated erythrocyte sedimentation rate (ESR) and C-reactive protein (CRP), but normal procalcitonin (PCT). Blood cultures grow methicillin-resistant Staphylococcus aureus (MRSA), which is resistant to gentamicin but sensitive to rifampin and vancomycin.
Diagnostic Test Results:

1. Erythrocyte sedimentation rate (ESR): Elevated
2. C-reactive protein (CRP): Elevated
3. Procalcitonin (PCT): Normal
4. Blood cultures: MRSA (resistant to gentamicin, sensitive to rifampin and vancomycin)

What is the most appropriate next step in the management of this patient?

- A) Initiate monotherapy with intravenous vancomycin
- B) Initiate combination therapy with intravenous vancomycin, rifampin, and a fluoroquinolone
- C) Initiate combination therapy with intravenous vancomycin and gentamicin
- D) Refer the patient for immediate surgical valve replacement

Correct Answer: B) Initiate combination therapy with intravenous vancomycin, rifampin, and a fluoroquinolone The patient presents with clinical and laboratory findings consistent with prosthetic valve endocarditis (PVE) caused by methicillin-resistant Staphylococcus aureus (MRSA). The treatment of staphylococcal PVE typically requires a multidrug regimen for 6–8 weeks, with rifampin playing a crucial role due to its ability to kill organisms adherent to foreign material, such as a prosthetic valve.

Monotherapy with intravenous vancomycin (Option A) is not sufficient for the treatment of staphylococcal PVE due to the risk of rifampin resistance emerging when it is used alone. Combination therapy with intravenous vancomycin and gentamicin (Option C) is not appropriate in this case because the MRSA isolate is resistant to gentamicin.

The inclusion of rifampin is important for its activity against biofilm-associated bacteria on the prosthetic valve. Since the MRSA isolate is resistant to gentamicin, another agent should be substituted. A fluoroquinolone can be used as an alternative to gentamicin in combination with vancomycin and rifampin, as it provides broad-spectrum coverage and has good biofilm penetration.

Immediate surgical valve replacement (Option D) may be necessary in cases of PVE with complications such as heart failure, uncontrolled infection, or abscess formation. However, there is no indication in the clinical scenario that the patient has any of these complications necessitating immediate surgery.

Therefore, the most appropriate next step in the management of this patient is to initiate combination therapy with intravenous vancomycin, rifampin, and a fluoroquinolone. This regimen addresses the need for a multidrug approach to treat MRSA PVE, prevents the emergence of rifampin resistance, and substitutes gentamicin with an alternative agent due to the isolate's resistance profile. The role of rifampin in the treatment of staphylococcal prosthetic valve endocarditis (PVE) is to enhance the antibacterial regimen due to its ability to kill organisms adherent to foreign material, such as a prosthetic valve. Rifampin is recommended as part of a multidrug regimen for 6–8 weeks, combined with intravenous anti-staphylococcal penicillin or cefazolin for methicillin-susceptible staphylococci, and intravenous glycopeptides or lipopeptides for methicillin-resistant staphylococci (MRSA), along with intravenous gentamicin during the first two weeks. Its use is strongly encouraged due to its activity on planktonic bacteria embedded in biofilms, which contributes to eradicating bacteria attached to foreign material, thereby reducing the risk of relapse. However, the use of rifampin has been associated with severe adverse events and potential interactions with a large number of drugs. Despite its recommended use in international guidelines, the evidence supporting the systematic use of rifampin-based combination therapy for staphylococcal PVE is not strong, and its effectiveness remains a subject of ongoing research and debate.

10.6 A 68-year-old Female with Pulmonary Edema and Large Vegetation

Case 157

A 68-year-old female with a history of mitral valve prolapse presents with a 3-week history of fevers, malaise, and progressive dyspnea. She was diagnosed with mitral valve bacterial endocarditis 1 week ago and has been receiving appropriate intravenous antibiotic therapy. Despite this, she has developed worsening dyspnea and is now experiencing orthopnea and paroxysmal nocturnal dyspnea. On examination, she is tachypneic with a respiratory rate of 28 breaths per minute, blood pressure is 110/70 mmHg, and heart rate is 115 bpm. A new grade 4/6 holosystolic murmur is heard at the apex radiating to the axilla. Chest X-ray reveals pulmonary edema, and transthoracic echocardiogram shows a large vegetation (15 mm) on the mitral valve with severe mitral regurgitation and a flail leaflet.
Diagnostic Test Results:

1. Respiratory rate: 28 breaths per minute
2. Blood pressure: 110/70 mmHg
3. Heart rate: 115 bpm
4. Chest X-ray: Pulmonary edema
5. Transthoracic echocardiogram: Large vegetation (15 mm) on the mitral valve, severe mitral regurgitation, flail leaflet

What is the most appropriate timing for surgical intervention in this patient?

- A) Emergent surgical intervention (same day)
- B) Urgent surgical intervention (within 1–2 days)
- C) Elective surgical intervention (earlier usually preferred)
- D) Continue medical management and re-evaluate in 1 week

Correct Answer: A) Emergent surgical intervention (same day) The patient presents with signs of severe acute mitral regurgitation secondary to bacterial endocarditis, as evidenced by the new holosystolic murmur, flail mitral valve leaflet, large vegetation on the mitral valve, and symptoms of heart failure including pulmonary edema. These findings place the patient at high risk for decompensation and indicate the need for immediate surgical intervention. Emergent surgical intervention (Option A) is indicated in cases of valve dysfunction with pulmonary edema or cardiogenic shock, which is consistent with the patient's presentation. The presence of severe mitral regurgitation with heart failure symptoms and evidence of a flail leaflet on echocardiography supports the need for same-day surgery to prevent further hemodynamic compromise and to improve the patient's chances of survival. Urgent surgical intervention (Option B) is typically reserved for patients with valve obstruction by vegetation, unstable prosthesis, or acute regurgitation with heart failure (NYHA class III or IV) without immediate life-threatening complications. While this patient does have severe regurgitation and heart failure symptoms, the presence of pulmonary edema necessitates a more immediate response. Elective surgical intervention (Option C) is considered for patients with progressive paravalvular regurgitation, persistent infection despite adequate antimicrobial therapy, or specific pathogens such as fungi or highly resistant bacteria. This patient's condition is too critical to delay surgery for an elective timing. Continuing medical management and re-evaluating in 1 week (Option D) is not appropriate given the patient's acute presentation with severe mitral regurgitation and heart failure. Delaying surgery could result in further clinical deterioration and increased risk of mortality. Therefore, the correct answer is emergent surgical intervention (same day), as the patient's clinical presentation and echocardiographic findings indicate a high risk of hemodynamic collapse without immediate surgical correction of the valve dysfunction.

10.7 Preventive Measures for Endocarditis- Mechanical Aortic Valve

Case 158

A 43-year-old male with a history of aortic valve replacement with a mechanical prosthesis two years ago is scheduled for a dental extraction due to a carious molar. He has no history of endocarditis and is currently asymptomatic. His only medication is warfarin for anticoagulation. On physical examination, his vital signs are stable, and a mechanical heart valve click is audible. There are no signs of infection or heart failure. His INR is within the therapeutic range.
Diagnostic Test Results:

1. Vital signs: Stable
2. Physical examination: Presence of mechanical heart valve click, no signs of infection or heart failure
3. INR: Within therapeutic range

What is the most appropriate next step in the management of this patient to prevent endocarditis related to the upcoming dental procedure?

- A) No antibiotic prophylaxis is necessary before the dental extraction.
- B) Administer oral amoxicillin for antibiotic prophylaxis 1 hour before the dental extraction.
- C) Prescribe a course of oral amoxicillin to be taken for 7 days starting the day after the dental extraction.
- D) Administer intravenous vancomycin for antibiotic prophylaxis 1 hour before the dental extraction.

Correct Answer: B) Administer oral amoxicillin for antibiotic prophylaxis 1 hour before the dental extraction. The patient has a mechanical heart valve, which places him in a high-risk category for endocarditis. According to the American Heart Association (AHA) guidelines, antibiotic prophylaxis is recommended for patients with certain high-risk cardiac conditions undergoing dental procedures that involve manipulation of gingival tissue or the periapical region of teeth or perforation of the oral mucosa.

Option A is incorrect because the patient has a prosthetic heart valve, which is an indication for antibiotic prophylaxis before dental procedures that have the potential to cause bacteremia.

Option B is correct. The AHA recommends that high-risk patients, such as those with prosthetic heart valves, receive a single dose of oral amoxicillin (2 grams in adults) approximately 1 hour before dental procedures to provide prophylaxis against endocarditis.

Option C is incorrect because the AHA guidelines recommend a single dose of antibiotic prophylaxis before the procedure, not a 7-day course of antibiotics after the procedure.

Option D is incorrect because intravenous vancomycin is reserved for patients who are unable to take oral medications or have an allergy to amoxicillin or penicillin. There is no indication in the clinical scenario that the patient has an allergy to amoxicillin or is unable to take oral medications.

Therefore, the most appropriate next step in the management of this patient is to administer oral amoxicillin for antibiotic prophylaxis 1 hour before the dental extraction to prevent endocarditis, as per the AHA guidelines for high-risk cardiac lesions. The mechanism of action of amoxicillin in preventing endocarditis involves two primary protective effects: bactericidal activity and inhibition of bacterial adherence to the thrombotic vegetation on injured heart valves.The contraindications for using amoxicillin in preventing endocarditis include hypersensitivity or anaphylactic reactions to penicillin antibiotics. Patients with a history of such reactions should not be given amoxicillin for endocarditis prophylaxis. Alternative antibiotics should be considered for these individuals.The alternative antibiotics for preventing endocarditis in patients with hypersensitivity to penicillin antibiotics include clindamycin, which is an acceptable alternative for patients who are allergic to penicillins. Other alternatives may include clarithromycin or azithromycin for those unable to take oral medications or who have an allergy to amoxicillin or penicillin.

10.8 Endocarditis Prophylaxis in a 61-year-old Female

Case 159

A 61-year-old female with a history of mitral valve repair with annuloplasty ring placement for severe mitral regurgitation is scheduled for a tooth extraction due to advanced periodontal disease. She reports a severe allergic reaction to penicillin in the past, which resulted in anaphylaxis. Her current medications include lisinopril, metoprolol, and furosemide. On physical examination, her blood pressure is 130/80 mmHg, heart rate is 68 bpm, and a mid-diastolic murmur is heard at the apex. She has no signs of active infection or heart failure. Her renal function is normal.
Diagnostic Test Results:

1. Blood pressure: 130/80 mmHg
2. Heart rate: 68 bpm
3. Physical examination: Mid-diastolic murmur at the apex, no signs of infection or heart failure
4. Renal function: Normal

Given the patient's history of a severe penicillin allergy and the need for endocarditis prophylaxis, what is the most appropriate antibiotic regimen to administer before her dental procedure?

- A) Amoxicillin: 2 g PO 1 hour before the procedure
- B) Ampicillin: 2 g IV within 1 hour before the procedure
- C) Clindamycin: 600 mg PO 1 hour before the procedure
- D) Cefazolin: 1 g IV 30 minutes before the procedure

Correct Answer: C) Clindamycin: 600 mg PO 1 hour before the procedure he patient has a high-risk cardiac lesion (mitral valve repair with annuloplasty ring) and is scheduled for a dental procedure that requires endocarditis prophylaxis. She has a documented severe allergy to penicillin, which contraindicates the use of amoxicillin (Option A) and ampicillin (Option B), both of which are beta-lactam antibiotics. Option C is correct. According to the American Heart Association (AHA) guidelines, for patients with a high-risk cardiac condition who are undergoing dental procedures and have a history of severe penicillin allergy (e.g., anaphylaxis), an alternative antibiotic such as clindamycin is recommended. The recommended dose is 600 mg taken orally 1 hour before the procedure. Option D is incorrect because cefazolin, a cephalosporin, is generally avoided in patients with a history of severe penicillin allergy due to the potential for cross-reactivity, especially in cases of anaphylaxis. Although the cross-reactivity rate is low, in a patient with a history of anaphylaxis to penicillin, it is safer to use a non-beta-lactam antibiotic.

Therefore, the most appropriate antibiotic regimen for this patient, considering her severe penicillin allergy and the need for endocarditis prophylaxis, is clindamycin 600 mg taken orally 1 hour before the dental procedure.

11 CARDIOLOGY QUESTIONS

1. A 61-year-old male presents to the emergency department with complaints of progressive shortness of breath, fatigue, and lower extremity swelling over the past few weeks. He has a history of untreated hypertension and diabetes mellitus. On physical examination, his blood pressure is 140/90 mmHg, heart rate is 110 bpm, and respiratory rate is 24 breaths per minute. Jugular venous pressure (JVP) is elevated and rises significantly with inspiration. Cardiac auscultation reveals distant heart sounds and a pericardial knock. ECG shows low voltage QRS complexes. Echocardiography demonstrates a thickened pericardium with constrictive physiology.

What is the most appropriate next step in the diagnosis or management of this patient?

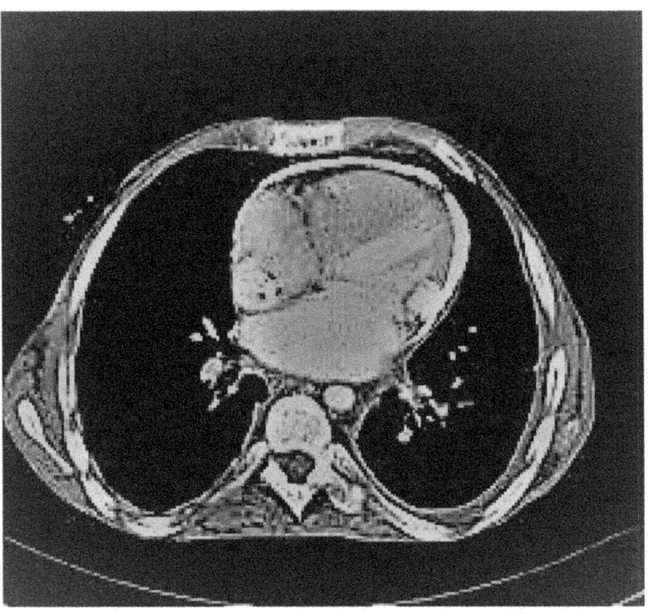

Figure 11.1: 61-year-old man

- A) Initiate diuresis with furosemide
- B) Perform cardiac catheterization

- C) Start empiric antibiotics for suspected infection
- D) Order cardiac MRI for further evaluation

2. A 65-year-old female presents to the cardiology clinic with complaints of worsening fatigue, abdominal distension, and lower extremity edema. She has a history of rheumatic fever in childhood. On physical examination, her blood pressure is 130/80 mmHg, heart rate is 90 bpm, and jugular venous pressure (JVP) is elevated with a prominent "a" wave and a slow "y" descent. Cardiac auscultation reveals a diastolic rumble at the lower left sternal border. Echocardiography shows thickened tricuspid valve leaflets with restricted motion and Doppler evidence of tricuspid stenosis. Question: What is the most appropriate next step in the diagnosis or management of this patient?

- A) Initiate anticoagulation therapy
- B) Perform exercise stress testing
- C) Order cardiac CT angiography
- D) Refer for surgical evaluation

3. A 60-year-old male presents to the cardiology clinic with complaints of increasing shortness of breath on exertion, fatigue, and palpitations. He has a history of hypertension and a prior myocardial infarction. On physical examination, his blood pressure is 140/90 mmHg, heart rate is 80 bpm, and a holosystolic murmur is heard at the apex that radiates to the axilla. ECG shows evidence of left ventricular hypertrophy. Echocardiography reveals severe mitral regurgitation with dilated left atrium and left ventricle. Question: What is the most appropriate next step in the diagnosis or management of this patient?

- A) Initiate medical therapy with beta-blockers
- B) Perform coronary angiography
- C) Refer for mitral valve repair or replacement
- D) Start anticoagulation therapy

4. A 42-year-old man with a history of hypertrophic cardiomyopathy presents with shortness of breath and chest pain. On physical examination, he is found to have a systolic murmur that is loudest at the left sternal border. What is the effect of the Valsalva maneuver on this murmur? Which of the following is the most appropriate answer?

- A. The murmur will become shorter and less intense.
- B. The murmur will become longer and louder.
- C. The murmur will not change in intensity or duration.
- D. The murmur will become softer and shorter.

5. A 33-year-old woman with a history of atrial septal defect (ASD) presents with shortness of breath and fatigue. On ECG, she is found to have incomplete right bundle branch block (RBBB). What is the most likely type of ASD? Which of the following is the most appropriate answer?

- A. Ostium primum defect
- B. Ostium secundum defect
- C. Sinus venosus defect
- D. None of the above

6. A 37-year-old man with a history of ventricular septal defect (VSD) presents with shortness of breath and fatigue. He has a Qp/Qs ratio of 1.5:1, but his pulmonary artery pressure and pulmonary vascular resistance are both below two-thirds of the systemic pressure and systemic resistance, respectively. Should he undergo percutaneous or surgical closure of his VSD? Which of the following is the most appropriate answer?

- A. No, he should not undergo percutaneous or surgical closure of his VSD.

- B. Yes, he should undergo percutaneous or surgical closure of his VSD.
- C. It is uncertain whether he should undergo percutaneous or surgical closure of his VSD.

7. A 51-year-old man with a history of tetralogy of Fallot presents to your office for a dental cleaning. He has never had antibiotic prophylaxis before dental procedures. Is antibiotic prophylaxis recommended for this patient? Which of the following is the most appropriate answer?

- A. Yes, antibiotic prophylaxis is recommended.
- B. No, antibiotic prophylaxis is not recommended.
- C. It is uncertain whether antibiotic prophylaxis is recommended.

8. A 53-year-old woman with a history of mitral stenosis presents with shortness of breath and fatigue. She has no other medical problems. What is the preferred procedure to manage her mitral stenosis? Which of the following is the most appropriate answer?

- A. Medical therapy
- B. Open surgical valvotomy
- C. Percutaneous balloon valvuloplasty
- D. Watchful waiting

9. A 71-year-old woman with a history of severe chronic primary mitral regurgitation (MR) presents with dyspnea on exertion. Her echocardiogram shows an LVEF of 55% and an end-systolic left ventricular diameter of 39 mm. Which of the following is the most appropriate treatment for this patient?

- A. Medical therapy with diuretics and ACE inhibitors
- B. Mitral valve repair
- C. Mitral valve replacement
- D. Transcatheter mitral valve repair
- E. Observation

10. A 75-year-old man presents with exertional dyspnea and syncope. Physical examination reveals a weak, delayed carotid pulse and a systolic murmur that is best heard at the second intercostal space on the right side. Which of the fol-lowing findings are most likely to be present on this patient's physical examination?

- A. Soft or absent A2
- B. S4
- C. Pulsus paradoxus
- D. Midsystolic click.
- E. Diastolic murmur

11. A 74-year-old man with severe aortic stenosis is being evaluated for transcatheter aortic valve replacement (TAVR). What are some of the potential complications associated with this procedure?

- A. Stroke
- B. Permanent pacemaker
- C. Paravalvular aortic regurgitation
- D. All of the above

12. A 62-year-old woman with chronic aortic regurgitation (AR) presents with dyspnea on exertion. She is currently taking a beta-blocker. What is the rationale for avoiding beta-blockers in patients with chronic AR?

- A. Beta-blockers can worsen heart failure.

- B. Beta-blockers can increase the risk of stroke.
- C. Beta-blockers can prolong the duration of diastole.
- D. Beta-blockers can decrease cardiac output.

13. A 56-year-old man with a history of mitral valve prolapse presents with fever, chills, and fatigue. He has no recent dental work or other known risk factors for endocarditis. What are the most likely causative microorganisms associated with his native-valve endocarditis (NVE)?

- A. Viridans streptococci
- B. Staphylococci
- C. HACEK organisms
- D. Streptococcus gallolyticus subspecies gallolyticus

14. A 79-year-old man with a history of pacemaker implantation presents with fever, chills, and fatigue. He had his pacemaker implanted 6 months ago. What are the most likely causative microorganisms associated with his CIED-related endocarditis?

- A. Viridans streptococci
- B. CoNS
- C. S aureus
- D. HACEK organisms

15. A 68-year-old man with a history of mitral valve prolapse presents with fever, chills, and fatigue. He has no recent dental work or other known risk factors for endocarditis. An MRI scan is performed, which reveals the presence of multiple clinically asymptomatic emboli. What is the prevalence of clinically asymptomatic emboli detected on MRI in pa-tients diagnosed with left-sided endocarditis?

- A. Under 5%
- B. 10-30%
- C. 5-10%
- D. 30-65%

16. A 67-year-old man with a history of mitral valve prolapse presents with fever, chills, and fatigue. He has no recent dental work or other known risk factors for endocarditis. A transesophageal echocardiogram (TEE) is performed, which is negative for any evidence of endocarditis. What is the next best step in management?

- A. Discharge the patient from the hospital
- B. Repeat the TEE examination in 7-10 days.
- C. Start antibiotic therapy.
- D. Refer the patient to a cardiologist for further evaluation.

17. A 64-year-old man with a history of prosthetic mitral valve replacement presents with fever, chills, and fatigue. He has no recent dental work or other known risk factors for endocarditis. An echocardiogram is performed, which reveals the presence of a vegetation on the prosthetic mitral valve. The patient is clinically stable and does not have any evidence of heart failure or other complications. What is the recommended duration of treatment for this patient?

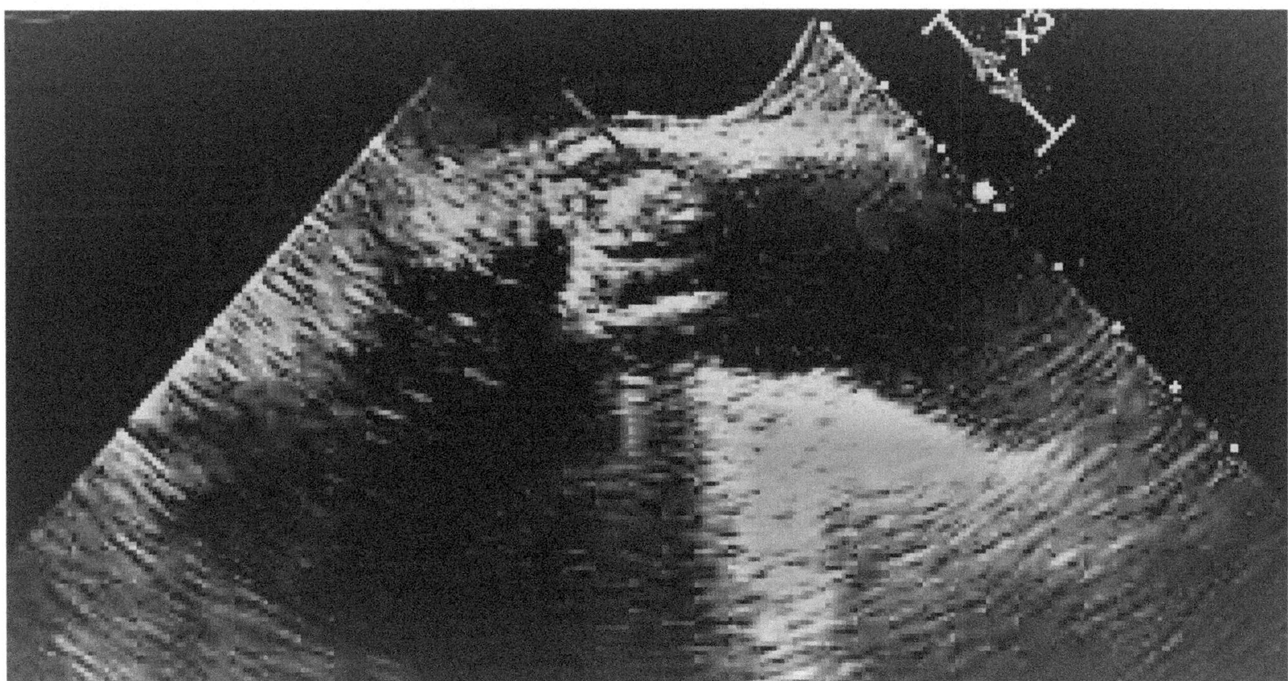

Figure 11.2: a vegetation on the prosthetic mitral valve

- A. 4 to 6 weeks
- B. 6 to 8 weeks
- C. 8 to 12 weeks
- D. 12 to 16 weeks

18. A 78-year-old woman with a history of dilated cardiomyopathy presents with dyspnea on exertion. She is currently in New York Heart Association (NYHA) class III heart failure. What is the role of aldosterone antagonist therapy in treating her condition?

- A. Aldosterone antagonist therapy is not indicated for patients with dilated cardiomyopathy.
- B. Aldosterone antagonist therapy may be considered for patients with dilated cardiomyopathy in NYHA class II heart failure.
- C. Aldosterone antagonist therapy is recommended for patients with dilated cardiomyopathy in NYHA class III heart failure.
- D. Aldosterone antagonist therapy is recommended for patients with dilated cardiomyopathy in NYHA class IV heart failure.

19. A 71-year-old man with a history of dilated cardiomyopathy presents with dyspnea on exertion. He is currently in NYHA class III heart failure. He has an LVEF of 30% and a QRS duration of 160 milliseconds. Is he a candidate for cardiac resynchronization therapy (CRT)?

- A. Yes, he is a candidate for CRT because he meets all of the criteria.
- B. No, he is not a candidate for CRT because his LVEF is above 35
- C. No, he is not a candidate for CRT because his QRS duration is below 150 milliseconds.
- D. It is unclear if he is a candidate for CRT because he does not have left bundle branch block.

20. A 69-year-old man with a history of systemic amyloidosis presents with dyspnea on exertion. He has no

prior histo-ry of heart disease. What are the expected imaging findings in this patient?

- A. Normal echocardiogram
- B. Dilated left ventricle with decreased ejection fraction.
- C. Bilateral atrial enlargement with speckled pattern in the ventricles
- D. Thickened pericardium with pericardial effusion

21. A 49-year-old man presents with exertional dyspnea and chest pain. On physical examination, you note a brisk carotid upstroke with pulsus bisferiens, an S4 sound, and a harsh systolic murmur along the left sternal border. What is the most likely diagnosis?

- A. Hypertrophic cardiomyopathy
- B. Mitral stenosis
- C. Aortic stenosis
- D. Mitral regurgitation

22. A 52-year-old man with hypertrophic cardiomyopathy presents with a history of syncope. He has no other cardiac risk factors. His echocardiogram shows a left ventricular wall thickness of 3.2 cm. What is the indication for an implantable cardioverter-defibrillator (ICD) in this patient?

- A. Syncope
- B. Left ventricular wall thickness of 3.2 cm
- C. Family history of sudden death
- D. All of the above

23. A 56-year-old man presents with a 2-week history of progressive dyspnea and fatigue. He has no other medical history. His physical examination is unremarkable. His laboratory tests show an elevated white blood cell count and an elevated troponin level. His chest X-ray shows cardiomegaly. His echocardiogram shows an enlarged left ventricle with decreased ejection fraction. What is the next best step in the management of this patient?

- A. Endomyocardial biopsy
- B. Start empiric antibiotic therapy.
- C. Refer the patient to a cardiologist for further evaluation.
- D. Discharge the patient home with close follow-up.

24. A 39-year-old man presents with chest pain. His ECG shows widespread ST elevation with reciprocal ST depression. He has no history of heart disease. What is the most likely diagnosis?

- A. Acute pericarditis
- B. Acute ST elevation myocardial infarction (STEMI)
- C. Early repolarization
- D. Arrhythmogenic right ventricular

25. A 52-year-old man presents with chest pain and a pericardial rub. His ECG shows diffuse ST elevation with reciprocal ST depression. He has no history of heart disease. What is the most appropriate management for this patient?

- A. Start aspirin and clopidogrel.
- B. Start heparin.
- C. Start colchicine.
- D. Discharge the patient home with close follow-up.

26. A 57-year-old man presents with chest pain and shortness of breath. His ECG shown, What is the significance of this finding?

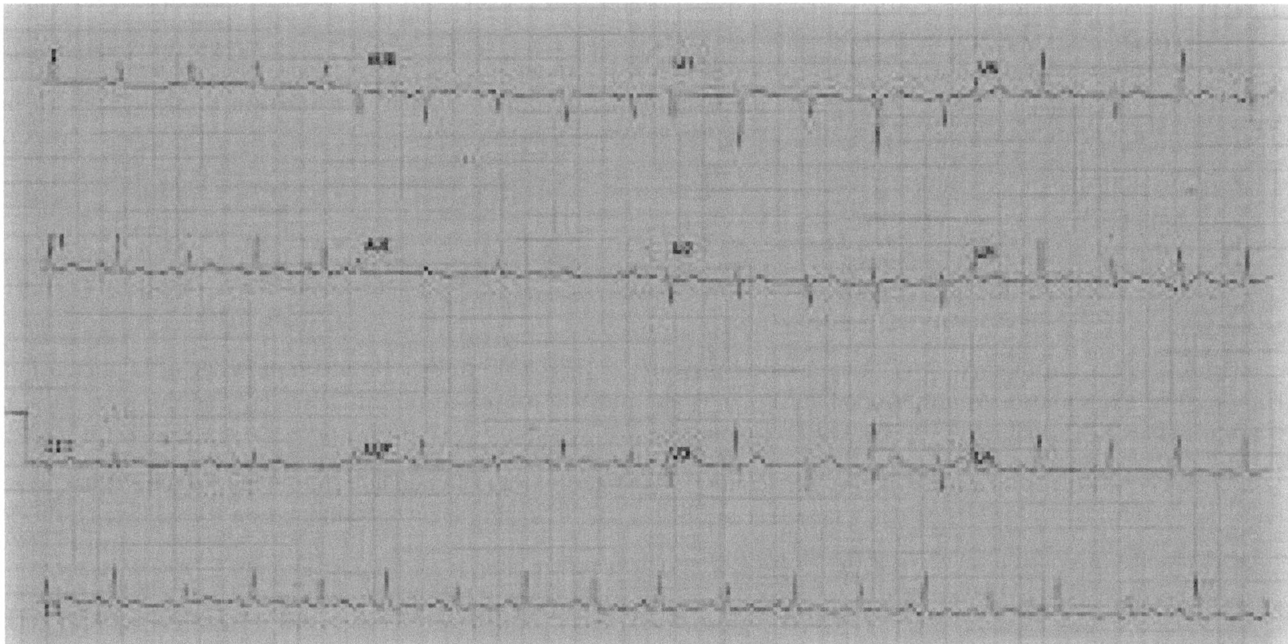

Figure 11.3: 57-year-old man

- A. Electrical alternans is a benign finding that is not associated with any significant pathology.
- B. Electrical alternans is a sign of cardiac tamponade.
- C. Electrical alternans is a sign of myocardial infarction.
- D. Electrical alternans is a sign of pericarditis.

27. A 67-year-old man presents with dyspnea on exertion and peripheral edema. He has no history of heart disease. His echocardiogram shows thickened pericardium with restricted diastolic filling. What is the next best step in the diagnosis of this patient?

- A. Cardiac catheterization
- B. Endomyocardial biopsy
- C. MRI
- D. CT

28. A 72-year-old man with hypertension presents with a serum creatinine level of 2.7 mg/dL. He is currently taking hydrochlorothiazide (HCTZ) for his hypertension. What is the next best step in his management?

- A. Increase the dose of HCTZ.
- B. Add a loop of diuretic to the regimen.
- C. Switch to a different thiazide diuretic.
- D. Discontinue HCTZ.

29. A 60-year-old man with hypertension is started on lisinopril. He also takes potassium chloride supplements for hypokalemia. What is the most important monitoring concern for this patient?

- A. Hypotension

- B. Hyperkalemia
- C. Renal insufficiency
- D. Hyperglycemia

30. A 25-year-old woman with chronic hypertension is planning to become pregnant. She is currently taking lisinopril for her hypertension. What is the most appropriate antihypertensive medication to switch her to in preparation for pregnancy?

- A. Methyldopa
- B. Labetalol
- C. Hydralazine
- D. Nifedipine

31. A 58-year-old man presents with a blood pressure of 220/120 mmHg. He has no history of hypertension. His physical examination is unremarkable. What is the most appropriate initial treatment for this patient? A. Nitroprusside B. Nicardipine C. Labetalol D. Enalaprilat

32. A 57-year-old man with a history of smoking, hypertension, and hypercholesterolemia presents with chest pain. He is referred to for an exercise stress test. Which of the following is a contraindication to exercise testing?

- A. Acute myocardial infarction (heart attack)
- B. Unstable angina
- C. Severe aortic stenosis
- D. Myocarditis or pericarditis
- E. Low exercise tolerance

33. A 58-year-old man with a history of smoking, hypertension, and hypercholesterolemia presents with chest pain. He is referred to for an exercise stress test. Which of the following is NOT a criterion for a positive exercise test?

- A. Chest pain or other symptoms that are consistent with angina.
- B. Diagnostic ST-segment changes on the ECG
- C. Failure to reach the target heart rate.
- D. A drop in blood pressure during exercise.
- E. A normal ECG

34. A 57-year-old man with a history of hypertension and diabetes presents with chest pain. He is prescribed a beta-blocker. Which of the following is a contraindication to beta-blockers?

- A. Congestive heart failure (CHF)
- B. Atrioventricular (AV) block
- C. Bronchospasm
- D. "Brittle" diabetes
- E. All of the above

35. A 55-year-old man with a history of coronary artery disease undergoes percutaneous coronary intervention (PCI) for a 50% stenosis of the left anterior descending artery. The procedure is performed with balloon dilatation alone. What is the rate of restenosis following this intervention?

- A. 10%
- B. 20%

- C. 30%
- D. 40%
- E. 50%

36. A 68-year-old man with a history of coronary artery disease presents with unstable angina. He has tried multiple medications, but his symptoms are not controlled. He has a left main coronary artery stenosis of 70% and a three-vessel disease. Which of the following is the most appropriate treatment for this patient?

- A. Percutaneous coronary intervention (PCI)
- B. Coronary artery bypass grafting (CABG)
- C. Medical therapy with nitrates and beta-blockers
- D. Medical therapy with calcium channel blockers
- E. Medical therapy with aspirin and clopidogrel

37. A 60-year-old man with a history of chronic stable angina presents to your clinic. He is currently taking medical therapy, but his symptoms are not well-controlled. He is considering PCI. Which of the following statements is most ac-curate?

- A. PCI is more effective than medical therapy in reducing the risk of MI or mortality in patients with chronic stable angina.
- B. PCI is more effective than medical therapy in providing relief from angina symptoms in patients with chronic stable angina.
- C. Medical therapy and PCI are equally effective in reducing the risk of MI or mortality in patients with chronic stable angina.
- D. Medical therapy and PCI are equally effective in providing relief from angina symptoms in patients with chronic stable angina.
- E. There is not enough evidence to determine which treatment is more effective in patients with chronic stable angina.

38. A 57-year-old man presents to the emergency department with chest pain. He has a history of ECG changes consistent with Prinzmetal's variant angina. Which of the following is the best way to confirm the diagnosis?

- A. Coronary angiography with provocative testing
- B. Coronary angiography without provocative testing
- C. Electrocardiography (ECG)
- D. Stress test
- E. Echocardiogram

39 A 61-year-old man presents to the emergency department with chest pain. He has a history of coronary artery dis-ease. His ECG shows ST-segment depression. What is the most likely diagnosis?

- A. NSTEMI
- B. STEMI
- C. Unstable angina
- D. Prinzmetal's variant angina
- E. Pericarditis

40. A 67-year-old man with a history of coronary artery disease presents to the emergency department with unstable angina. He is taken to the cardiac catheterization laboratory for percutaneous coronary intervention (PCI). Which of the following is the recommended therapy for this patient?

- A. Tirofiban
- B. Eptifibatide
- C. Abciximab
- D. Aspirin
- E. Clopidogrel

41. A 61-year-old man with a history of coronary artery disease presents to the emergency department with chest pain. He has a troponin level that is elevated, but his ECG does not show ST-segment elevation. He is currently receiving medical therapy for his chest pain, but his pain is not controlled. Which of the following is the most appropriate man-agement strategy for this patient?

- A. Immediate invasive strategy
- B. Selective invasive strategy
- C. Conservative medical therapy
- D. Observation

42. A 63-year-old man with a history of coronary artery disease presents to the emergency department with chest pain. He has a troponin level that is elevated, but his ECG does not show ST-segment elevation. He does not have any of the criteria for immediate invasive strategy. He does, however, have diabetes mellitus, renal insufficiency, and reduced left ventricular systolic function. Which of the following is the most appropriate management strategy for this patient?

- A. Immediate invasive strategy
- B. Selective invasive strategy
- C. Delayed invasive strategy.
- D. Conservative medical therapy

43. A 58-year-old man with a history of coronary artery disease presents to the emergency department with chest pain. He has an ECG that shows abnormal Q waves in leads V1-V2. What is the most likely diagnosis?

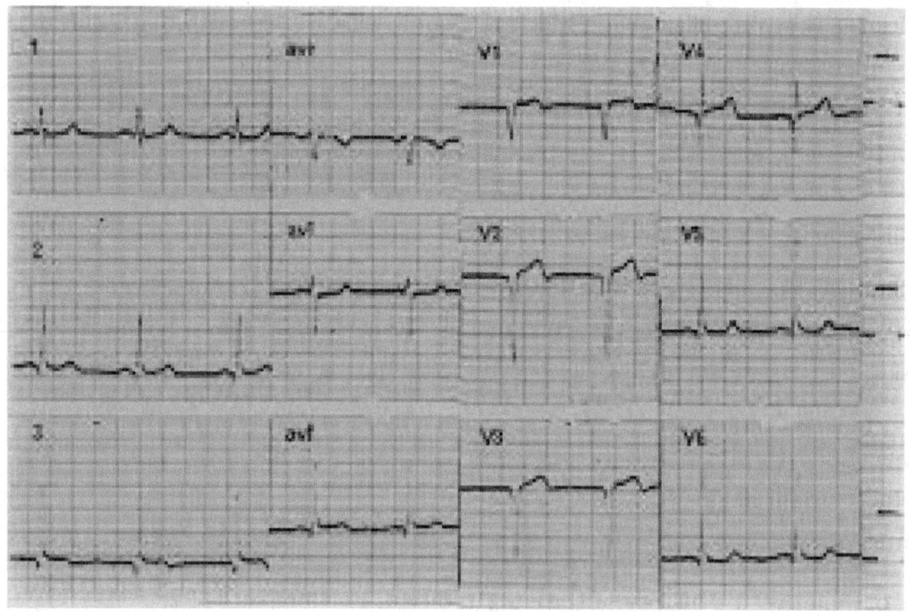

Figure 11.4: 58-year-old

- A. Anterolateral MI
- B. Inferior MI
- C. Apical MI
- D. True posterior MI
- E. Non-specific ST-T changes

44. A 56-year-old man with a history of coronary artery disease presents to the emergency department with chest pain. He has an ECG that shows ST-segment elevation in the anterior leads. The nearest PCI center is 150 minutes away. Which of the following is the most appropriate treatment option for this patient?

- A. Immediate PCI
- B. Intravenous fibrinolysis
- C. Medical therapy with aspirin and clopidogrel
- D. Observation

45. A 59-year-old man with a history of coronary artery disease presents to the emergency department with chest pain. He has an ECG that shows ST-segment elevation in the anterior leads. He is also in hemodynamically unstable ventricular tachycardia. What is the most appropriate treatment option for this patient?

- A. Immediate electrical countershock
- B. Intravenous fibrinolysis
- C. Medical therapy with aspirin and clopidogrel
- D. Observation

46. A 71-year-old man with a history of coronary artery disease presents to the emergency department with chest pain. He has an ECG that shows ST-segment elevation in the anterior leads. He is also in acute heart failure. Which of the fol-lowing is the most appropriate initial therapy for this patient?

- A. Furosemide
- B. Oxygen
- C. Nitrates
- D. Digitalis
- E. All of the above

47. A 65-year-old man with a history of coronary artery disease presents to the emergency department with chest pain. He has an ECG that shows ST-segment elevation in the anterior leads. He is also in cardiogenic shock. His systolic blood pressure is 80 mmHg, and his pulmonary capillary wedge pressure (PCWP) is 25 mmHg. What treatment options are available to maintain his systolic blood pressure above 90 mmHg and reduce his PCWP?

- A. Norepinephrine
- B. Dopamine
- C. Intraaortic balloon counterpulsation (IABP)
- D. All of the above

48. A 62-year-old man with a history of coronary artery disease presents to the emergency department with chest pain. He has an ECG that shows ST-segment elevation in the anterior leads. He is also hypothetical. His systolic blood pres-sure is 80 mmHg, and his heart rate is 120 beats per minute. An echocardiogram shows that he has a right ventricular MI. What is the treatment for his hypotension? A. Intravenous fluids B. Vasopressors C. Intraaortic balloon counterpulsation D. Mechanical ventilation

49. A 66-year-old man with a history of coronary artery disease presents to the emergency department with

palpitations. He has an ECG that shows atrial flutter with a ventricular rate of 120 beats per minute. What is the initial treatment for this patient?

- A. Beta blockers
- B. Verapamil
- C. Diltiazem
- D. Digoxin
- E. All of the above

50. A 75-year-old man with a history of coronary artery disease presents to the emergency department with palpitations. He has an ECG that shows Torsade de pointes. What is the treatment for this patient?

- A. Intravenous magnesium
- B. Overdrive pacing
- C. Isoproterenol
- D. Lidocaine
- E. All of the above

51. A 61-year-old man with a history of coronary artery disease presents to the emergency department with palpitations. He has an ECG that shows supraventricular tachycardia with aberrant ventricular conduction. The ventricular rate is 200 beats per minute. What is the treatment for this patient?

- A. Beta blockers
- B. Verapamil
- C. Diltiazem
- D. Digoxin
- E. Electrical cardioversion

52. A 69-year-old man with a history of coronary artery disease presents to the cardiologist with complaints of fatigue and lightheadedness. He has an ECG that shows sinus bradycardia with a heart rate of 40 beats per minute. He is also taking digoxin for his heart condition. What is the Class I indication for pacemaker implantation in this patient?

- A. Sinus bradycardia with a heart rate of 40 beats per minute
- B. Sinus bradycardia with symptoms
- C. Sinus bradycardia with symptoms that are refractory to medical therapy.
- D. Sinus bradycardia with symptoms that are refractory to medical therapy and are associated with an increased risk of syncope.
- E. All of the above

53. A 61-year-old man with a history of coronary artery disease presents to the emergency department with complaints of lightheadedness. He has an ECG that shows Mobitz II AV block with a 2:1 conduction pattern. What is the most appropriate next step in management?

- A. Observation
- B. Medications to increase the heart rate.
- C. Permanent pacemaker implantation
- D. Electrophysiology study

54. A 59-year-old man with a history of coronary artery disease presents to the cardiologist with complaints

of palpitations and lightheadedness. He has an ECG that shows atrial fibrillation. What is the best approach to managing his AFib?

- A. Rhythm control with cardioversion
- B. Rate control with beta-blockers
- C. Rate control with calcium channel blockers
- D. Ibutilide

55. A 65-year-old man with a history of coronary artery disease and hypertension presents to the cardiologist with com-plaints of palpitations and lightheadedness. He has an ECG that shows chronic atrial fibrillation. He also has a history of rheumatic mitral stenosis. What is the best approach to managing his AFib?

- A. Rate control with beta-blockers
- B. Rate control with calcium channel blockers
- C. Rhythm control with cardioversion
- D. Anticoagulation with warfarin

56. A 67-year-old woman with a history of heart failure presents to the emergency department with complaints of nau-sea, vomiting, and visual disturbances. She is also taking digoxin for her heart condition. What is the most appropriate next step in management?

- A. Discontinue digoxin and monitor her symptoms.
- B. Administer atropine intravenously.
- C. Administer digoxin-specific antibody fragments.
- D. Admit to the hospital for observation.

57. A 81-year-old man with a history of heart failure presents to the cardiologist with complaints of shortness of breath and fatigue. He has an ejection fraction of 30% and is already taking the maximum tolerated dose of beta-blockers. What is the next best treatment option for this patient?

- A. Ivabradine
- B. Digoxin
- C. Ranolazine
- D. Hydralazine/isosorbide dinitrate
- E. Dobutamine

58. 63-year-old man with a history of diabetes mellitus presents to the emergency department with complaints of fever, shortness of breath, and altered mental status. He is found to be hypotensive and tachycardic. His initial laboratory workup shows leukocytosis and elevated serum lactate levels. His chest X-ray shows a diffuse infiltrate. What is the most appropriate vasopressor agent to initiate in this patient?

- A. Dopamine
- B. Norepinephrine
- C. Epinephrine
- D. Vasopressin
- E. Milrinone

59. A 68-year-old man presents to the emergency department with chest pain and shortness of breath. He is found to have a type A aortic dissection. What is the most appropriate initial treatment for this patient?

- A. Sodium nitroprusside

- B. Metoprolol
- C. Verapamil
- D. Diltiazem
- E. Hydralazine

60. A 55-year-old man with hypercholesterolemia is being evaluated for treatment. Which of the following is the most likely benefit of interventions aimed at lowering his LDL-C levels?

- A. Reduced risk of myocardial infarction
- B. Reduced risk of stroke.
- C. Reduced risk of overall mortality
- D. All of the above
- E. None of the above

61.A 38-year-old woman presents to the emergency department with chest pain that has lasted for 2 hours. She has no significant past medical history. An electrocardiogram shows no ST-segment elevations. Her troponin level is elevated. She undergoes a cardiac catheterization, which reveals no obstructive coronary disease. Her left ventricular function is found to be depressed. Which of the following is the most appropriate next step to confirm a potential diagnosis?

- A. Cardiac Magnetic Resonance Imaging (MRI)
- B. Pulmonary Function Tests
- C. Abdominal Ultrasound
- D. Chest X-ray
- E. Carotid Doppler Ultrasound

62. A patient with a left bundle branch block (LBBB) and poor exercise tolerance presents for evaluation of chest pain. Which of the following diagnostic tests is most appropriate?

- (A) Exercise stress test
- (B) Echocardiogram
- (C) Coronary CTA
- (D) Pharmacologic stress test with perfusion imaging
- (E) Cardiac catheterization

63. A 56-year-old man presents to the emergency department with chest pain that has been intermittent over the past few days. The pain is not associated with exertion and does not radiate. He has a family history of early coronary artery disease (CAD), hypertension, and hyperlipidemia. His chest pain is somewhat atypical, but given his risk factors, he has an intermediate probability of CAD. Which of the following is the most appropriate next step to exclude coronary disease?

- A. Cardiac Magnetic Resonance Imaging (MRI)
- B. Exercise Stress Test
- C. Coronary CT Angiography
- D. Cardiac Catheterization
- E. Echocardiogram

64.A 67-year-old man with a history of hypertension and hyperlipidemia presents with chest pain on exertion. He undergoes an exercise stress test, which is stopped after 7 minutes due to angina. His BP does not augment with exercise, and his ECG at 7 minutes into recovery shows diffuse ST depressions ¿2 mm and an ST elevation in aVR. Which of the following is the next most appropriate step in management?

- (A) Admit to the hospital for further monitoring
- (B) Perform coronary angiography
- (C) Start beta blocker therapy
- (D) Order a nuclear stress test
- (E) Refer to a cardiologist for follow-up

65.A 62-year-old man presents with a history of chest pain that occurs with exertion and is relieved by rest. His exercise stress test shows evidence of ischemia in a single territory, confirming the diagnosis of coronary artery disease (CAD). Assuming he is already on low-dose aspirin , what would be the next best step in management?

- A. Initiate -blocker and statin
- B. Proceed to coronary angiography
- C. Optimize lipid-lowering therapy only
- D. Consider coronary revascularization
- E. Perform a transthoracic echocardiogram

66. A 68-year-old man undergoes cardiac catheterization and receives a stent in his right coronary artery. Immediately after the procedure, he develops hypotension and a rapidly expanding hematoma at the access site. What is the most appropriate next step in management?

- (A) Start aspirin and P2Y12 inhibitor therapy
- (B) Administer blood products empirically
- (C) Order a CT of the abdomen
- (D) Apply manual compression to the access site
- (E) Consult the cardiologist

67. A 59-year-old male underwent stent placement for management of an acute coronary syndrome 10 months ago. He is currently on dual antiplatelet therapy with aspirin and clopidogrel. The patient now has severe knee pain and is considered for a knee replacement surgery. What is the best management of the patient's medication regimen considering the impending surgery?

- A. Continue dual antiplatelet therapy and proceed with knee replacement.
- B. Temporarily discontinue clopidogrel and proceed with knee replacement.
- C. Replace clopidogrel with intravenous P2Y12 inhibitor cangrelor.
- D. Continue dual antiplatelet therapy and delay knee replacement until 12 months have passed since stent placement.
- E. Conduct stress testing to guide the duration of dual antiplatelet therapy.

68. A 62-year-old male presents to the emergency department with intermittent chest pain over the last few days. He has a past medical history of hypertension and hyperlipidemia. His vitals are stable and his initial EKG and troponin levels are normal. His Thrombolysis in Myocardial Infarction (TIMI) score is 2. What is the most appropriate next step in the management of this patient?

- A. Initiate conservative therapy with aspirin, -blocker, and nitrates as needed, followed by noninvasive risk stratification (stress testing) to help determine if coronary angiography is appropriate, provided the patient remains asymptomatic.
- B. Perform immediate diagnostic angiography with the intent to revascularize.
- C. Perform early (within 24 hours) diagnostic angiography with the intent to revascularize.
- D. Immediately initiate dual antiplatelet therapy and proceed to coronary angiography.

- E. Initiate high dose statin therapy and order a coronary CT angiogram.

69. A patient with suspected acute coronary syndrome (ACS) is being evaluated for the appropriate timing of angiography. Which of the following is the most appropriate timing for angiography in this patient?

- A. within 6 hours
- Within 24 hours
- C.Within 48 hours
- D. Within 72 hours
- E.Immediately

70. A patient presents with a late presentation of a larger territory myocardial infarction (MI), especially of the anterior wall. He develops a harsh holosystolic murmur at the lower sternal border, especially in the presence of a palpable systolic thrill. What is the next best step in management?

- A. Initiate afterload reducing agents
- B. Start right heart catheterization
- C. Begin interventions with an intra-aortic balloon pump
- D. Urgent transthoracic echocardiography
- E. Wait and observe for further symptoms

71. Which of the following is the first-line therapy for vasospastic angina?

- A. Aspirin
- B. Beta-blocker
- C. Calcium channel blocker
- D. Nitrate
- E. None of the above

72. A 69-year-old woman is hospitalized due to severe shortness of breath. She has a history of congestive heart failure and has recently been diagnosed with sepsis. Despite being on inotropic support, her cardiac output remains reduced. Additionally, she is hypotensive and requires a vasopressor to maintain her systemic vascular resistance at a low end of normal. What is the most likely classification of her shock state?

- A. Mixed—cardiogenic and distributive
- B. Cardiogenic shock
- C. Distributive shock
- D. Obstructive shock
- E. Hypovolemic shock

73. A 68-year-old woman presents with symptoms suggestive of a heart failure exacerbation. She has acute kidney injury with normal mentation, normal perfusion, and normal pulse pressure. She has had a limited response to oral diuretics. What is the most appropriate next step in her management?

- A. Administer intravenous crystalloid.
- B. Administer intravenous furosemide.
- C. Start intravenous inotropic agents.
- D. Initiate renal replacement therapy.
- E. Arrange for an urgent cardiac transplantation.

74. What is a major risk of the intra-aortic balloon pump?

- A. Decreased aortic regurgitation
- B. Increased aortic regurgitation
- C. Decreased afterload
- D. Increased cardiac output
- E. None of the above

75. Which of the following medications is recommended for patients with heart failure with preserved ejection fraction (HFpEF) to reduce the risk of rehospitalization for HF?

- A. ACE inhibitor
- B. Phosphodiesterase type 5 inhibitor
- C. Aspirin
- D. Spironolactone
- E. SGLT2i

76. A patient is presented in cardiogenic shock due to profound acute decompensated heart failure (HF). The patient's condition is not improving with the current treatment plan. What would be the next appropriate step?

- A. Increase the dose of pressor
- B. Increase the dose of dobutamine
- C. Insert a percutaneous left ventricular assist device (eg, Impella or Tandem Heart)
- D. Use an intra-aortic balloon pump
- E. Continue with the current treatment plan

77. A 48-year-old male with a history of significant alcohol and cocaine use presents with symptoms of dilated cardiomyopathy. He also has recent influenza infection. Cardiac MRI does not support a diagnosis of acute myocarditis. His ejection fraction (EF) is significantly decreased. What is the most appropriate next step in management?

- A. Initiate guideline-directed medical therapy, advise abstinence from alcohol and cocaine, and repeat transthoracic echocardiogram in 1 month.
- B. Initiate angiotensin-converting enzyme (ACE) inhibitor and -blocker; repeat transthoracic echocardiogram in 3 months.
- C. Perform a myocardial biopsy to determine the cause of the systolic dysfunction.
- D. Immediate placement of a primary prevention implantable cardiac defibrillator.
- E. Arrange for immediate referral for heart transplant evaluation.

78. What is the most likely diagnosis in a patient with low voltages on ECG and thick ventricular walls on transthoracic echocardiogram?

- A. Amyloidosis
- B. Sarcoidosis
- C. Long-standing hypertension
- D. Hypertrophic cardiomyopathy
- E. None of the above

79. A 52-year-old woman presents with a history of mitral valve prolapse. Echocardiography reveals an ejection fraction (EF) of 45% and a left ventricular end-systolic dimension (LVESD) of 42 mm. She is asymptomatic and without evidence of congestion. What should be the next step in the management of this patient's condition?

- A. Start furosemide
- B. Repeat echocardiography in 6 months
- C. Refer for mitral valve surgery
- D. Start ambulatory ECG monitoring
- E. Start beta-blocker therapy

80. A patient with a mechanical aortic valve and atrial fibrillation needs to have dental surgery. Which of the following is the best anticoagulation management strategy?

- A. Continue coumadin and monitor INR closely.
- B. Stop coumadin and start heparin 24 hours before surgery.
- C. Stop coumadin now and bridge with unfractionated heparin.
- D. Start a novel oral anticoagulant (NOAC) 24 hours before surgery.
- E. None of the above.

81. A 27-year-old woman with rheumatic mitral stenosis presents at 20 weeks gestation with symptoms of New York Heart Association (NYHA) class III heart failure. What is the best management strategy?

- A. Continue medical management and monitor closely.
- B. Schedule surgical mitral valve replacement.
- C. Perform percutaneous mitral balloon valvuloplasty (PMBV).
- D. Refer for PMBV as anatomy allows.
- E. Terminate the pregnancy.

82. A patient presents with distant heart sounds, elevated jugular vein pulsation, and hypotension, suggestive of Beck's triad. What is the most appropriate initial treatment step?

- A. Perform an emergent transthoracic echocardiogram
- B. Initiate pericardiocentesis
- C. Give 500 mL fluid bolus
- D. Conduct a pulmonary embolism CT scan
- E. Create a pericardial window

83. A 62-year-old man presents with a history of radiation therapy. He is found to have a jugular venous pulsation that does not decrease with inspiration and signs and symptoms of right-sided heart failure with clear lungs. An echocardiogram reveals respirophasic variation. What is the most likely diagnosis?

- A. Restrictive cardiomyopathy
- B. Constrictive pericarditis
- C. Acute myocarditis
- D. Dilated cardiomyopathy
- E. Hypertrophic cardiomyopathy

84. A 47-year-old man with no prior cardiovascular history presents with a blood pressure of 135/85 mmHg. What is the best management strategy?

- A. Calculating his atherosclerotic cardiovascular disease (ASCVD) risk score and, if ¿10%, starting an antihypertensive agent now.
- B. Starting an antihypertensive agent now.
- C. Monitoring his blood pressure closely and following up in 3 months.

- D. Recommending lifestyle changes only.
- E. None of the above.

85. 54-year-old woman with a history of type 2 diabetes mellitus visits your clinic for a routine check-up. She has been managing her diabetes with metformin. Recent laboratory results indicate the presence of microalbuminuria. Her blood pressure today is 150/90 mmHg. You decide to start her on antihypertensive therapy. Which of the following should be your first choice?

- A. Amlodipine (Calcium channel blocker)
- B. Hydrochlorothiazide (Diuretic)
- C. Metoprolol (Beta-blocker)
- D. Lisinopril (ACE inhibitor)
- E. Losartan (Angiotensin II receptor blocker)

86. A 69-year-old man presents to the emergency department with severe chest pain and blood pressure of 220/130 mmHg. He is tachycardic with a heart rate of 110 beats per minute. Chest X-ray shows a widened mediastinum. What is the best initial management strategy?

- A. Oral labetalol
- B. Intravenous labetalol
- C. Intravenous nitroglycerin
- D. Intravenous nitroprusside
- E. Intravenous esmolol

87. A 26-year-old woman presents with severe hypertension. On physical examination, an abdominal bruit is noted. What is the most appropriate next step in her diagnostic evaluation?

- A. MR angiography (MRA) of the renal arteries
- B. Duplex ultrasound of the renal arteries
- C. Noncontrast CT scan of the abdomen
- D. Renal angiography
- E. Percutaneous transluminal renal angioplasty

88. A 73-year-old man with a 5.2 cm abdominal aortic aneurysm (AAA) is referred to you for management. He has no symptoms related to the AAA. The AAA has grown by 0.5 cm in the past 6 months. What is the best management strategy?

- A. Observe the AAA with serial imaging.
- B. Start antihypertensive therapy to slow the growth of the AAA.
- C. Perform surgical repair of the AAA.
- D. Perform endovascular aneurysm repair (EVAR) of the AAA.
- E. None of the above.

89. A 26-year-old man presents with sudden onset severe chest and back pain. He stands at 6 feet 5 inches tall, with long arms and fingers, a high-arched palate, and a pectus excavatum deformity. On physical examination, you note a diastolic murmur and bilateral pulmonary rales. His blood pressure is elevated at 160/90 mmHg. Given this presentation, what would be the most appropriate next step in management?

- A. Administer a high-flow oxygen therapy
- B. Initiate anticoagulation treatment

- C. Prescribe analgesics for pain control
- D. Arrange for urgent surgical intervention
- E. Begin treatment with antihypertensive medications

90. A 37-year-old man presents with intermittent fevers, a recent history of a target-shaped rash, and travel to an endemic area for Lyme disease. He is hemodynamically unstable with a heart rate of 40 beats per minute and complete heart block with a slow escape rhythm. What is the best management strategy?

- A. Administer intravenous atropine.
- B. Perform transesophageal echocardiogram (TEE).
- C. Start intravenous antibiotics for Lyme disease and observe.
- D. Place a transvenous temporary pacemaker.
- E. Implant a permanent pacemaker.

91. A 72-year-old man with chronic obstructive pulmonary disease (COPD) presents with shortness of breath and a heart rate of 130 beats per minute. His ECG shows an irregular rhythm with three distinct P-wave morphologies. What is the most likely diagnosis?

- A. Atrial fibrillation
- B. Multifocal atrial tachycardia
- C. Atrioventricular nodal reentrant tachycardia
- D. Wolff-Parkinson-White syndrome

92. A 33-year-old patient presents to the emergency department with palpitations and dizziness. An ECG shows evidence of a pre-excitation syndrome, likely Wolff-Parkinson-White (WPW) syndrome, and he has now developed a rapid supraventricular tachycardia. What is the most appropriate initial management in this case?

- A) Adenosine
- B) Digoxin
- C) Direct current cardioversion
- D) Procainamide
- E) No treatment necessary

93. A 54-year-old woman with no prior cardiac history is admitted with pneumonia and started on broad-spectrum antibiotics. She suddenly goes into cardiac arrest with polymorphic ventricular tachycardia. Her ECG shows a pseudo-RBBB pattern with ST-segment elevation in V1 to V3. What is the most likely cause of her arrhythmia?

- A. Brugada syndrome
- B. Long QT interval
- C. Arrhythmogenic right ventricular cardiomyopathy
- D. Ischemia
- E. Left bundle branch block

94. A 52-year old woman with a history of hypertension presents with her fourth episode of monomorphic ventricular tachycardia over the past 2 months despite adequate medical therapy including -blockers, mexiletine, and amiodarone. Her most recent coronary angiogram suggests that her ventricular tachycardia is not driven by ischemia. What is the next most appropriate step in care?

- A. Increase dosage of -blockers
- B. Change mexiletine to another antiarrhythmic drug

- C. Initiate anticoagulation therapy
- D. Perform radiofrequency ablation
- E. Schedule for implantation of a cardiac defibrillator

95. A 68-year-old woman with a history of hypertension and atrial fibrillation (AF) presents with shortness of breath and fatigue. On examination, she is tachycardic with a heart rate of 130 beats per minute and her blood pressure is 160/90 mmHg. Transthoracic echocardiography (TTE) shows a dilated left ventricle with an ejection fraction of 30%. What is the best management strategy?

- A. Increase her heart rate control medications.
- B. Start her on anticoagulation.
- C. Perform transesophageal echocardiogram (TEE); if no left atrial thrombus, perform cardioversion.
- D. Refer her for ablation of her AF.
- E. None of the above.

96. A 68-year old man with a history of ischemic cardiomyopathy presents with new-onset atrial fibrillation (AF). Which medication would be the most appropriate for the management of his condition?

- A. Amiodarone
- B. Flecainide
- C. Propafenone
- D. Diltiazem
- E. Metoprolol

97. A 72-year old woman presents to the emergency department following a mechanical fall. She has a life-threatening traumatic intracranial hemorrhage and is on both aspirin and apixaban. What would be the most appropriate intervention to manage her condition?

- A. Andexanet alfa
- B. Idarucizumab
- C. Fresh frozen plasma
- D. Vitamin K
- E. Platelet transfusion

98. A 69-year-old woman with rheumatic mitral stenosis and atrial fibrillation (AF) is currently taking warfarin for stroke prevention. She asks you about the possibility of switching to a direct-acting oral anticoagulant (DOAC). What is your response?

- A. DOACs are safe and effective alternatives to warfarin for stroke prevention in patients with AF and rheumatic mitral stenosis.
- B. DOACs are not indicated for stroke prevention in patients with AF and rheumatic mitral stenosis.
- C. DOACs are safe and effective alternatives to warfarin for stroke prevention in patients with AF and rheumatic mitral stenosis, but they require more frequent monitoring than warfarin.
- D. DOACs are safe and effective alternatives to warfarin for stroke prevention in patients with AF and rheumatic mitral stenosis, but they are more expensive than warfarin.
- E. DOACs are safe and effective alternatives to warfarin for stroke prevention in patients with AF and rheumatic mitral stenosis, but they are not as effective as warfarin in preventing thromboembolism.

99. A 58-year-old man presents with hypotension and elevated neck veins 6 hours after pacemaker implantation. He is also noted to have a blunted Y descent in his jugular veins. What is the most likely diagnosis?

- A. Pacemaker syndrome
- B. Lead perforation leading to cardiac tamponade
- C. Pacemaker-mediated tachycardia
- D. Flash pulmonary edema
- E. None of the above

100. A 63-year-old male patient presents with a fever, positive blood cultures showing S. aureus, and erythema around his pacemaker site. Despite a negative transesophageal echocardiogram (TEE), he has staphylococcal bacteremia. What would be the most appropriate treatment plan for this patient?

- A. Continue oral antibiotics
- B. Continue intravenous antibiotics
- C. Plan for pacemaker system removal
- D. Valve surgery
- E. Increase dosage of current medication

101.A 46-year-old man presents to the emergency department with sharp, central chest pain that worsens on lying down and improves on sitting forward. He also reports a low-grade fever. His ECG is shown below. Which of the following is the most likely diagnosis?

1.png

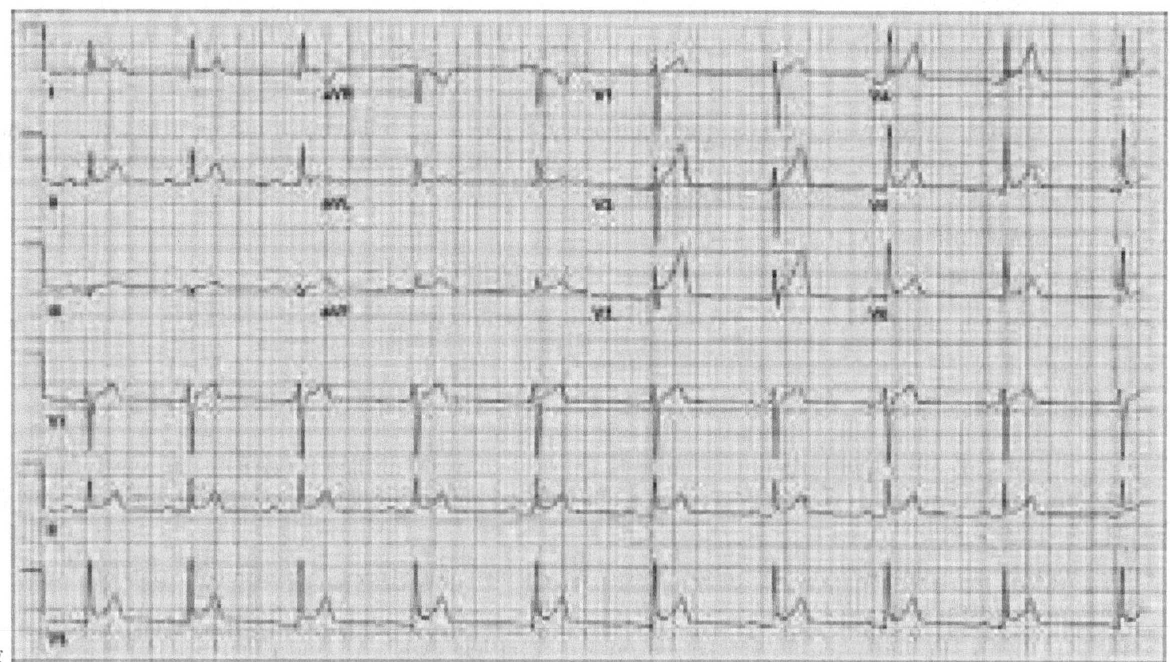

Figure 11.5: ECG of the patient

- A. Myocardial infarction
- B. Pulmonary embolism
- C. Pneumonia
- D. Pericardial effusion
- E. Acute pericarditis

102. A 53-year-old woman with a history of depression and anxiety presents to the clinic for a routine check-up. She is currently taking fluoxetine for her depression and lorazepam for her anxiety. She has no complaints and her physical examination is unremarkable. An ECG is performed as part of her routine check-up, Which of the following is the most appropriate next step in management?

QT.png 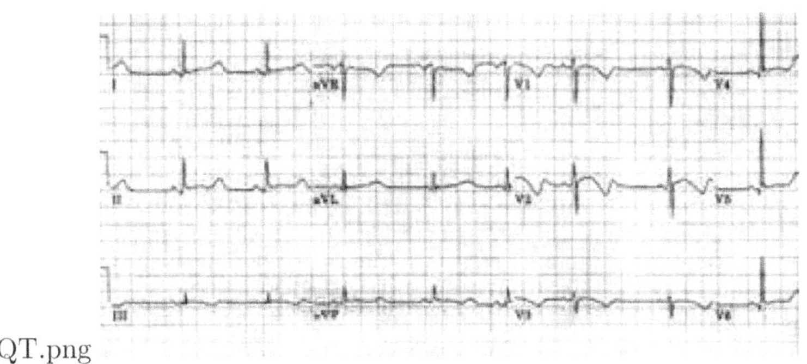

Figure 11.6: A 53-year-old woman ECG

- A. Discontinue fluoxetine and lorazepam immediately
- B. Start her on a beta-blocker
- C. Monitor her QT interval regularly
- D. Start her on a calcium channel blocker
- E. Refer her for an implantable cardioverter-defibrillator (ICD)

103. A 68-year-old man with a history of hypertension and type 2 diabetes presents to the emergency department with generalized weakness and muscle cramps. His medications include hydrochlorothiazide and metformin. His blood pressure is 140/90 mmHg, pulse is 80 beats per minute, and other vital signs are stable. Laboratory tests reveal a serum potassium level of 2.8 mEq/L (normal: 3.5-5.0 mEq/L). An ECG is performed, which is most likely to show which of the following?

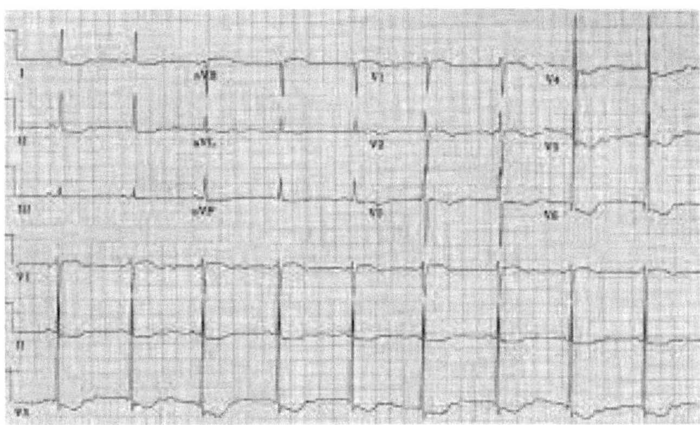

Figure 11.7: A 68-year-old man ECG

- A. T-wave flattening or inversion
- B. QRS widening
- C. ST-segment elevation
- D. PR segment elevation
- E. Absence of P waves

104. A 60-year-old man with a history of chronic kidney disease and hypertension presents to the emergency department with palpitations and weakness. His medications include lisinopril and amlodipine. His blood pressure is 130/80 mmHg, pulse is 90 beats per minute, and other vital signs are stable. Laboratory tests reveal a serum potassium level of 6.2 mEq/L (normal: 3.5-5.0 mEq/L). An ECG is performed, Which of the following is the most appropriate initial step in management?

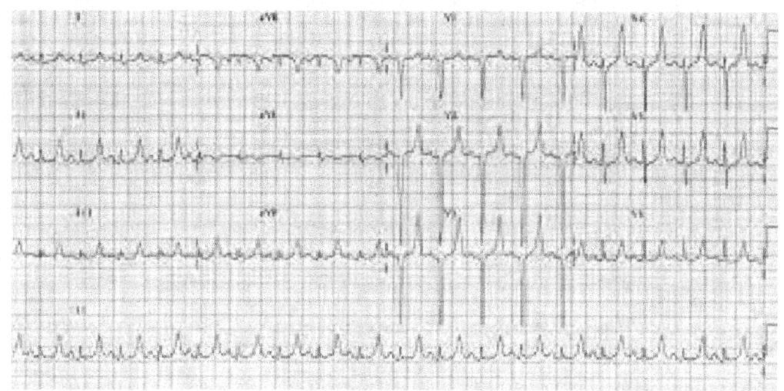

Figure 11.8: A 60-year-old man ECG

- A. Administer sodium polystyrene sulfonate
- B. Start him on a loop diuretic
- C. Administer intravenous calcium gluconate
- D. Discontinue lisinopril
- E. Start him on a beta-blocker

105. A 63year-old woman with a history of thyroidectomy for thyroid carcinoma presents to the emergency department with muscle twitches and spasms. She also reports numbness and tingling around her mouth and fingertips. Her blood pressure is 120/80 mmHg, pulse is 80 beats per minute, and other vital signs are stable. Laboratory tests reveal a serum calcium level of 6.8 mg/dL (normal: 8.5-10.2 mg/dL). An ECG is performed, which is most likely to show which of the following?

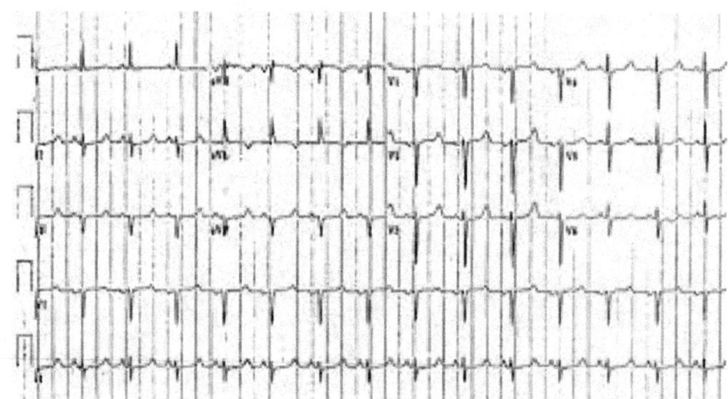

Figure 11.9: A 63year-old woman with a history of thyroidectomy

- A. Prolonged QT interval
- B. ST-segment elevation
- C. Shortened PR interval
- D. Absence of P waves
- E. QRS widening

106. A 67-year-old man with a history of hyperparathyroidism presents to the emergency department with constipation, polyuria, and confusion. His blood pressure is 140/90 mmHg, pulse is 80 beats per minute, and other vital signs are stable. Laboratory tests reveal a serum calcium level of 12.0 mg/dL (normal: 8.5-10.2 mg/dL). An ECG is performed, which is most likely to show which of the following findings?

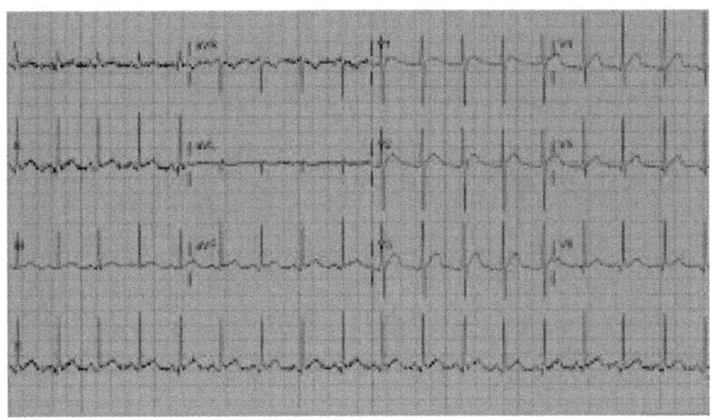

Figure 11.10: A 67-year-old man ECG

- A. Prolonged QT interval
- B. Shortened QT interval
- C. Prominent U waves
- D. PR segment elevation
- E. QRS narrowing

107. A 63-year-old man with a history of hypertension and smoking presents to the emergency department with severe chest pain radiating to his left arm. His blood pressure is 150/90 mmHg, pulse is 90 beats per minute, and other vital signs are stable. An ECG is performed, which of the following is the most likely diagnosis?

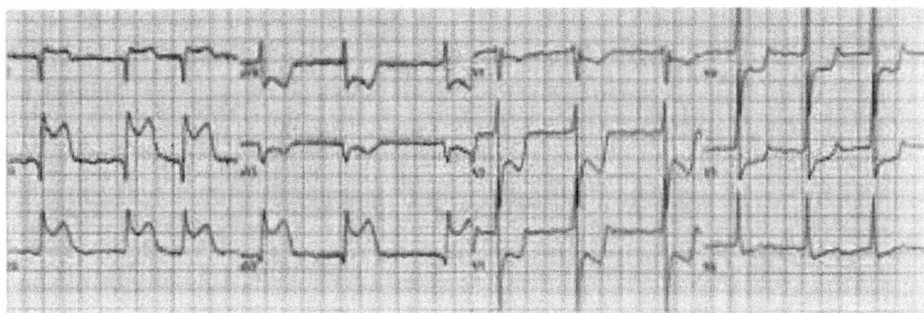

Figure 11.11: A 63-year-old man ECG

- A. Anterior ST-elevation myocardial infarction
- B. Pericarditis
- C. Inferior ST-elevation myocardial infarction
- D. Stable angina
- E. Unstable angina

108. A 61-year-old man with a history of ischemic heart disease suddenly collapses. On examination, he has no central pulse. The ECG shown here , What is the most appropriate initial management?

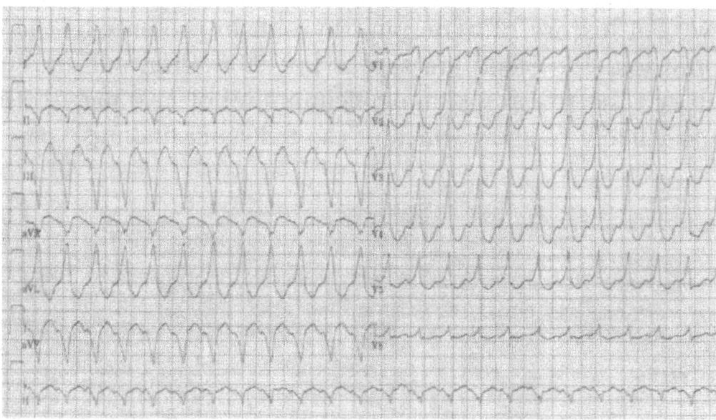

Figure 11.12: 67 year old

- A. Administer intravenous beta-blockers
- B. Begin chest compressions and prepare for defibrillation
- C. Administer intravenous amiodarone
- D. Perform immediate DC cardioversion
- E. Administer intravenous fluids

109. A 34-year-old woman presents to the emergency department with a sudden onset of palpitations. She has no history of heart disease but has been experiencing high levels of stress and anxiety recently. Her heart rate is 150 beats per minute, and the ECG shown here. What is the most likely diagnosis and initial treatment?

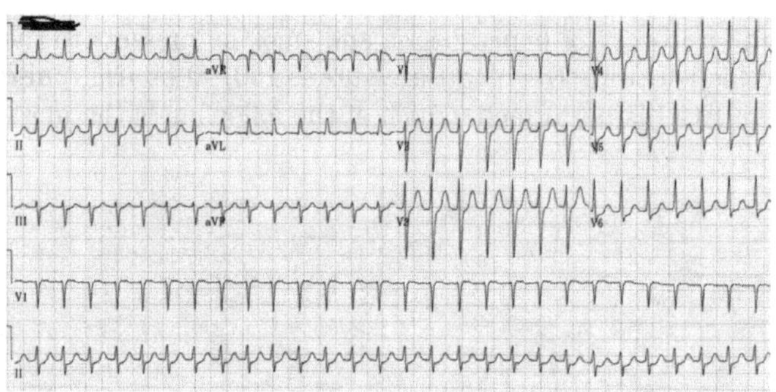

Figure 11.13: 34-year-old woman

- A. Sinus tachycardia; treat with beta-blockers
- B. Atrial flutter; treat with electrical cardioversion
- C. Ventricular tachycardia; treat with defibrillation
- D. Junctional supraventricular tachycardia (SVT); treat with vagal maneuvers and adenosine
- E. Atrial fibrillation; treat with anticoagulation

110. A 59-year-old man with a history of renal disease requiring dialysis presents to the emergency department. He missed his last dialysis session due to feeling dizzy and unwell. His ECG shown. What is the most likely diagnosis and immediate treatment?

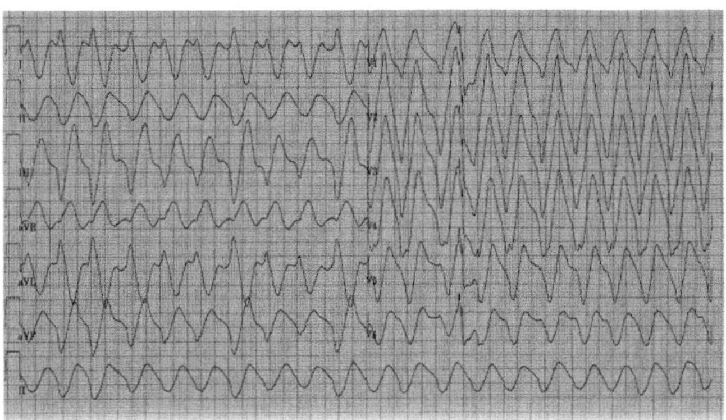

Figure 11.14: A 59-year-old man

- A. Hypokalemia; treat with oral potassium supplements
- B. Hyperkalemia; treat with calcium gluconate, insulin and dextrose, and urgent dialysis
- C. Hypocalcemia; treat with intravenous calcium
- D. Hypercalcemia; treat with intravenous fluids and furosemide
- E. Hyponatremia; treat with hypertonic saline

111. A 21-year-old man with a history of fainting episodes collapses during a basketball match. His ECG shown . What is the most likely diagnosis and the initial treatment?

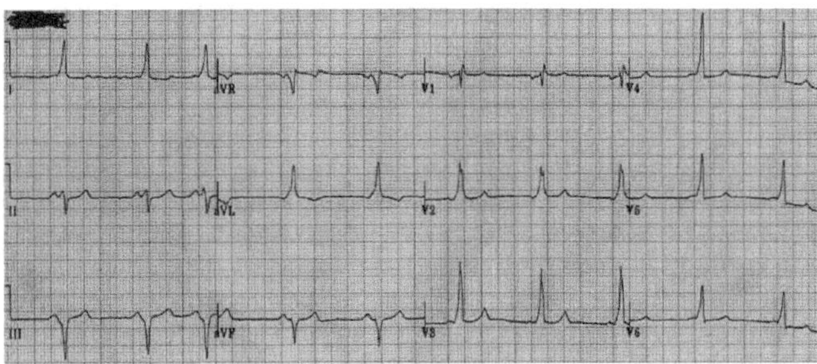

Figure 11.15: A 21-year-old

- A. Atrial fibrillation; treat with electrical cardioversion
- B. Ventricular tachycardia; treat with defibrillation
- C. Wolff-Parkinson-White (WPW) syndrome; treat with catheter ablation
- D. Long QT syndrome; treat with beta-blockers
- E. Brugada syndrome; treat with an implantable cardioverter-defibrillator (ICD).

112.A 56-year-old smoker presents with tight epigastric pain. His ECG shown, what is the most likely diagnosis and the initial treatment?

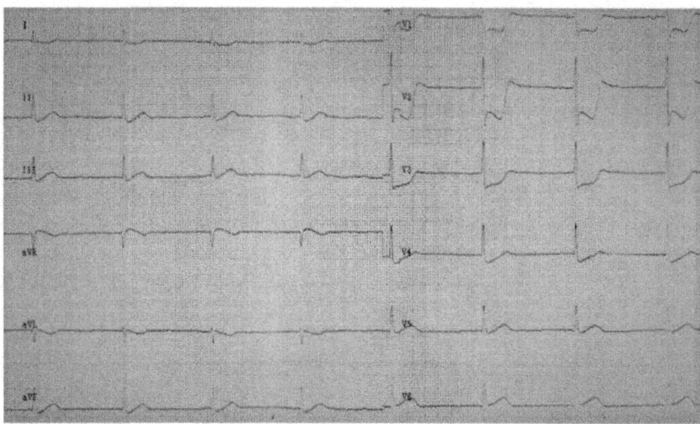

Figure 11.16: 56-year-old smoker

- A. Anterior myocardial infarction; treat with percutaneous coronary intervention (PCI)
- B. Posterior myocardial infarction; treat with thrombolytic therapy
- C. Posterior myocardial infarction; treat with percutaneous coronary intervention (PCI)
- D. Anterior myocardial infarction; treat with thrombolytic therapy
- E. Pericarditis; treat with nonsteroidal anti-inflammatory drugs (NSAIDs)

113. A 51-year-old man presents with a collapse. He has been recently unwell with a chest infection for which he has been prescribed clarithromycin. He also takes medication for his hayfever. His ECG shown, what is the most likely diagnosis and the initial treatment?

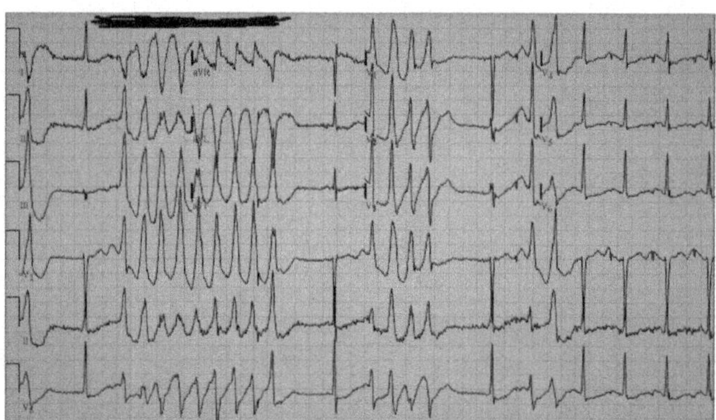

Figure 11.17: 51-year-old man

- A. Ventricular fibrillation; treat with defibrillation
- B. Atrial fibrillation; treat with electrical cardioversion
- C. Torsades de pointes; treat with intravenous magnesium
- D. Supraventricular tachycardia; treat with adenosine
- E. Sinus tachycardia; treat with beta-blockers

114.A 39-year-old man presents with palpitations after a weekend of heavy drinking. His ECG shown, what is the most likely diagnosis and the initial treatment?

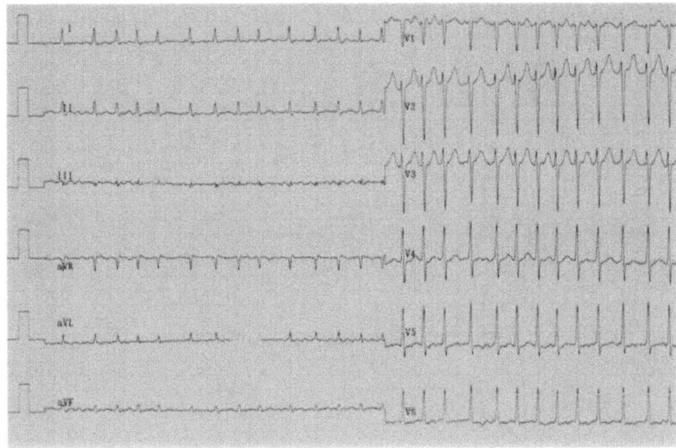

Figure 11.18: 39-year-old man

- A. Sinus tachycardia; treat with beta-blockers
- B. Atrial fibrillation; treat with rate control and anticoagulation
- C. Ventricular fibrillation; treat with defibrillation
- D. Supraventricular tachycardia; treat with adenosine
- E. Atrial flutter; treat with electrical cardioversion

115. A 42-year-old man presents with palpitations and shortness of breath after a weekend of heavy drinking. His ECG shown,what is the diagnosis and the initial treatment?

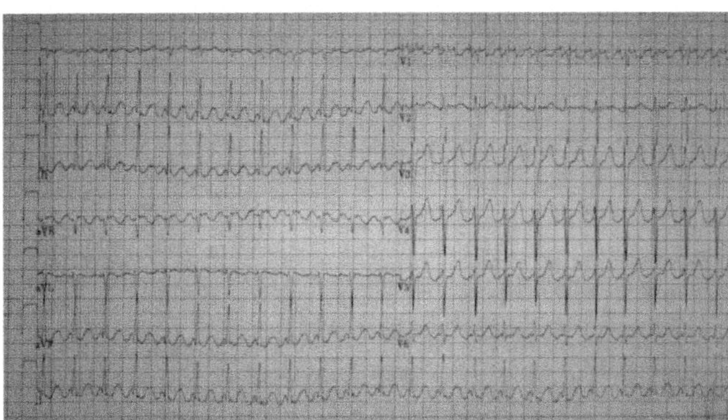

Figure 11.19: A 42-year-old man

- A. Atrial fibrillation; treat with rate control and anticoagulation
- B. Atrial flutter; treat with electrical cardioversion
- C. Ventricular tachycardia; treat with defibrillation
- D. Supraventricular tachycardia; treat with adenosine
- E. Sinus tachycardia; treat with beta-blockers

116. A 62-year-old man presents with occasional episodes of dizziness and syncope in the past. His ECG shown, what is the most likely diagnosis and the initial treatment?

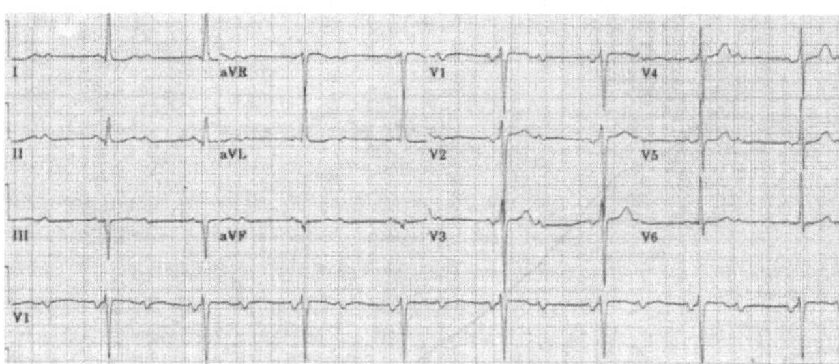

Figure 11.20: 62-year-old man

- A. Sinus bradycardia; treat with atropine
- B. Mobitz type 1 second-degree AV block; treat with observation
- C. Mobitz type 2 second-degree AV block; treat with pacemaker implantation
- D. Third-degree AV block; treat with pacemaker implantation
- E. Supraventricular tachycardia; treat with adenosine

117.A 71-year-old woman presents with episodes of dizziness and fatigue. Her ECG shows a regular atrial rate, but the ventricular rate is slower and not associated with the P waves. What is the most likely diagnosis and the initial treatment?

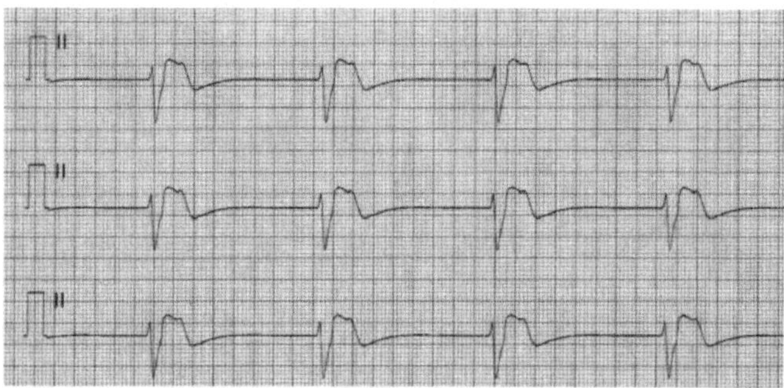

Figure 11.21: 71-year-old woman

- A. First-degree AV block; treat with observation
- B. Mobitz type 1 second-degree AV block; treat with observation
- C. Mobitz type 2 second-degree AV block; treat with pacemaker implantation
- D. Third-degree AV block; treat with pacemaker implantation
- E. Supraventricular tachycardia; treat with adenosine

118. A 77-year-old man presents with episodes of dizziness and occasional fainting. His ECG shown. What is the most likely diagnosis and the initial treatment?

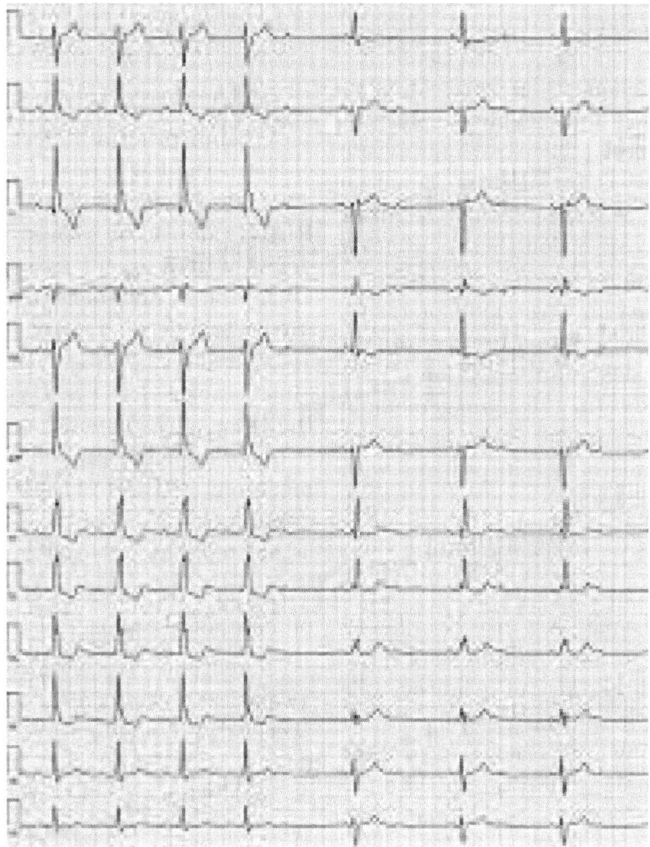

Figure 11.22: 77-year-old man

- A. First-degree AV block; treat with observation
- B. Mobitz type 1 second-degree AV block; treat with observation
- C. Mobitz type 2 second-degree AV block; treat with pacemaker implantation
- D. Trifascicular block; treat with pacemaker implantation
- E. Supraventricular tachycardia; treat with adenosine

11.1 ANSWERS

1.The correct answer is B) Perform cardiac catheterization.

In this clinical scenario, the patient's presentation with symptoms of heart failure, elevated JVP with Kussmaul's sign, pericardial knock on auscultation, and echocardiographic findings suggestive of constrictive pericarditis indicate the need for further evaluation with cardiac catheterization. Cardiac catheterization can help confirm the diagnosis by demonstrating equalization of diastolic pressures in all cardiac chambers, characteristic of constrictive pericarditis. Initiating diuresis with furosemide (option A) may provide symptomatic relief but does not address the underlying cause. Starting empiric antibiotics for suspected infection (option C) is not indicated in the absence of clear evidence of infection. Ordering cardiac MRI for further evaluation (option D) may be helpful in some cases but is not the most appropriate next step when constrictive pericarditis is strongly suspected based on clinical and echocardiographic findings.

2. The correct answer is D) Refer for surgical evaluation.

In this clinical scenario, the patient's history of

rheumatic fever, symptoms of right heart failure, physical examination findings of an elevated JVP with classic features of tricuspid stenosis (prominent "a" wave and slow "y" descent), and echocardiographic evidence support the diagnosis of tricuspid stenosis. The next appropriate step would be to refer the patient for surgical evaluation for possible intervention such as tricuspid valve repair or replacement. Initiating anticoagulation therapy (option A) may be considered in certain cases of valvular heart disease but is not the primary management for tricuspid stenosis. Performing exercise stress testing (option B) and ordering cardiac CT angiography (option C) are not indicated as the next steps in the management of tricuspid stenosis. Referral for surgical evaluation is crucial to assess the need for intervention in patients with significant tricuspid stenosis.

3. The correct answer is C) Refer for mitral valve repair or replacement.

In this clinical scenario, the patient's history of hypertension, prior myocardial infarction, symptoms of heart failure, physical examination findings of a holosystolic murmur at the apex radiating to the axilla, ECG evidence of left ventricular hypertrophy, and echocardiographic confirmation of severe mitral regurgitation indicate the need for further management. The most appropriate next step would be to refer the patient for mitral valve repair or replacement to address the severe mitral regurgitation. Initiating medical therapy with beta-blockers (option A) may help manage symptoms but does not address the underlying cause of severe mitral regurgitation. Performing coronary angiography (option B) may be considered to assess coronary artery disease but is not the primary management for severe mitral regurgitation. Starting anticoagulation therapy (option D) is not indicated as the first-line management in this scenario. Referral for mitral valve repair or replacement is crucial to improve outcomes in patients with severe mitral regurgitation.

4. The correct answer is B. The murmur will become longer and louder.

The Valsalva maneuver is a test that is used to assess the heart and lungs. It involves bearing down as if to have a bowel movement, which increases the pressure in the chest. This can have a number of effects on heart murmurs. In patients with hypertrophic cardiomyopathy, the Valsalva maneuver can cause the systolic murmur to become longer and louder. This is because the increased pressure in the chest can cause the mitral valve to close more tightly, which allows less blood to leak back into the left atrium during systole. This results in a louder murmur. The other answer choices are not as appropriate. The murmur will not change in intensity or duration in most patients. The murmur may become softer and shorter in patients with mitral valve prolapse.

5. The correct answer is A. Ostium primum defect.

Ostium primum defect is a type of ASD that is located in the lower part of the atrial septum. It is often associated with left-axis deviation on ECG. Incomplete RBBB can also be seen in patients with ostium primum defect, but it is not as common as left-axis deviation. Ostium secundum defect is a type of ASD that is located in the middle of the atrial septum. It is not typically associated with left-axis deviation or incomplete RBBB. Sinus venosus defect is a type of ASD that is located near the entry of the superior vena cava into the right atrium. It is not typically associated with left-axis deviation or incomplete RBBB. The other answer choices are not as appropriate. None of the other types of ASD are typically associated with left-axis deviation or incomplete RBBB.

6. The correct answer is B. Yes, he should undergo percutaneous or surgical closure of his VSD.

Percutaneous or surgical closure of VSD is indicated for patients who exhibit symptoms or experience volume overload, provided that irreversible pulmonary vascular disease is not present. This patient has a Qp/Qs ratio of 1.5:1, which is above the normal range of 1.0:1. This suggests that he is experiencing volume overload. Additionally, his pulmonary artery pressure and pulmonary vascular resistance are both below two-thirds of the systemic pressure and systemic resistance, respectively. This suggests that he does not have irreversible pulmonary vascular disease. Therefore, he should undergo percutaneous or surgical closure of his VSD. The other answer choices are not as appropriate. No, he should not undergo percutaneous or surgical closure of his VSD is not the correct answer because the patient is experiencing symptoms and volume overload. It is uncertain whether he should undergo percutaneous or surgical closure of his VSD is not the correct answer because the patient meets the criteria for closure of his VSD.

7. The correct answer is A. Yes, antibiotic prophylaxis is recommended.

Tetralogy of Fallot is a congenital heart defect that includes a ventricular septal defect, a right ventricular outflow tract obstruction, an overriding aorta, and right ventricular hypertrophy. This defect can cause a right-to-left shunt, which means that blood can flow from the right side of the heart to the left side of the heart. This can increase the risk of bacteria in the bloodstream from attaching to the heart valves and causing infective endocarditis. The American Heart Association recommends antibiotic prophylaxis for dental procedures in patients with tetralogy of Fallot. This is because the dental procedure can cause bacteremia, which is the presence of bacteria in the bloodstream. Antibiotic prophylaxis can help to prevent the bacteria from attaching to the heart valves and causing infective endocarditis. The other answer choices are not as appropriate. No, antibiotic prophylaxis is not recommended, but is not the correct answer because the patient has a congenital heart defect that increases the risk of infective endocarditis. It is uncertain whether antibiotic prophylaxis is recommended that is not the correct answer because the patient has a congenital heart defect that increases the risk of infective endocarditis.

8. The correct answer is C. Percutaneous balloon valvuloplasty.

Percutaneous balloon valvuloplasty is a minimally invasive procedure that is used to open a narrowed mitral valve. This procedure is usually performed under local anesthesia and does not require a large incision. Percutaneous balloon valvuloplasty is the preferred procedure for the management of uncomplicated mitral stenosis because it is less invasive and has a shorter recovery time than open surgical valvotomy. Open surgical valvotomy is a more invasive procedure that is performed under general anesthesia. This procedure involves making a large incision in the chest and opening the mitral valve with a scalpel. Open surgical valvotomy is typically only used if percutaneous balloon valvuloplasty is not an option. Medical therapy is not a long-term solution for mitral stenosis. Medical therapy can be used to relieve symptoms, but it will not open the mitral valve. Watchful waiting is not an appropriate option for this patient because she is already experiencing symptoms.

9. The patient is symptomatic with severe MR and has evidence of progressive left ventricular dysfunction. In cases where patients exhibit symptoms or experience progressive left ventricular dysfunction, such as a left ventricular ejection fraction (LVEF) below 60% or an end-systolic left ventricular diameter equal to or greater than 40 mm, surgical valve repair or replacement is considered an appropriate course of action. It is important to take into account valve repair as a potential treatment option for patients who are asymptomatic but have severe chronic mitral regurgitation (MR) and exhibit recent onset atrial fibrillation (AF), pulmonary hypertension, or a progressive decline in left ventricular ejection fraction (LVEF) or an increase in left ventricular end-systolic diameter on consecutive imaging. In this case, the patient's LVEF is still within the normal range, so valve repair is a viable option. Medical therapy with diuretics and ACE inhibitors may be used to manage the patient's symptoms, but it will not address the underlying problem of mitral regurgitation. Transcatheter mitral valve repair is a newer procedure that may be an option for some patients, but it is not yet as widely available as valve repair. Observation is not a reasonable option for this patient, as she is already symptomatic.

10. The answer to this question is A. Soft or absent A2.

This is because as the aortic valve narrows, it becomes more difficult for blood to flow out of the heart. This can cause the A2 heart sound to become softer or even absent. The other answer choices are also possible findings in patients with aortic stenosis, but they are not as specific as a soft or absent A2. For example, S4 is a heart sound that is often heard in patients with aortic stenosis, but it can also be heard in other conditions. Pulsus paradoxus is a decrease in systolic blood pressure during inspiration that is often seen in patients with severe heart failure, but it is not a specific finding for aortic stenosis. Midsystolic click is a heart sound that is often heard in patients with mitral valve prolapse, but it is not a finding in aortic stenosis. Diastolic murmur is a heart sound that is often heard in patients with aortic regurgitation, but it is not a finding in aortic stenosis.

11. The answer to this question is D. All of the above.

TAVR is a minimally invasive procedure, but it is not without risks. The most common complications associated with TAVR are stroke, the need for a permanent pacemaker, and paravalvular aortic regurgitation. Stroke occurs in about 1% of patients undergoing TAVR, and the need for a permanent pacemaker occurs in about 10% of patients. Paravalvular aortic regurgitation is a complication that occurs when there is a leak around the new valve. This can lead to heart failure and other complications. Other potential complications of TAVR include bleeding, infection, and vascular complications. However, these complications are less common than stroke, the need for a permanent pacemaker, and paravalvular aortic regurgitation.

12.The answer to this question is C. Beta-blockers can prolong the duration of diastole.

This is because beta-blockers work by slowing down the heart rate. A slower heart rate means that there is more time for blood to fill the left ventricle during diastole. In patients with chronic AR, this can lead to an increase in the amount of blood that regurgitates back into the left ventricle during diastole. This can worsen heart failure symptoms and increase the risk of stroke. The other answer choices are also possible reasons why beta-blockers should be avoided in patients with chronic AR, but they are not as likely as the prolongation of diastole. For example, beta-blockers can worsen heart failure by decreasing cardiac output. However, this is not as likely to happen in patients with chronic AR as it is in patients with other types of heart failure. Beta-blockers can also increase the risk of stroke by slowing down the heart rate. However, this risk is also relatively low in patients with chronic AR.

13. The answer to this question is A. Viridans streptococci.

Viridans streptococci are the most common causative microorganisms associated with NVE. They are found in the oral cavity and can enter the bloodstream through small breaks in the gums or other oral tissues. The other answer choices are also possible causative microorganisms for NVE, but they are less common than viridans streptococci. For example, staphylococci are another common causative microorganism for NVE, but they are more likely to be seen in patients who have a history of intravenous drug use or other risk factors for infection. HACEK organisms are a group of bacteria that are less common than viridans streptococci or staphylococci, but they can still cause NVE. Streptococcus gallolyticus subspecies gallolyticus is a less common causative microorganism for NVE, but it is more likely to be seen in patients who have colon cancer or polyp.

14. The answer to this question is C. S aureus.

S aureus is the most common causative microorganism associated with CIED-related endocarditis. It is found on the skin and can enter the bloodstream through small breaks in the skin. CoNS are also a common causative microorganism for CIED-related endocarditis. They are found in the skin and mucous membranes. Viridans streptococci and HACEK organisms are less common causative microorganisms for CIED-related endocarditis. The other answer choices are also possible causative microorganisms for CIED-related endocarditis, but they are less common than S aureus or CoNS. For example, viridans streptococci are another common causative microorganism for CIED-related endocarditis, but they are more likely to be seen in patients who have a history of dental work or other risk factors for infection. HACEK organisms are a group of bacteria that are less common than S aureus or CoNS, but they can still cause CIED-related endocarditis.

15. The answer to this question is D. 30-65%.

This is according to research findings that have revealed the presence of clinically asymptomatic emboli in approximately 30-65% of individuals diagnosed with left-sided endocarditis. The other answer choices are also possible prevalence rates for clinically asymptomatic emboli detected on MRI in patients diagnosed with left-sided endocarditis, but they are less likely than 30-65%. For example, 10-30% is the prevalence rate for clinically asymptomatic emboli detected on CT scans in patients diagnosed with left-sided endocarditis. 5-10% is the prevalence rate for clinically asymptomatic emboli detected on echocardiography in patients diagnosed with left-sided endocarditis. ¡5% is the prevalence rate for clinically asymptomatic emboli detected on physical examination in patients diagnosed with left-sided endocarditis.

16. The answer to this question is B. Repeat the TEE examination in 7-10 days.

This is because a negative TEE result does not definitively rule out the diagnosis of endocarditis, especially if there is a high likelihood of the disease. Repeating the TEE examination can help to confirm or rule out the diagnosis. The other answer choices are also possible next steps in management, but they are less likely than repeating the TEE examination. For example, discharging the patient from the hospital is not a reasonable option if there is a high likelihood of endocarditis. Starting with antibiotic therapy is a possible option, but it should only be done if there is a high likelihood of endocarditis, and the patient is symptomatic. Referring the patient to a cardiologist for further evaluation is a possible option, but it is not the best next step in management if the patient is already being seen by a cardiologist.

17. The answer to this question is B. 6 to 8 weeks.

This is because staphylococcal PVE is typically managed through a multidrug regimen lasting for a duration of 6 to 8 weeks. The other answer choices are also possible durations of treatment for staphylococcal PVE, but they are less likely than 6 to 8 weeks. For example, 4 to 6 weeks is the recommended duration of treatment for non-staphylococcal PVE. 8 to 12 weeks is the recommended duration of treatment for staphylococcal PVE that is complicated by heart failure or other complications. 12 to 16 weeks is the recommended duration of treatment for staphylococcal PVE that is methicillin resistant.

18. The answer to this question is A. Hypertrophic cardiomyopathy.

The correct answer is C. Aldosterone antagonist therapy is recommended for patients with dilated cardiomyopathy in NYHA class III heart failure.

Aldosterone antagonists, such as spironolactone or eplerenone, are recommended in patients with NYHA class II-IV heart failure and who have symptoms of the condition, according to the American Heart Association and the American College of Cardiology. These medications have been shown to reduce both morbidity and mortality in these patients.

In the case of the patient described, who has dilated cardiomyopathy and is in NYHA class III heart failure, aldosterone antagonist therapy would be a recommended part of her treatment plan.This is because aldosterone antagonists have been shown to improve symptoms and survival in patients with dilated cardiomyopathy. The other answer choices are also possible roles of aldosterone antagonist therapy in treating dilated cardiomyopathy, but they are less likely than for patients with NYHA class III heart failure. For example, aldosterone antagonist therapy is not indicated for patients with dilated cardiomyopathy who are not symptomatic. Aldosterone antagonist therapy may be considered for patients with dilated cardiomyopathy in NYHA class II heart failure, but it is not as effective as for patients in NYHA class III heart failure. Aldosterone antagonist therapy is not recommended for patients with dilated cardiomyopathy in NYHA class IV heart failure, as it has not been shown to be effective in this group of patients.

19. The answer to this question is A.

The patient meets all of the criteria for CRT, including heart failure of class III-IV severity, LVEF below 35%, and an extended QRS duration. Therefore, he is a candidate for CRT. The other answer choices are also possible, but they are less likely than for patients who meet all of the criteria for CRT. For example, a patient with LVEF above 35% is not a candidate for CRT. A patient with QRS duration below 150 milliseconds is not a candidate for CRT, unless they have left bundle branch block. A patient without left bundle branch block may still be a candidate for CRT, but it is less likely than for patients with left bundle branch block.

20. The answer to this question is C.

Bilateral atrial enlargement with speckled pattern in the ventricles. This is because infiltrative diseases, such as amyloidosis, can cause restrictive cardiomyopathy. Restrictive cardiomyopathy is characterized by a thickened myocardium that does not relax properly, which can lead to diastolic dysfunction and heart failure. The imaging findings of restrictive cardiomyopathy include bilateral atrial enlargement and a speckled pattern in the ventricles. The speckled pattern is caused by amyloid deposits in the myocardium. The other answer choices are also possible imaging findings in patients with heart disease, but they are less likely than bilateral atrial enlargement with speckled pattern in the ventricles. For example, a normal echocardiogram is not expected in a patient with restrictive cardiomyopathy. A dilated left ventricle with decreased ejection fraction is more likely to be seen in patients with dilated cardiomyopathy. A thickened pericardium with pericardial effusion is more likely to be seen in patients with constrictive pericarditis.

21. The answer to this question is A. Hypertrophic cardiomyopathy.

This is because the physical examination findings described are characteristic of hypertrophic cardiomyopathy. The brisk carotid upstroke with pulsus bisferiens is caused by the increased stroke volume that occurs in hypertrophic cardiomyopathy. The S4 sound is caused by the late diastolic closure of the mitral valve that occurs in hypertrophic cardiomyopathy. The harsh systolic murmur along the left sternal border is caused by the turbulent flow of blood through the narrowed left ventricular outflow tract that occurs in hypertrophic cardiomyopathy. The blowing murmur indicative of mitral regurgitation at the apex is caused by the backflow of blood through the mitral valve that occurs in hypertrophic cardiomyopathy. The other answer choices are also possible diagnoses, but they are less likely than hypertrophic cardiomyopathy. For example, mitral stenosis is characterized by a diastolic murmur that is heard best at the apex. Aortic stenosis is characterized by a systolic murmur that is heard best at the second right intercostal space. Mitral regurgitation is characterized by a holosystolic murmur that is heard best at the apex. 22.The answer to this question is D. All of the above.

This is because all of the factors listed are indications for an ICD in patients with hypertrophic cardiomyopathy. Syncope is a risk factor for sudden death in patients with hypertrophic cardiomyopathy. Left ventricular wall thickness of 3.2 cm is considered significant and is a risk factor for sudden death. Family history of sudden death is a risk factor for sudden death in patients with hypertrophic cardiomyopathy. The other answer choices are also possible indications for an ICD in patients with hypertrophic cardiomyopathy, but they are less likely than all of the factors listed. For example, nonsustained ventricular tachycardia (VT) is a risk factor for sudden death, but it is less likely than syncope in patients with hypertrophic cardiomyopathy. Exertional hypotension is a risk factor for sudden death, but it is less likely than left ventricular wall thickness of 3.2 cm in patients with hypertrophic cardiomyopathy.

23. The answer to this question is B. Start empiric antibiotic therapy.

This is because the patient's symptoms and laboratory findings are consistent with myocarditis. However, the diagnosis of myocarditis cannot be made definitively without endomyocardial biopsy. In most cases, the diagnosis of myocarditis can be made through non-invasive diagnostic methods, such as laboratory tests, imaging studies, and clinical evaluation. However, in this case, the patient's symptoms and laboratory findings are so suggestive of myocarditis that it is reasonable to start empiric antibiotic therapy while awaiting the results of the endomyocardial biopsy. The other answer choices are also possible next steps in the management of this patient, but they are less likely than starting empiric antibiotic therapy. For example, endomyocardial biopsy is not commonly used in the diagnostic evaluation of myocarditis and would only be performed if the diagnosis was uncertain after non-invasive testing. Refer the patient to a cardiologist for further evaluation is a reasonable next step, but it is not as likely as starting empiric antibiotic therapy in this case. Discharge the patient home with close follow-up is not a reasonable next step, as the patient's symptoms and laboratory findings are suggestive of a serious condition.

24. The answer to this question is A. Acute pericarditis.

This is because the ECG findings of widespread ST elevation with reciprocal ST depression are characteristic of acute pericarditis. In contrast, the ECG findings of acute STEMI are typically characterized by upwardly convex ST elevations accompanied by reciprocal ST depression in leads opposite to the affected area. Additionally, PR depression is not typically observed in acute pericarditis, but it is often seen in acute STEMI. T wave inversions may manifest in both acute pericarditis and acute STEMI, but they typically occur after the ST elevations have resolved in acute pericarditis. The other answer choices are also possible diagnoses, but they are less likely than acute pericarditis. For example, early repolarization is a benign condition that can cause ECG changes that mimic acute pericarditis. However, the ECG findings of early repolarization are typically seen in young, healthy individuals and are not associated with chest pain. ARVC is a rare genetic disorder that can cause ECG changes that mimic acute pericarditis. However, ARVC is typically associated with other symptoms, such as syncope and palpitations.

25. The answer to this question is C. Start colchicine.

This is because the administration of anticoagulants in cases of acute pericarditis is generally not recommended due to the potential risk of pericardial hemorrhage. Colchicine is a medication that is used to treat acute pericarditis and is not associated with the same risk of pericardial hemorrhage. The other answer choices are also possible treatments for acute pericarditis, but they are less likely than colchicine. For example, aspirin and clopidogrel are antiplatelet medications that can help to prevent the formation of blood clots. However, they can also increase the risk of pericardial hemorrhage. Heparin is an anticoagulant that can help to prevent the formation of blood clots. However, it is also associated with the risk of pericardial hemorrhage. Discharge the patient home with close follow-up is not a reasonable management option for this patient, as he has chest pain and a pericardial rub.

26.The answer to this question is B. Electrical alternans is a sign of cardiac tamponade.

This is because the swinging motion of the heart that causes electrical alternans is a consequence of the increased pressure in the pericardial sac that occurs in cardiac tamponade. The other answer choices are also possible interpretations of electrical alternans, but they are less likely than cardiac tamponade. For example, electrical alternans can be a benign finding that is not associated with any significant pathology. However, it is more likely to be a sign of cardiac tamponade in a patient with chest pain and shortness of breath. Myocardial infarction and pericarditis can also cause electrical alternans, but they are less likely than cardiac tamponade in this patient.

27. The answer to this question is A. Cardiac catheterization.

This is because cardiac catheterization is the most definitive way to diagnose constrictive pericarditis. During cardiac catheterization, the physician can measure the diastolic pressures in all chambers of the heart. If the diastolic pressures are equalized, then this is a sign of constrictive pericarditis. Additionally, the ventricular pressure tracings in constrictive pericarditis exhibit a characteristic "dip and plateau" appearance. The other answer choices are also possible diagnostic tests for constrictive pericarditis, but they are less definitive than cardiac catheterization. For example, endomyocardial biopsy can be used to diagnose constrictive pericarditis, but it is not as sensitive as cardiac catheterization. MRI and CT can also be used to diagnose constrictive pericarditis, but they are not as specific as cardiac catheterization.

28. The answer to this question is B. Add a loop diuretic to the regimen.

This is because the serum creatinine level of 2.7 mg/dL is above the level at which thiazides are typically effective. Loop diuretics are more potent than thiazides and can be effective in patients with higher serum creatinine levels. The other answer choices are also possible management options for this patient, but they are less likely than adding a loop diuretic. For example, increasing the dose of HCTZ may be effective in some patients, but it is less likely to be effective in a patient with a serum creatinine level of 2.7 mg/dL. Switching to a different thiazide diuretic may also be effective, but it is less likely to be effective than adding a loop diuretic. Discontinue HCTZ is not a reasonable management option for this patient, as he is currently taking HCTZ for his hypertension.

29. The answer to this question is B. Hyperkalemia.

This is because ACE inhibitors and ARBs can cause hyperkalemia, and potassium supplements and potassium-sparing diuretics can further increase the risk of hyperkalemia. The other answer choices are also possible monitoring concerns for this patient, but they are less likely than hyperkalemia. For example, hypotension is a possible side effect of ACE inhibitors and ARBs, but it is less likely in a patient who is also taking potassium supplements. Renal insufficiency is a possible side effect of ACE inhibitors and ARBs, but it is less likely in a patient who is otherwise healthy. Hyperglycemia is not a side effect of ACE inhibitors or ARBs.

30. The answer to this question is A. Methyldopa.

This is because methyldopa is the most commonly used antihypertensive medication in pregnancy. It is safe for both the mother and the fetus, and it has been shown to be effective in controlling blood pressure. The other answer choices are also possible antihypertensive medications that can be used in pregnancy, but they are less commonly used than methyldopa. For example, labetalol and hydralazine are also safe for use in pregnancy, but they are not as effective as methyldopa in controlling blood pressure. Nifedipine is a calcium channel blocker that is safe for use in pregnancy, but it is not as commonly used as methyldopa because it can cause fetal tachycardia.

31. The answer to this question is A. Nitroprusside.

This is because nitroprusside is the most effective antihypertensive agent for the treatment of hypertensive crisis. It is a short-acting agent that can be titrated to achieve the desired blood pressure response. The other answer choices are also possible antihypertensive agents that can be used for the treatment of hypertensive crisis, but they are not as effective as nitroprusside. For example, nicardipine and labetalol are also short-acting agents, but they are not as potent as nitroprusside. Enalaprilat is a longer-acting agent, but it takes longer to start working than nitroprusside. Hydralazine is a short-acting agent, but it can cause reflex tachycardia.

32. The correct answer is A.

Acute myocardial infarction is a contraindication to exercise testing because it is a condition in which the blood supply to the heart muscle is suddenly blocked. Exercise testing could worsen the condition and could lead to further damage to the heart muscle. The other answer choices are not contraindications to exercise testing. Unstable angina is a condition in which the patient experiences chest pain that is not relieved by rest or medication. However, exercise testing can be used to diagnose unstable angina and to determine the severity of the condition. Severe aortic stenosis is a narrowing of the aortic valve, which prevents blood from flowing smoothly from the heart to the rest of the body. However, exercise testing can be used to assess the patient's cardiovascular function and to determine the need for surgery. Myocarditis is an inflammation of the heart muscle. However, exercise testing can be used to diagnose myocarditis and to determine the severity of the condition. Pericarditis is an inflammation of the sac that surrounds the heart. However, exercise testing can be used to diagnose pericarditis and to determine the severity of the condition. Low exercise tolerance is the inability to exercise for a significant period of time due to a medical condition. However, exercise testing can be modified to accommodate patients with low exercise tolerance.

33. The correct answer is E.

A normal ECG is not a criterion for a positive exercise test. A positive exercise test is a sign that the patient may have coronary artery disease. However, a normal ECG does not rule out coronary artery disease. There are many patients with coronary artery disease who have a normal ECG. The other answer choices are all criteria for a positive exercise test. Chest pain or other symptoms that are consistent with angina are a sign that the patient is experiencing ischemia, which is a lack of blood flow to the heart muscle. Diagnostic ST-segment changes on the ECG are changes in the electrical activity of the heart that can be seen on an ECG. These changes are typically seen in patients with coronary artery disease. Failure to reach the target heart rate is a sign that the patient is not getting enough exercise. This could be due to a number of factors, such as poor exercise tolerance or a medical condition. A drop in blood pressure during exercise is a sign that the heart is not getting enough blood flow. This could be due to coronary artery disease or another medical condition.

34. The correct answer is E.

All of the above are contraindications to beta-blockers. Here are some additional details about the contraindications to beta-blockers: Congestive heart failure (CHF) is a condition in which the heart cannot pump blood effectively. Beta-blockers can worsen CHF by making the heart beat slower and weaker. Atrioventricular (AV) block is a condition in which the electrical signals that control the heart's rhythm are not transmitted properly. Beta-blockers can worsen AV block by slowing down the heart rate. Bronchospasm is a narrowing of the airways that can make it difficult to breathe. Beta-blockers can worsen bronchospasm by relaxing the airways. "Brittle" diabetes is a type of diabetes that is difficult to control. Beta-blockers can worsen "brittle" diabetes by making it more difficult to control blood sugar levels.

35. The rate of restenosis following balloon dilatation alone during PCI is approximately 30-45%.

This is because balloon dilatation can cause damage to the inner lining of the artery, which can lead to the formation of scar tissue. This scar tissue can narrow the artery again, resulting in restenosis. The other answer choices are incorrect. The rate of restenosis is lower than 10% in patients who undergo PCI with stenting. The rate of restenosis is higher than 50% in patients who have a high-risk lesion, such as a lesion that is heavily calcified or that has a long segment of stenosis. 36. The patient in this question has severe coronary artery disease (CAD) that is not responsive to medical treatment. He also has a left main coronary artery stenosis, which is a high-risk lesion that is associated with a high risk of death. In this case, CABG is the most appropriate treatment because it provides a more durable and effective way to improve blood flow to the heart. The other answer choices are incorrect. PCI is not a good option for this patient because his lesions are not suitable for this procedure. Medical therapy with nitrates and beta-blockers, calcium channel blockers, aspirin, and clopidogrel may help to control the patient's symptoms, but they will not provide a long-term solution to his CAD.

37.The answer is B.

PCI is more effective than medical therapy in providing relief from angina symptoms in patients with chronic stable angina. The available evidence shows that PCI does not reduce the risk of MI or mortality in patients with chronic stable angina. However, it does provide more effective relief from angina symptoms than medical therapy. This is because PCI opens up the narrowed coronary arteries, which improves blood flow to the heart. The other answer choices are incorrect. Medical therapy is not as effective as PCI in providing relief from angina symptoms. There is not enough evidence to determine which treatment is more effective in reducing the risk of MI or mortality in patients with chronic stable angina.

38.The answer is A.

Coronary angiography with provocative testing. Prinzmetal's variant angina is a type of angina that is caused by coronary artery vasospasm. This means that the coronary arteries narrow, which restricts blood flow to the heart. The diagnosis of Prinzmetal's variant angina can be confirmed by coronary angiography with provocative testing. This involves injecting a drug, such as acetylcholine, that can trigger coronary artery vasospasm. If the patient experiences chest pain and ECG changes consistently with Prinzmetal's variant angina, then the diagnosis is confirmed. The other answer choices are incorrect. Coronary angiography without provocative testing is not as sensitive for diagnosing Prinzmetal's variant angina. ECG, stress test, and echocardiogram can be used to support the diagnosis of Prinzmetal's variant angina, but they cannot confirm the diagnosis. 39. The answer is A. NSTEMI. NSTEMI and STEMI are both types of heart attacks, but they are distinguished by their ECG findings. In NSTEMI, the ECG shows ST-segment depression or T-wave inversion, but there is no ST-segment elevation. In STEMI, the ECG shows ST-segment elevation. The other answer choices are incorrect. Unstable angina is a condition that is similar to NSTEMI, but it does not involve the death of heart muscle tissue. Prinzmetal's variant angina is a type of angina that is caused by coronary artery vasospasm. Pericarditis is an inflammation of the pericardium, which is the sac that surrounds the heart.

40. The answer is A. Tirofiban.

High-risk unstable patients who undergo PCI are at an increased risk of developing a heart attack or stroke. In order to reduce this risk, these patients are often given an intravenous glycoprotein IIb/IIIa antagonist. Glycoprotein IIb/IIIa antagonists work by blocking the binding of platelets together, which helps to prevent the formation of blood clots. Tirofiban and eptifibatide are two of the most commonly used glycoprotein IIb/IIIa antagonists. Tirofiban is administered as a loading dose of 25 g/kg/min followed by a maintenance dose of 0.15 g/kg/min. Eptifibatide is administered as a loading dose of 180 g/kg followed by an infusion of 2 g/kg/min. The other answer choices are incorrect. Aspirin and clopidogrel are antiplatelet agents, but they are not as effective as glycoprotein IIb/IIIa antagonists in preventing heart attacks and strokes in high-risk unstable patients who undergo PCI.

41. The answer is A. Immediate invasive strategy.

Patients with NSTE-ACS who exhibit refractory angina, indications of heart failure or the development or exacerbation of mitral regurgitation, hemodynamic instability, recurrent angina or ischemia during periods of rest or with minimal exertion despite intensive medical treatment, and sustained episodes of ventricular tachycardia or ventricular fibrillation should be managed with an immediate invasive strategy. This means that they should undergo coronary angiography and revascularization as soon as possible. The other answer choices are incorrect. Selective invasive strategy is a management strategy that is used for patients with NSTE-ACS who do not meet the criteria for immediate invasive strategy. Conservative medical therapy is a management strategy that is used for patients with NSTE-ACS who do not meet the criteria for either immediate invasive strategy or selective invasive strategy. Observation is management strategies that is used for patients with NSTE-ACS who are stable and do not meet the criteria for any of the other management strategies.

42. The answer is C. Delayed invasive strategy.

Patients with NSTE-ACS who do not meet the criteria for immediate invasive strategy but have additional factors such as diabetes mellitus, renal insufficiency, reduced left ventricular systolic function, early postinfarction angina, a history of percutaneous coronary intervention within the past 6 months, prior coronary artery bypass graft surgery, or a GRACE risk score between 109 and 140 or a TIMI risk score of 2 or higher should be managed with a delayed invasive strategy. This means that they should undergo coronary angiography and revascularization after a period of observation and medical therapy. The other answer choices are incorrect. Immediate invasive strategy is a management strategy that is used for patients with NSTE-ACS who meet the criteria for immediate invasive strategy. Selective invasive strategy is a management strategy that is used for patients with NSTE-ACS who do not meet the criteria for immediate invasive strategy but do not have any of the additional factors listed above. Conservative medical therapy is a management strategy that is used for patients with NSTE-ACS who do not meet the criteria for either immediate invasive strategy or selective invasive strategy.

43. The answer is C. Apical MI.

Abnormal Q waves in leads V1-V2 are most commonly seen in apical MI. This is because the apical region of the heart is supplied by the left anterior descending artery (LAD), which is the most common site of coronary artery disease. The other answer choices are incorrect. Anterolateral MI typically involves leads I, aVL, V5, and V6. Inferior MI typically involves leads II, III, and aVF. True posterior MI is a rare type of MI that typically involves leads V1-V2. Non-specific ST-T changes can be seen in a variety of conditions, including MI, ischemia, and electrolyte imbalances. 44. The answer is B. Intravenous fibrinolysis. In patients with STEMI, the goal is to restore blood flow to the affected heart muscle as quickly as possible. If PCI is not available or if the delay between initial medical contact and PCI is more than 120 minutes, intravenous fibrinolysis is a viable treatment option. Intravenous fibrinolysis works by breaking up the blood clot that is blocking the coronary artery. The other answer choices are incorrect. Immediate PCI is the preferred treatment option for STEMI, but it is not available in this case. Medical therapy with aspirin and clopidogrel is a good option for patients who are not candidates for fibrinolysis, but it is not as effective as fibrinolysis in restoring blood flow to the heart muscle. Observation is not a recommended treatment option for STEMI.

45. The answer is A. Immediate electrical countershock.

Hemodynamically unstable ventricular tachycardia is a life-threatening arrhythmia that requires immediate treatment. for this arrhythmia. The recommended discharge for this procedure is an unsynchronized discharge of 200-300 J, or 50% less if a biphasic device is being used. The other answer choices are incorrect. Intravenous fibrinolysis is not a recommended treatment for hemodynamically unstable ventricular tachycardia. Medical therapy with aspirin and clopidogrel is a good option for patients who are not candidates for electrical countershock, but it is not as effective in treating this arrhythmia. Observation is not a recommended treatment option for hemodynamically unstable ventricular tachycardia.

46. The answer is E. All of the above.

The primary treatment for acute CHF post MI involves the administration of diuretics, such as furosemide, intravenously at a dosage of 10-20 mg. Inhaled oxygen and vasodilators, specifically nitrates, are recommended. Nitrates can be administered orally, topically, or intravenously, unless the patient is experiencing hypotension, indicated by a systolic blood pressure below 100 mmHg. The therapeutic efficacy of Digitalis in the context of acute myocardial infarction is generally limited. Diuretics help to reduce fluid overload, which is a major cause of CHF. Oxygen helps to improve oxygen delivery to the heart muscle. Nitrates help to dilate the blood vessels, which can improve blood flow to the heart muscle. Digitalis can help to strengthen the heart muscle, but it is not as effective as diuretics, oxygen, and nitrates in treating acute CHF.

47. The answer is D. All of the above.

Cardiogenic shock is a life-threatening condition that occurs when the heart is unable to pump enough blood to meet the body's needs. In cardiogenic shock, the systolic blood pressure is typically below 90 mmHg and the PCWP is elevated. There are a number of treatment options available for cardiogenic shock. These include the administration of vasopressors such as norepinephrine or dopamine, the use of intraaortic balloon counterpulsation

(IABP), and mechanical ventilation. Vasopressors work by constricting the blood vessels, which increases the blood pressure. IABP works by inflating a balloon in the aorta during diastole, which increases the blood pressure during this phase of the cardiac cycle. Mechanical ventilation helps to improve the oxygen delivery to the tissues. The choice of treatment for cardiogenic shock depends on the severity of the condition and the patient's individual circumstances. In general, the goal of treatment is to maintain a systolic blood pressure above 90 mmHg and reduce the PCWP.

48. The answer is A. Intravenous fluids.

Right ventricular MI can cause hypotension because the right ventricle is unable to pump blood effectively. This can lead to a decrease in cardiac output and a decrease in blood pressure. The treatment for hypotension caused by right ventricular MI is the administration of intravenous fluids. This will increase the volume of blood in the circulation and help to improve cardiac output.Vasopressors and intraaortic balloon counterpulsation may also be used to treat hypotension caused by right ventricular MI. However, these treatments are typically used only if intravenous fluids are not effective. Mechanical ventilation is not typically used to treat hypotension caused by right ventricular MI. However, it may be used if the patient is also in cardiogenic shock.

49. The answer is E. All of the above.

Atrial flutter is a type of arrhythmia that occurs when the heart's atria (the upper chambers of the heart) beat very fast. This can cause the heart's ventricles (the lower chambers of the heart) to beat too fast, which can lead to symptoms such as palpitations, shortness of breath, and chest pain. The initial treatment for atrial flutter is to slow down the heart rate. This can be done with medications such as beta blockers, verapamil, diltiazem, or digoxin. These medications work by blocking the effects of adrenaline and noradrenaline, which are hormones that speed up the heart rate. If the patient is stable, the doctor may then consider trying to convert the heart back to normal sinus rhythm (NSR). This can be done with electrical cardioversion or with chemical cardioversion. Electrical cardioversion involves using a shock to the heart to stop the atrial flutter and start the heart beating normally again. Chemical cardioversion involves giving the patient a medication that will stop the atrial flutter and start the heart beating normally again.

50. The answer is E. All of the above.

Torsade de pointes is a type of arrhythmia that can be life-threatening. It occurs when the heart's ventricles beat very rapidly and irregularly. This can cause the heart to quiver, which can lead to a loss of consciousness or even death. The treatment for Torsade de pointes is to stop the arrhythmia and to prevent it from happening again. The first step is to give the patient intravenous magnesium. Magnesium helps to stabilize the heart's rhythm. If the magnesium is not effective, the doctor may then try overdrive pacing or the use of isoproterenol. Overdrive pacing involves using a pacemaker to artificially increase the heart rate. Isoproterenol is a medication that increases the heart rate. If the patient is still in Torsade de pointes after these treatments, the doctor may then give the patient lidocaine. Lidocaine is a medication that slows down the heart rate. Torsade de pointes are frequently linked to an extended QT interval, which may arise from congenital factors or drug-induced causes.

51. The answer is E. Electrical cardioversion.

Supraventricular tachycardia with aberrant ventricular conduction is a type of arrhythmia that occurs when the heart's atria beat very fast and the heart's ventricles beat irregularly. This can cause the heart to quiver, which can lead to a loss of consciousness or even death. The treatment for supraventricular tachycardia with aberrant ventricular conduction depends on the patient's individual circumstances. In general, the goal of treatment is to stop the arrhythmia and to prevent it from happening again. If the patient is stable, the doctor may try to slow down the heart rate with medications such as beta blockers, verapamil, diltiazem, or digoxin. However, if the patient is not stable or if the ventricular rate is very high, the doctor may need to use electrical cardioversion to stop the arrhythmia. Electrical cardioversion involves using a shock to the heart to stop the arrhythmia and start the heart beating normally again. In this case, the patient has a ventricular rate of 200 beats per minute, which is very high. Therefore, the doctor will likely recommend electrical cardioversion to stop the arrhythmia.

52. The answer is E. All of the above.

The Class I indications for pacemaker implantation in patients with SA node dysfunction are those that are considered to be the most clear-cut and for which there is the strongest evidence of benefit. These indications include Sinus bradycardia with a heart rate of ¡40 beats per minute: This is the most common indication for pacemaker implantation in patients with SA node dysfunction. Sinus bradycardia is a slow heart rate that can cause symptoms such as fatigue, lightheadedness, and syncope. Sinus bradycardia with symptoms: Even if the heart rate is ¿40 beats per minute, if the patient is symptomatic, a pacemaker may be indicated. Symptoms can include fatigue, lightheadedness, and syncope. Sinus bradycardia with symptoms that are refractory to medical therapy: If the patient is taking medications to treat their sinus bradycardia and the symptoms are not improving, a pacemaker may be indicated. Sinus bradycardia with symptoms that are refractory to medical therapy and are associated with an increased risk of syncope: If the patient is taking medications to treat their sinus bradycardia and the symptoms are not improving and the patient is at an increased risk of syncope, a pacemaker may be indicated.

53. The answer is C. Permanent pacemaker implantation.

Mobitz II AV block is a type of heart block that occurs when there is a delay in the conduction of electrical impulses from the atria to the ventricles. This can cause the heart rate to slow down and can lead to symptoms such as lightheadedness, syncope, and chest pain. Mobitz II AV block is a more serious type of heart block than Mobitz I AV block. This is because in Mobitz II AV block, the PR interval is not constant, which can lead to sudden progression to complete heart block. Complete heart block is a condition in which the atria and ventricles are no longer synchronized, which can lead to a very slow heart rate and can be life-threatening. The treatment for Mobitz II AV block is permanent pacemaker implantation. This is because pacemakers can help to regulate the heart rate and prevent sudden progression to complete heart block. In this case, the patient has Mobitz II AV block with a 2:1 conduction pattern. This means that for every two atrial beats, there is only one ventricular beat. This is a serious condition, and the patient should be referred to for permanent pacemaker implantation. The other answer choices are not appropriate for this patient. Observation is not appropriate because the patient is symptomatic. Medications to increase the heart rate may be helpful in some cases, but they are not a long-term solution. Electrophysiology study is a test that can be used to diagnose and evaluate heart block, but it is not necessary in this case.

54. The answer is B. Rate control with beta-blockers.

Atrial fibrillation (AFib) is a type of arrhythmia that occurs when the heart's atria (the upper chambers of the heart) beat very fast and irregularly. This can cause the heart's ventricles (the lower chambers of the heart) to beat too fast, which can lead to symptoms such as palpitations, shortness of breath, and chest pain. The two main approaches to managing AFib are rhythm control and rate control. Rhythm control aims to restore and maintain a normal heart rhythm, usually through medications or procedures such as cardioversion. Rate control seeks to keep the heart rate within a certain range, typically between 60 and 100 beats per minute. In this case, the patient is symptomatic with AFib. Therefore, the best approach is to manage his AFib with rate control. Beta-blockers are a good choice for rate control in patients with AFib because they can slow down the heart rate and reduce the risk of complications such as stroke. The other answer choices are not appropriate for this patient. Rhythm control with cardioversion is not an appropriate option for this patient because he is symptomatic. Rate control with calcium channel blockers is not an appropriate option because calcium channel blockers can worsen heart failure. Ibutilide is a medication that can be used to convert AFib to a normal heart rhythm, but it is not appropriate for patients who are not hemodynamically stable.

55. The answer is E. All of the above.

Atrial fibrillation (AFib) is a type of arrhythmia that occurs when the heart's atria (the upper chambers of the heart) beat very fast and irregularly. This can cause the heart's ventricles (the lower chambers of the heart) to beat too fast, which can lead to symptoms such as palpitations, shortness of breath, and chest pain. The patient in this case has a number of risk factors for stroke, including chronic atrial fibrillation, rheumatic mitral stenosis, and hypertension. Therefore, he should be managed with a combination of rate control, rhythm control, and anticoagulation therapy. Rate control with beta-blockers or calcium channel blockers is important to slow down the heart rate and reduce the risk of complications such as stroke. Rhythm control with cardioversion may be used to restore a normal heart rhythm, but it is not always successful. Anticoagulation therapy with warfarin or a direct oral anticoagulant is important to reduce the risk of stroke. The other answer choices are not appropriate for this patient. Rate control with digoxin is not an appropriate option because digoxin can worsen heart failure. Rhythm control with ibutilide is not an appropriate option because ibutilide can cause serious side effects such as heart block.

56. The answer is C. Administer digoxin-specific antibody fragments.

Digitalis toxicity is a serious condition that can occur when a patient takes too much digoxin. Symptoms of digitalis toxicity can include nausea, vomiting, visual disturbances, confusion, and heart arrhythmias. The treatment for digitalis toxicity depends on the severity of the symptoms. In mild cases, the doctor may recommend discontinuing digoxin and monitoring the patient's symptoms. In more severe cases, the doctor may administer atropine intravenously or digoxin-specific antibody fragments. Digoxin-specific antibody fragments are a specific antidote for digoxin toxicity. They work by binding to digoxin in the bloodstream and preventing it from binding to its receptors in the heart. This can help to reverse the symptoms of digitalis toxicity. In this case, the patient is experiencing nausea, vomiting, and visual disturbances. These are all symptoms of digitalis toxicity. Therefore, the most appropriate next step in management is to administer digoxin-specific antibody fragments. The other answer choices are not appropriate for this patient. Discontinue digoxin and monitoring her symptoms is not an appropriate option because the patient is already experiencing symptoms of digitalis toxicity. Administering atropine intravenously may help to improve the heart rate, but it will not address the underlying cause of the toxicity. Admitting to the hospital for observation is a good option, but it is not the most appropriate next step in management.

57.The answer is A. Ivabradine.

Ivabradine is a medication that is used to treat heart failure. It works by slowing down the heart rate. This can help to improve the heart's ability to pump blood and reduce the symptoms of heart failure. In this case, the patient has a history of heart failure and an ejection fraction of 30%. He is already taking the maximum tolerated dose of beta-blockers. Therefore, the next best treatment option for this patient is ivabradine. The other answer choices are not appropriate for this patient. Digoxin is a medication that is used to treat heart failure, but it is not as effective as ivabradine in slowing down the heart rate. Ranolazine is a medication that is used to treat angina, but it is not as effective as ivabradine in treating heart failure. Hydralazine/isosorbide dinitrate is a combination medication that is used to treat heart failure, but it is not as effective as ivabradine in slowing down the heart rate. Dobutamine is a medication that is used to treat heart failure, but it is not as effective as ivabradine in improving the heart's ability to pump blood.

58.The answer is B. Norepinephrine.

Sepsis is a life-threatening condition that occurs when the body's response to an infection damages its own tissues and organs. Septic shock is a severe form of sepsis that is characterized by low blood pressure, high heart rate, and low oxygen levels. The treatment for septic shock includes fluids, antibiotics, and vasopressors. Vasopressors are medications that are used to raise blood pressure. Norepinephrine is a vasopressor that is generally preferred over dopamine as the first-line vasopressor agent in the treatment of septic shock. This is because norepinephrine is more selective for alpha-adrenergic receptors, which leads to a more pronounced increase in blood pressure. Dopamine, on the other hand, also activates beta-adrenergic receptors, which can lead to tachycardia and arrhythmias. In addition, norepinephrine has been shown to be more effective than dopamine in reducing mortality in patients with septic shock. The other answer choices are not as appropriate as norepinephrine in this case. Dopamine is a less selective vasopressor that can lead to tachycardia and arrhythmias. Epinephrine is a more potent vasopressor than norepinephrine, but it can also lead to tachycardia and arrhythmias. Vasopressin is a vasopressor that is often used in conjunction with norepinephrine, but it is not as effective as norepinephrine as a single agent. Milrinone is a medication that is used to improve cardiac function, but it is not a vasopressor.

59. The answer is A. Sodium nitroprusside.

Aortic dissection is a serious condition in which the wall of the aorta tears. This can cause blood to flow between the layers of the aorta, creating a false lumen. The false lumen can then expand and rupture, which can be fatal.The treatment for aortic dissection aims to stabilize the patient and prevent the dissection from progressing. This includes the following: Lowering blood pressure: This is done to reduce the pressure inside the aorta and prevent the dissection from expanding. Blood pressure is typically lowered to a target of 100-120 mmHg. Controlling heart rate: Heart rate is controlled to a rate of 60-80 beats per minute. This helps to reduce the workload on the heart and prevent the dissection from progressing. Preventing clot formation: Clots can form in the false lumen and block blood flow to the organs. This can be prevented by using medications such as heparin or aspirin. In the case of a type A aortic dissection, the initial treatment is to lower blood pressure with sodium nitroprusside. This is a medication that relaxes the blood vessels and lowers blood pressure. Metoprolol, verapamil, and diltiazem are also beta-blockers that can be used to lower blood pressure. However, they are not as effective as sodium nitroprusside in the acute setting. Hydralazine is a direct vasodilator that should not be used in patients with aortic dissection because it can increase the risk of aortic rupture. Once the patient's blood pressure is stabilized, other treatments may be considered, such as surgery or endovascular repair.

60. The answer is D, all of the above.

Interventions aimed at significantly lowering LDL-C levels in individuals with hypercholesterolemia can reduce the risk of cardiovascular disease, such as myocardial infarction and stroke, as well as overall mortality. This has been shown in numerous clinical trials, including the landmark Framingham Heart Study. The reason why interventions aimed at lowering LDL-C levels are so effective is because LDL cholesterol is a major risk factor for cardiovascular disease. LDL cholesterol is known as "bad" cholesterol because it can build up in the arteries and form plaques. These plaques can narrow the arteries, making it difficult for blood to flow through them. This can lead to a heart attack or stroke. By lowering LDL-C levels, interventions can help to reduce the risk of these complications. In addition, interventions can also help to improve overall cardiovascular health. For example, they can help to reduce the risk of heart failure and peripheral vascular disease.

61.The correct answer is : A. Cardiac Magnetic Resonance Imaging (MRI).

This patient's clinical presentation suggests a non–ST-elevation myocardial infarction (NSTEMI), yet her cardiac catheterization shows no obstructive coronary disease . This condition, known as myocardial infarction with no obstructive coronary artery disease (MINOCA), is more commonly seen in women. Patients with MINOCA continue to be at risk for major adverse cardiac events, thus it is crucial to investigate alternative causes for the patient's symptoms. Coronary films should be reviewed for any missed dissections, plaque erosion/disruption, emboli, or spasms. Additionally, assessing left ventricular (LV) function is a key step in evaluating such patients. In this case, the patient exhibits depressed LV function and elevated troponin levels. One possible diagnosis to consider given these findings is myocarditis, an inflammation of the myocardium that can result in impaired heart function and elevated cardiac biomarkers. Cardiac MRI is a non-invasive diagnostic tool that is particularly useful in the diagnosis of myocarditis, as it can reveal characteristic patterns of myocardial inflammation and edema. Therefore, it is the most appropriate next step to confirm the diagnosis in this patient. Other options listed, such as pulmonary function tests, abdominal ultrasound, chest X-ray, and carotid Doppler ultrasound, are less relevant in this clinical scenario as they do not directly aid in diagnosing the potential cause of this patient's symptoms.

62. Correct answer: D

Exercise stress testing is not recommended for patients with LBBB because the ECG changes associated with ischemia may be masked by the LBBB pattern. Echocardiography and coronary CTA can be used to evaluate for structural heart disease, but they cannot reliably diagnose ischemia. Cardiac catheterization is the most definitive test for diagnosing coronary artery disease, but it is invasive and should only be performed if the other noninvasive tests are inconclusive. Pharmacologic stress testing with perfusion imaging is the best diagnostic test for this patient. It is a noninvasive test that can reliably diagnose ischemia in patients with LBBB. The most common pharmacologic stress agents are dobutamine and adenosine. These agents dilate the coronary arteries and increase myocardial blood flow. If the patient has coronary artery disease, the areas of the heart that are supplied by the diseased arteries will not receive enough blood flow during stress, and this will show up on the perfusion images. LBBB causes a widening of the QRS complex on the ECG. This can make it difficult to see the ECG changes associated with ischemia. Pharmacologic stress testing with perfusion imaging is a noninvasive and accurate test for diagnosing ischemia in patients with LBBB. It is also relatively safe and well-tolerated. The most common risks of pharmacologic stress testing are mild and temporary, such as headache, flushing, and shortness of breath. More serious side effects, such as chest pain, arrhythmias, and heart attack, are rare. Patients with severe heart failure, unstable angina, or recent myocardial infarction should not undergo pharmacologic stress testing with perfusion imaging.

63.The correct answer is : C. Coronary CT Angiography.

In this patient who has atypical chest pain along with risk factors for coronary artery disease (CAD), a coronary CT angiography is a reasonable test to exclude coronary disease. It provides information about the anatomy of the coronary arteries as well as any stenoses. With its high negative predictive value, it can effectively rule out CAD in patients with an intermediate risk. If positive findings are observed, they may need to be confirmed with a coronary angiogram. Though Cardiac MRI can be used to examine the cardiac structure and function, it is not optimal in an emergency room setting due to the length of the test. Exercise stress testing can evaluate functional capacity and provoke symptoms with exercise, but this patient's chronic knee pain may limit his ability to reach 85% of the maximum predicted heart rate, thus limiting the test's diagnostic ability. Cardiac catheterization, while definitive, is invasive and usually reserved for when non-invasive tests are inconclusive or the patient is at high risk. An Echocardiogram is used mainly for assessing the heart's function and structure but is less sensitive and specific for detecting CAD. Therefore, given this patient's intermediate risk and the need for a relatively quick and reliable diagnostic method, a coronary CT angiography is the most appropriate next step.

64. Correct answer: B

The patient in this vignette has a high-risk stress test for several reasons. He achieved only 4 METs before stopping due to angina, his BP did not augment with exercise, and his ECG at 7 minutes into recovery showed diffuse ST depressions ¿2 mm and an ST elevation in aVR. These findings are highly concerning for significant coronary artery disease (CAD). Coronary angiography is the most definitive test for diagnosing CAD. It involves injecting a contrast dye into the coronary arteries and then taking X-rays to see how the blood flows through the arteries. Once the diagnosis of CAD is confirmed, coronary angiography can also be used to guide treatment, such as stenting or bypass surgery. The other options are not the best next steps in management. Admitting to the hospital for further monitoring is not necessary unless the patient is unstable or has other symptoms or findings that suggest an acute coronary syndrome. Starting beta blocker therapy is not enough to treat the underlying CAD. Ordering a nuclear stress test would not be as definitive as coronary angiography in this setting. Referring to a cardiologist for follow-up is appropriate, but the cardiologist would likely recommend coronary angiography as the next step in management.

65.The correct answer is: A. Initiate -blocker and statin.

This patient presents with a syndrome consistent with stable angina. Once CAD is confirmed, optimal medical therapy should be initiated, which includes low-dose aspirin, -blockers, and statin therapy. Coronary angiography (option B) is typically reserved for patients with refractory symptoms despite optimal medical therapy or those with high-risk stress test findings such as low ejection fraction, severe ischemia in more than one territory, or exercise-induced arrhythmias. While optimizing lipid-lowering therapy (option C) is also important, it's not the only therapy needed. Medical management of CAD requires a combination of antiplatelet, antihypertensive, and lipid-lowering medications. Coronary revascularization (option D) is usually considered after a trial of optimized medical therapy in patients with moderate to severe ischemia and in the absence of left main disease on coronary CT angiography, as per the ISCHEMIA trial. A transthoracic echocardiogram (option E) can identify structural heart disease but is not the next step in the management of this patient's CAD. Therefore, the next best step in managing this patient's CAD would be to initiate -blocker and statin therapy, hence, the correct answer is option A.

66.Correct answer: D

Access site bleeding is a known complication of cardiac catheterization. The first step in managing active hemorrhage is manual compression of the access site. This should be done by pressing firmly on the common femoral artery, just above the groin. If manual compression is not successful, surgical or percutaneous intervention may be necessary. Starting aspirin and P2Y12 inhibitor therapy would not be helpful in the acute setting, as these medications take time to work. Administering blood products empirically may be necessary if the patient is hemodynamically unstable, but this should be done in consultation with a hematologist. Ordering a CT of the abdomen may be necessary to evaluate for hemoperitoneum, but this should be done after the bleeding has been controlled.

67. Correct Answer: B. Temporarily discontinue clopidogrel and proceed with knee replacement.

Patients who undergo stent placement for managing an acute coronary syndrome are at a higher risk for stent thrombosis and recurrent myocardial infarction. In such cases, dual antiplatelet therapy is recommended for a minimum of 12 months, regardless of the stent type. However, in this case, the patient's severe knee pain necessitates a knee replacement surgery, which may increase the risk of bleeding if dual antiplatelet therapy is continued. The optimal approach would be to temporarily discontinue clopidogrel, which is part of the dual antiplatelet therapy, to permit the knee replacement surgery. The use of intravenous P2Y12 inhibitor cangrelor (option C) is not typically indicated for elective procedures and is more applicable for semi-urgent procedures in patients at high risk of stent thrombosis. Continuing dual antiplatelet therapy and delaying the knee replacement (option D) may not be feasible due to the patient's severe knee pain. Lastly, there is no role for stress testing to guide the duration of dual antiplatelet therapy (option E). Therefore, option B is the most appropriate choice in this scenario.

68. The correct answer is A.

Initiate conservative therapy with aspirin, -blocker, and nitrates as needed, followed by noninvasive risk stratification (stress testing) to help determine if coronary angiography is appropriate, provided the patient remains asymptomatic. The patient in the question is presenting with symptoms suggestive of unstable angina. However, his TIMI score is low (2), indicating a low risk of adverse events. In such cases, a conservative strategy involving optimal medical treatment, followed by noninvasive risk stratification to assess the need for coronary angiography is typically recommended. This strategy is preferred over immediate or early diagnostic angiography for low-risk patients who remain asymptomatic on medical therapy.

69. The correct answer is B.

Within 24 hours. For high-risk patients with elevated troponin, ST-segment changes, or high Global Registry of Acute Coronary Events (GRACE) score (¿140), early angiography within 24 hours is recommended[1]. Lower-risk patients (e.g., those without the above features, but with diabetes, chronic kidney disease, percutaneous coronary intervention in the past 6 months, prior coronary artery bypass grafting, or left ventricular ejection fraction ¡40%) can undergo angiography within 72 hours. Patients with refractory or recurrent angina or hemodynamic or electrical instability should undergo angiography immediately.

70.The correct answer is D. Urgent transthoracic echocardiography. The patient's presentation is suggestive of a ventricular septal defect, a mechanical complication that can develop after a myocardial infarction (MI), particularly in larger territory MIs and late presentations. The harsh holosystolic murmur at the lower sternal border, especially in the presence of a palpable systolic thrill, is pathognomonic for a ventricular septal defect. The diagnosis of a ventricular septal defect is typically made by a transthoracic echocardiogram, making option D the best next step in management. Although an increase of venous oxygen saturation between the right atrium and the pulmonary artery (PA) by right heart catheterization can be suggestive of a ventricular septal defect, it is not the first step in diagnosing this condition. Afterload reducing agents (option A) and interventions such as intra-aortic balloon pump (option C) can help decrease left to right shunting through the ventricular septal defect as a bridge to surgery but these interventions are done after the diagnosis is established. Waiting and observing for further symptoms (option E) is not appropriate in this scenario as the patient's condition requires urgent attention.

71. Answer: C. Calcium channel blocker

Vasospastic angina, also known as Prinzmetal angina, is a type of angina that is caused by a narrowing of the coronary arteries due to spasm. This spasm can be triggered by a variety of factors, including cold weather, stress, and smoking. Calcium channel blockers are the first-line therapy for vasospastic angina because they work to relax the smooth muscles in the coronary arteries, preventing spasm and widening the arteries to improve blood flow. Nitrates can also be effective in treating vasospastic angina, but they are less desirable as a first-line therapy because they can lead to nitrate tolerance, which means that they become less effective over time. Beta-blockers, particularly nonselective beta-blockers, can actually precipitate vasospasm and should therefore be avoided in patients with vasospastic angina.Aspirin should be used with caution in patients with vasospastic angina, as it can inhibit prostacyclin production at high doses, which can also precipitate vasospasm. Therefore, the correct answer is C. Calcium channel blocker.

72. The correct answer is A. Mixed—cardiogenic and distributive.

The patient's hypotension is indicative of a mixed shock state, including both cardiogenic (as evidenced by reduced cardiac output despite inotropic support due to diminished left ventricle [LV] function) and distributive (evidenced by low end of normal systemic vascular resistance but on vasopressor) shock. In pure cardiogenic shock and cardiac tamponade, we would typically expect high filling pressures. In pure distributive shock in a patient with sepsis, we would expect a normal or high cardiac output. Thus, this patient's clinical picture is most consistent with a mixed cardiogenic and distributive shock state.

73. The correct answer is B. Administer intravenous furosemide.

This patient's symptoms of heart failure exacerbation and acute kidney injury are likely due to cardiorenal syndrome, which is often driven by factors such as venous congestion. The initial treatment of choice in such cases is diuresis, which should not only improve the patient's symptoms of congestion but also likely improve her creatinine levels. Intravenous crystalloid, choice A, would likely worsen her heart failure exacerbation. Intravenous inotropic agents, choice C, are not indicated unless the patient's cardiac output is significantly reduced, which does not appear to be the case here. Renal replacement therapy, choice D, would not address the underlying cause of her symptoms, which is the heart failure exacerbation. Finally, urgent cardiac transplantation, choice E, is a drastic measure that would not be considered as an initial treatment in this scenario. Given her limited response to oral diuretics, it is possible that she is experiencing poor gut absorption due to bowel edema. Therefore, the most appropriate next step in her management is to administer intravenous furosemide or another intravenous diuretic, hence choice B is the correct answer.

74. Answer: B. Increased aortic regurgitation

One of the major risks of the intra-aortic balloon pump is that inflation during diastole can increase preexisting aortic regurgitation. This is because the inflated balloon partially obstructs the aortic valve, making it more difficult for the valve to close completely during diastole. Aortic aneurysms and aortic regurgitation are relative contraindications to balloon pump placement because they increase the risk of complications from the procedure. Therefore, the correct answer is B. Increased aortic regurgitation.

75. Answer: D. Spironolactone

Spironolactone is a mineralocorticoid receptor antagonist that is recommended for patients with HFpEF to reduce the risk of rehospitalization for HF. This is based on the results of the TOPCAT trial, which showed that spironolactone reduced the risk of HF hospitalization by 11% in patients with HFpEF. ACE inhibitors, phosphodiesterase type 5 inhibitors, and aspirin have not been shown in clinical trials to reduce the risk of HF hospitalization in patients with HFpEF. Trials of SGLT2i in HFpEF patients are ongoing. Therefore, the correct answer is D. Spironolactone.

76. answer: C.

Insert a percutaneous left ventricular assist device (eg, Impella or Tandem Heart) This patient is in cardiogenic shock due to profound acute decompensated HF. Increasing the dose of the pressor would not address his cardiogenic shock. Similarly, increasing the dose of dobutamine is unlikely to be sufficient and could risk further end-organ damage. An intra-aortic balloon pump is also unlikely to offer adequate support. A percutaneous left ventricular assist device can provide up to 5 L/min cardiac output and would be the next best step, as it can provide the necessary support to improve the patient's condition. It should be noted, however, that randomized trials supporting the use of assist devices are currently lacking, so their use should be carefully considered in the context of the patient's overall health and other treatment options.

77.Correct Answer: B. Initiate angiotensin-converting enzyme (ACE) inhibitor and -blocker; repeat transthoracic echocardiogram in 3 months.

This patient's systolic heart failure may be related to his influenza infection or his alcohol and cocaine use. Regardless of the cause, the first step in management should be to start guideline-directed medical therapy, including an ACE inhibitor and a -blocker, to promote positive left ventricle (LV) remodeling and possibly improve his EF. Additionally, he should be advised to abstain from alcohol and cocaine use, which can contribute to systolic dysfunction. A repeat transthoracic echocardiogram should be performed in 3 months to assess for recovery of function. One month may be too soon to expect significant improvement. If his LV function remains significantly impaired at that time, consideration can be given to placement of an implantable cardiac defibrillator for primary prevention of sudden cardiac death. A myocardial biopsy is not indicated in this case, as it is typically pursued in cases of hemodynamic or electrical instability when the pathology is expected to change the management. Immediate placement of a defibrillator or referral for transplant evaluation would be premature at this stage, as there is a reasonable expectation for recovery in LV function with appropriate therapy and lifestyle modifications.

78. Answer: A. Amyloidosis

Amyloidosis is a condition in which abnormal proteins are deposited in the organs and tissues of the body. This can damage the organs and tissues, including the heart. A classic ECG finding in cardiac amyloidosis is low voltages, despite thick ventricular walls on echocardiogram. This is because the amyloid deposits can interfere with the conduction of electrical signals through the heart. Sarcoidosis is another type of infiltrative cardiomyopathy, but it does not typically cause increased left ventricle (LV) wall thickness. Patients with sarcoidosis may have patchy involvement of the heart, which can lead to a variety of ECG abnormalities, but not typically low voltages. Long-standing hypertension and hypertrophic cardiomyopathy can both cause LV wall thickening, but they do not typically cause low voltages on ECG. Therefore, the most likely diagnosis in a patient with low voltages on ECG and thick ventricular walls on transthoracic echocardiogram is amyloidosis. Additional diagnostic tests for cardiac amyloidosis include:

- Serum and urine protein electrophoresis
- Quantification of serum free light chain ratio
- Possible fat pad biopsy
- Cardiac MRI

79. The correct answer is: C. Refer for mitral valve surgery.

Patients with chronic severe primary mitral regurgitation due to mitral valve prolapse should be referred for mitral valve replacement if they have an EF between 30% and 60% or a LVESD ¿40 mm, regardless of symptom status. In this case, the patient has an EF of 45% and LVESD of 42mm, meeting the criteria for referral. She has no evidence of congestion, so furosemide (Choice A) is not indicated. Since she already has an indication for mitral valve intervention, additional testing with ambulatory ECG monitoring (Choice D) or repeat echocardiography (Choice B) is not indicated. Beta-blocker therapy (Choice E) is not the primary intervention for her condition. Therefore, referral for mitral valve surgery (Choice C) is the most appropriate next step.

80. Answer: C. Stop coumadin now and bridge with unfractionated heparin.

Patients with mechanical heart valves are at high risk for thromboembolism, so it is important to maintain anticoagulation during and after surgery. Coumadin is a vitamin K antagonist that takes several days to reach its full therapeutic effect. Therefore, it is necessary to bridge patients from coumadin to heparin before surgery. Unfractionated heparin is a parenteral anticoagulant that has a rapid onset of action. It is the preferred bridging anticoagulant for patients with mechanical heart valves because it is effective and has a relatively low risk of hemorrhage. NOACs are contraindicated in patients with mechanical heart valves because they are not as effective at preventing thromboembolism in this population. Therefore, the best anticoagulation management strategy for this patient is to stop coumadin now and bridge with unfractionated heparin. The heparin should be started 24 hours before surgery and continued until the patient is back on coumadin with a therapeutic INR. The patient's INR should be checked at least 24 hours before surgery to ensure that it is within the therapeutic range. The patient's heparin dosage should be adjusted based on their INR. The patient should be monitored closely for signs of bleeding and thrombosis.

81. Answer: D. Refer for PMBV as anatomy allows.

Rheumatic mitral stenosis is a common valvular heart disease in pregnant women, and it can pose a significant risk to both the mother and the fetus. The increased cardiac output and blood volume of pregnancy can lead to decompensation of mitral stenosis and the development of heart failure. In pregnant women with moderate-to-severe mitral stenosis and heart failure, PMBV is the preferred treatment modality. PMBV is a minimally invasive procedure that can widen the mitral valve opening and improve cardiac function. It is safe and effective in pregnant women, and it can be performed at any stage of pregnancy. Surgical mitral valve replacement is a more invasive procedure and is typically reserved for pregnant women with severe mitral stenosis who do not respond to PMBV or who have other medical conditions that make PMBV high-risk. Termination of pregnancy is only recommended in pregnant women with severe mitral stenosis and heart failure who are not candidates for PMBV or surgery. Therefore, the best management strategy for this patient is to refer her for PMBV as anatomy allows. The patient's mitral valve anatomy should be assessed by echocardiography to determine if she is a candidate for PMBV. The patient's cardiac function and symptoms should be closely monitored during pregnancy. The patient should be counseled about the risks and benefits of PMBV and surgery.

82. Answer-C. Give 500 mL fluid bolus

The patient's presentation is suggestive of tamponade, which is characterized by Beck's triad (distant heart sounds, elevated jugular vein pulsation, and hypotension). The initial treatment for suspected tamponade involves volume expansion, hence the administration of a 500 mL fluid bolus. This is done while formulating a diagnostic and therapeutic plan. Performing an emergent transthoracic echocardiogram (Option A) is crucial to measure the size and location of the effusion, but it is typically done after initial fluid resuscitation. Similarly, initiating a pericardiocentesis (Option B) usually requires confirmation of the effusion's location and size, which is best done after volume expansion and echocardiogram. A pulmonary embolism CT scan (Option D) would not be the first step, as the history and physical are primarily suggestive of a pericardial effusion. A pericardial window (Option E) might be needed for posterior effusions not amenable to pericardiocentesis, but it's not the first step in management.

83.The correct answer is B. Constrictive pericarditis.

Constrictive pericarditis may occur in 1% to 2% of cases following pericarditis. In patients with tuberculosis, bacterial infections, neoplasm, or, as in this case, exposure to radiation therapy, the risk of developing constrictive pericarditis is higher. This condition occurs when there is adhesion between the visceral and parietal pericardium, resulting in a rigid pericardium limiting diastolic filling and increasing venous pressures. The limitation of venous return occurs only after the rapid filling stage following the opening of the tricuspid valve. These patients often present with the Kussmaul sign, which manifests as a jugular venous pulsation that does not decrease with inspiration. Sometimes, a pericardial knock may be present. ECG may show low voltages, but constrictive pericarditis does not cause conduction disease, which is more commonly seen with restrictive cardiomyopathy. Clinically, patients often have signs and symptoms of right-sided heart failure on examination with clear lungs. Diagnostically, a transthoracic echocardiogram reveals respirophasic variation, where during inspiration there is increased flow seen across the tricuspid valve and decreased flow across the mitral valve. Other findings include expiratory hepatic vein flow reversal. On simultaneous left and right heart catheterization, there is equalization of the ventricular end-diastolic pressures between the right and left ventricles and discordance of the right ventricular and left ventricular pressure peaks during the respiratory cycle.

84. Answer: A. Calculating his ASCVD risk score and, if ¿10%, starting an antihypertensive agent now.

The 2017 ACC/AHA blood pressure guidelines recommend starting antihypertensive therapy for adults with stage 1 hypertension (blood pressure of 130-139/80-89 mmHg) if they have clinical cardiovascular disease or a calculated ASCVD risk score of ¿10%. ASCVD risk scores are calculated using a variety of factors, including age, sex, race/ethnicity, blood pressure, cholesterol levels, smoking status, and diabetes status. For this patient, it is important to calculate his ASCVD risk score to determine whether he should start antihypertensive therapy now. If his ASCVD risk score is ¿10%, then antihypertensive therapy should be initiated. If his ASCVD risk score is ¡10%, then lifestyle changes should be recommended and his blood pressure should be monitored closely. Follow-up in 3 months is appropriate to assess his blood pressure response to lifestyle changes and to determine if antihypertensive therapy is needed. The patient should be counseled on the importance of lifestyle changes, such as weight loss, healthy diet, exercise, and smoking cessation. The patient should be instructed to monitor his blood pressure at home and to keep a record of his readings. The patient should be scheduled for follow-up in 3 months to assess his blood pressure response and to determine if antihypertensive therapy is needed.

85.The correct answer is: D. Lisinopril (ACE inhibitor)

First-line antihypertensives include ACE inhibitors, calcium channel blockers, and diuretics. However, the choice of which antihypertensive to initiate depends on the presence of comorbidities. In patients with diabetes mellitus who have microalbuminuria, it's recommended to start with an ACE inhibitor, barring any contraindications. ACE inhibitors have been shown to provide specific renal benefits in diabetic patients, such as reducing proteinuria and slowing the progression of diabetic nephropathy, hence their first-line status in this patient population. Options A, B, C, and E may also be used to manage hypertension but they are not the first-line choice in this specific clinical scenario.

86. Answer: B. Intravenous labetalol

This patient is experiencing a hypertensive emergency complicated by aortic dissection. Aortic dissection is a life-threatening condition in which the inner layer of the aorta tears, allowing blood to flow between the layers of the aorta. This can lead to rupture of the aorta and death. Hypertensive emergency is defined as a severe elevation in blood pressure (greater than 220/120 mmHg) that is associated with end-organ damage. In this patient, the aortic dissection is evidence of end-organ damage. The goal of initial management is to rapidly lower blood pressure and heart rate to reduce the risk of aortic rupture. Intravenous labetalol is a beta-blocker with alpha-blocking properties. It is the preferred initial agent for hypertensive emergency complicated by aortic dissection. Labetalol blocks both beta-adrenergic and alpha-adrenergic receptors, resulting in a decrease in heart rate, blood pressure, and systemic vascular resistance. Oral labetalol is not preferred in this setting because it takes longer to take effect. Intravenous nitroglycerin is a vasodilator that can lead to reflex tachycardia, which is undesirable in this patient. Intravenous nitroprusside and esmolol are also vasodilators, but they are not preferred over labetalol in this setting because they do not provide the same degree of heart rate control. The patient should be admitted to the intensive care unit for close monitoring and management. After initial blood pressure and heart rate control, imaging studies such as a computed tomography (CT) scan or transesophageal echocardiogram (TEE) should be performed to confirm the diagnosis of aortic dissection and determine the extent of the dissection. Once the diagnosis is confirmed, the patient should be treated with definitive therapy, such as endovascular repair or open surgery.

87. The correct answer is: A. MR angiography (MRA) of the renal arteries.

In this young patient with severe hypertension and an abdominal bruit, renal artery stenosis secondary to fibromuscular dysplasia should be strongly suspected. An MRA of the renal arteries would be a reasonable first step in her diagnostic evaluation. Although a duplex ultrasound (option B) can be considered, it cannot definitively exclude fibromuscular dysplasia. A noncontrast CT scan (option C) will not visualize the vasculature adequately. In some instances, direct visualization with renal angiography (option D) may be required if clinical suspicion remains high, but a diagnosis cannot be made noninvasively. For patients with confirmed fibromuscular dysplasia in whom BP cannot be controlled, percutaneous transluminal renal angioplasty (option E) should be considered. However, these are subsequent steps after initial diagnosis, making option A the most appropriate initial step.

88. Answer: C. Perform surgical repair of the AAA.

The guidelines for the management of AAAs are based on the size and rate of growth of the aneurysm. Surgical repair is recommended for AAAs that are 5.5 cm in size or those that are growing at a rate of ¿0.5 cm/y. In this patient, the AAA is 5.2 cm in size and has grown by 0.5 cm in the past 6 months. Therefore, the best management strategy is to perform surgical repair of the AAA. EVAR is a less invasive alternative to open surgical repair, but it is not recommended for all patients with AAAs. EVAR is typically reserved for patients who are considered to be high risk for open surgery. The patient's risk factors for cardiovascular disease should be assessed and managed. The patient should be counseled on the risks and benefits of surgical repair. The patient should be prepared for surgery and managed postoperatively.

89.The correct answer is D. Arrange for urgent surgical intervention.

This patient's physical characteristics strongly suggest Marfan syndrome, a connective tissue disorder that makes him susceptible to aortic dissection. The acute chest and back pain, diastolic murmur suggestive of aortic regurgitation, and new signs of heart failure (bilateral pulmonary rales) are concerning for a proximal aortic dissection (type A). Type A dissections are a surgical emergency and require urgent intervention. In contrast, distal aortic dissections (type B) may be managed medically by decreasing the rate of change of pressure in the aorta over time (dP/dt) and targeting a heart rate of less than 60 beats per minute and a central systolic blood pressure less than 120 mmHg. While patients with Marfan syndrome are indeed at increased risk for pneumothorax, this patient's clinical presentation is much more consistent with aortic dissection, thus necessitating urgent surgical intervention.

90. Answer: D. Place a transvenous temporary pacemaker.

This patient has a clinical syndrome concerning for early disseminated Lyme disease, which can include complete heart block due to Lyme carditis. His hemodynamic instability is a contraindication to observation alone. Atropine is a temporary treatment for bradycardia that works by blocking the vagus nerve, which slows the heart rate. However, it is not a definitive treatment for complete heart block. TEE is an imaging test that can be used to assess cardiac function and to rule out other causes of heart block, such as structural heart disease. However, it is not necessary to perform TEE before placing a temporary pacemaker in a hemodynamically unstable patient with complete heart block. Intravenous antibiotics are the definitive treatment for Lyme disease, but they may not resolve the heart block completely. Therefore, a temporary pacemaker is needed to support the patient's heart rate while the antibiotics take effect. A permanent pacemaker is not immediately indicated in this patient because the heart block may resolve following a course of antibiotics. However, if the heart block does not resolve, a permanent pacemaker may be necessary. Therefore, the best management strategy is to place a transvenous temporary pacemaker.

91. Answer: B. Multifocal atrial tachycardia

The ECG findings in this patient are consistent with multifocal atrial tachycardia (MAT). MAT is an arrhythmia characterized by an irregular rhythm with three or more distinct P-wave morphologies. It is most commonly seen in patients with chronic lung disease, such as COPD.The other answer choices are less likely. Atrial fibrillation (AF) is an arrhythmia characterized by chaotic atrial activation, resulting in the absence of distinct P waves on ECG. Atrioventricular nodal reentrant tachycardia (AVNRT) and Wolff-Parkinson-White syndrome (WPW) are arrhythmias characterized by reentry through the atrioventricular node. These arrhythmias may have a retrograde P wave on ECG, but they typically have a regular rhythm. The treatment of MAT depends on the underlying cause and the severity of the patient's symptoms. In patients with COPD, treatment of the underlying lung disease is often sufficient to resolve the MAT. In other cases, medications such as beta-blockers, calcium channel blockers, or digoxin may be used to control the heart rate. If the MAT is severe or does not respond to medical therapy, ablation of the ectopic foci may be considered.

92.The correct answer is: D. Procainamide. In patients with WPW syndrome, a rapid supraventricular tachycardia can conduct through both the atrioventricular node and the accessory pathway. If a medication is administered that purely blocks the atrioventricular node, there is a risk that the rhythm might travel exclusively down the accessory pathway and degenerate into ventricular fibrillation. For this reason, procainamide is the drug of choice as it will stabilize the atrial rhythm. Digoxin (Choice B) and adenosine (Choice A) will primarily target the atrioventricular node and are therefore contraindicated. Direct current cardioversion (Choice C) may eventually be required, but it is not emergent at this time if the patient is stable. Not treating the condition (Choice E) is not an option as it could lead to serious complications.

93. Answer: B. Long QT interval

The most likely cause of this patient's arrhythmia is an acquired long QT syndrome. Long QT syndrome is a condition in which the heart takes longer than normal to recharge between beats. This can lead to a variety of arrhythmias, including polymorphic ventricular tachycardia. Acquired long QT syndrome can be caused by a number of factors, including medications, electrolyte imbalances, and underlying medical conditions. In this patient, the most likely cause is the broad-spectrum antibiotics she is taking. Many antibiotics can prolong the QT interval, and this risk is increased in patients with other risk factors, such as female sex and hypokalemia. The other answer choices are less likely. Brugada syndrome is a rare genetic disorder that causes sudden cardiac death. It is typically associated with a different ECG pattern (type 1 Brugada pattern) and is more common in young men. Arrhythmogenic right ventricular cardiomyopathy is another rare condition that can cause sudden cardiac death. It is typically associated with monomorphic ventricular tachycardia and is more common in middle-aged men. Ischemia can cause polymorphic ventricular tachycardia, but this is more common in patients with underlying cardiovascular disease. Left bundle branch block is a conduction disorder that can be associated with ischemia, but it is not a direct cause of ventricular tachycardia. The treatment of acquired long QT syndrome is to discontinue any QT-prolonging medications and to correct any electrolyte imbalances. If the patient is hemodynamically unstable, cardioversion or defibrillation may be necessary. In some cases, medications such as beta-blockers or magnesium may be used to shorten the QT interval and prevent further arrhythmias. It is important to be aware of the medications that can prolong the QT interval and to use them with caution in patients with risk factors for long QT syndrome. It is also important to correct any electrolyte imbalances, such as hypokalemia, which can increase the risk of long QT syndrome.

94.The correct answer is: D. Perform radiofrequency ablation.

The patient presents with recurrent ventricular tachycardia, which has been occurring despite being on adequate medical therapy (-blockers, mexiletine, amiodarone). Her most recent coronary angiogram suggests that her ventricular tachycardia is not driven by ischemia. This indicates that the current medical therapy is not providing sufficient control of her arrhythmia. Option A is incorrect because simply increasing the dosage of -blockers may not address the underlying issue, as the patient's ventricular tachycardia has been recurring despite being on -blockers already. Option B is incorrect as changing mexiletine to another antiarrhythmic drug may not be effective, given that the patient's ventricular tachycardia is not responding to the current antiarrhythmic medications. Option C is incorrect as anticoagulation therapy is typically used for prevention of thromboembolic events in disorders such as atrial fibrillation or deep vein thrombosis, and it does not address the issue of recurrent ventricular tachycardia. Option E is incorrect because while implantation of a cardiac defibrillator can be useful in preventing sudden death from ventricular tachycardia, it does not treat or prevent the recurrence of the arrhythmia itself. Radiofrequency ablation (Option D) is a procedure that uses radio waves to destroy small areas of heart tissue that may be causing your heart's rhythm problems. This can be an effective therapy for recurrent ventricular tachycardia or ventricular tachycardia storm, making it the most appropriate next step in care for this patient.

95. Answer: C.

Perform transesophageal echocardiogram (TEE); if no left atrial thrombus, perform cardioversion. This patient has a tachycardia-induced cardiomyopathy, which is a reversible form of heart failure that can occur in patients with chronic tachycardia. The goal of treatment is to restore sinus rhythm and to control the heart rate. In this patient, increasing her heart rate control medications is unlikely to be sufficient to improve her left ventricular function. Starting her on anticoagulation is important to prevent thromboembolism, but it will not reverse her cardiomyopathy. Ablation of AF is a procedure that can be used to treat AF, but it is typically not recommended as a first-line therapy in patients with tachycardia-induced cardiomyopathy. Therefore, the best management strategy is to perform a TEE to rule out a left atrial thrombus. If there is no thrombus, then cardioversion can be performed to restore sinus rhythm. Once the patient is in sinus rhythm, her left ventricular function is likely to improve.

96.The correct answer is: A. Amiodarone.

The patient has new-onset AF and a history of an ischemic cardiomyopathy. Both flecainide (option B) and propafenone (option C) are class Ic antiarrhythmic drugs and can be useful for the management of AF. However, class Ic drugs are contraindicated in patients with ischemia or structural heart disease because they can potentially worsen the condition. Although amiodarone (option A) has potential side effects, it can be used to maintain sinus rhythm in patients with structural heart disease. Amiodarone is a class III antiarrhythmic drug and is often used in patients with AF, especially those with structural heart disease. It acts by prolonging the action potential duration and refractory period in all cardiac tissues, thereby making it effective for both ventricular and supraventricular arrhythmias. A nondihydropyridine calcium channel blocker such as diltiazem (option D) may be helpful for rate control but is not typically considered to be an antiarrhythmic therapy and is contraindicated in heart failure (HF) as it might cause a decrease in cardiac output, exacerbating symptoms in patients with HF. Option E, metoprolol, is a -blocker that may be used for rate control in AF but it does not typically convert AF to sinus rhythm or prevent future episodes of AF. Therefore, it is less suitable than amiodarone in this context.

97. The correct answer is: A. Andexanet alfa.

This patient presents with a life-threatening traumatic intracranial hemorrhage following a mechanical fall. She is on both aspirin and apixaban, which increases her risk of bleeding. In the acute setting, reversal of the effect of both agents would be indicated with both platelet transfusion and andexanet alfa. Andexanet alfa (option A) is a recombinant factor Xa protein that reverses the effect of factor Xa inhibitors, including apixaban. This would be the most appropriate immediate intervention to manage her condition. Option B, Idarucizumab, is a monoclonal antibody that reverses the effect of the direct thrombin inhibitor dabigatran, not a factor Xa inhibitor like apixaban. Fresh frozen plasma (option C) contains all factors in the soluble coagulation system and can be utilized to restore factor deficiencies in patients who are bleeding or are planned to undergo procedures. However, it wouldn't be as effective or rapid in reversing the effects of apixaban as andexanet alfa. Vitamin K (option D) will reverse the effects of warfarin but not a factor Xa inhibitor like apixaban. Option E, Platelet transfusion, is also necessary given her use of aspirin, which inhibits platelet function. However, this alone would not reverse the anticoagulant effect of the apixaban.

98. Answer: B.

DOACs are not indicated for stroke prevention in patients with AF and rheumatic mitral stenosis. DOACs are not indicated for stroke prevention in patients with AF and rheumatic mitral stenosis because they have not been studied in this population and may not be as effective as warfarin. Warfarin remains the only recommended oral anticoagulant for stroke prevention in patients with AF and rheumatic mitral stenosis. Patients with rheumatic mitral stenosis are at very high risk for stroke. DOACs have been shown to be effective for stroke prevention in patients with AF without rheumatic mitral stenosis. DOACs have a lower risk of intracranial hemorrhage than warfarin. DOACs require less frequent monitoring than warfarin. Overall, DOACs are not indicated for stroke prevention in patients with AF and rheumatic mitral stenosis.

99.Answer: B. Lead perforation leading to cardiac tamponade

The patient's clinical presentation is most consistent with cardiac tamponade secondary to pacemaker lead perforation. Cardiac tamponade is a condition in which fluid accumulates in the pericardium, the sac that surrounds the heart. This can put pressure on the heart and make it difficult to pump blood effectively. Pacemaker lead perforation is a complication of pacemaker implantation that can occur when the lead perforates the heart wall. This can lead to bleeding into the pericardium and cardiac tamponade. The other answer choices are less likely. Pacemaker syndrome is a condition that can occur in patients with pacemakers that are not programmed properly. It is characterized by a feeling of pulsation in the neck and a decrease in blood pressure when the patient stands up. Pacemaker-mediated tachycardia is a type of arrhythmia that can occur in patients with pacemakers. It is characterized by a rapid, irregular heart rate. Flash pulmonary edema is a condition that can occur in patients with acute heart failure. It is characterized by a sudden onset of shortness of breath and cough. The diagnosis of cardiac tamponade is based on the patient's clinical presentation and imaging studies. Echocardiography is the most useful imaging study for diagnosing cardiac tamponade. It can show the presence of pericardial fluid and the collapse of the right atrium and right ventricle during diastole. The treatment of cardiac tamponade is to remove the fluid from the pericardium. This can be done with a pericardiocentesis, which is a minimally invasive procedure. In some cases, open heart surgery may be necessary. The prevention of pacemaker lead perforation is to use caution during pacemaker implantation and to avoid implanting pacemakers in patients with thin heart walls.

100. The correct answer is: C. Plan for pacemaker system removal.

This patient's presentation suggests pacemaker infection. The presence of fever, positive blood cultures growing S. aureus, and erythema around his device site are all indicative of this. Despite not having evidence of endocarditis on TEE, the presence of staphylococcal bacteremia necessitates definitive therapy with system removal. Options A (Continue oral antibiotics) and B (Continue intravenous antibiotics) would be inadequate therapy in this case. Even though antibiotics can treat the bacteremia, they cannot completely eradicate the infection that is likely attached to the pacemaker device. Option D (Valve surgery) is not appropriate as the patient does not have evidence of endocarditis. Finally, simply increasing the dosage of the current medication (option E) would not be sufficient to treat the source of infection - the infected pacemaker system. Therefore, the most appropriate treatment plan would be to remove the pacemaker system (option C).

101. The correct answer is E. Acute pericarditis.

The patient's symptoms and ECG findings are consistent with acute pericarditis. The classic ECG findings in pericarditis include PR segment depression, which is caused by inflammation of the pericardium interfering with electrical conduction between the atria and ventricles, and ST-segment elevation, which can be caused by irritation of the epicardium, the outer layer of the heart. Electrical alternans, seen in about 50% of cases of pericarditis, is caused by the swinging of the heart within the pericardial sac, which changes the distance between the electrodes and the heart muscle.

A. Myocardial infarction: While this can cause ST-segment elevation, it would also typically cause Q waves and T-wave inversion, which are not present in this case. B. Pulmonary embolism: This condition can cause chest pain and shortness of breath, but it would not typically cause an ECG with the findings seen in this case. C.

Pneumonia: This can cause chest pain and fever, but it would not typically cause an ECG with the findings seen in this case. D. Pericardial effusion: This can cause ST-segment elevation, but it would not typically cause PR segment depression. Therefore, based on the patient's symptoms and ECG findings, acute pericarditis is the most likely diagnosis.

102. The correct answer is C. Monitor her QT interval regularly.

The patient's ECG shows a prolonged QT interval, which can increase the risk of a serious heart rhythm disorder called Torsades de Pointes (TdP). This can lead to fainting or even sudden death. Both fluoxetine and lorazepam can cause QT prolongation, but the risk is generally low and these medications are important for managing her mental health conditions.

Therefore, the most appropriate next step in management is to monitor her QT interval regularly, especially since she is taking medications that can prolong the QT interval. If her QT interval continues to increase or if she develops symptoms of TdP (such as fainting), then further action may be needed, such as adjusting her medications or considering other treatments.

The other options are less likely:

A. Discontinue fluoxetine and lorazepam immediately: This could worsen her mental health conditions and is not necessary unless her QT interval is significantly prolonged or she has symptoms of TdP. B. Start her on a beta-blocker: Beta-blockers can be used to treat some heart conditions, but they are not the first-line treatment for a prolonged QT interval without other heart conditions. D. Start her on a calcium channel blocker: Calcium channel blockers can be used to treat some heart conditions, but they are not the first-line treatment for a prolonged QT interval without other heart conditions. E. Refer her for an implantable cardioverter-defibrillator (ICD): An ICD can be used to treat serious heart rhythm disorders, but it is not necessary unless she has a very high risk of sudden cardiac death, such as a significantly prolonged QT interval with symptoms of TdP.

103. The correct answer is A. T-wave flattening or inversion.

The patient's symptoms and laboratory tests are consistent with hypokalemia, which is a common side effect of thiazide diuretics like hydrochlorothiazide. Hypokalemia can disrupt the electrical activity of the heart, leading to characteristic changes on an ECG. Early changes in hypokalemia often include T-wave flattening or slight inversion, typically seen in leads II, III, and aVF initially, and mild ST-segment depression, usually occurring in leads V5 and V6.

The other options are less likely:

B. QRS widening: This indicates prolonged conduction through the ventricles and is seen in extreme cases of hypokalemia, not typically at the level seen in this patient. C. ST-segment elevation: This is not a typical finding in hypokalemia. D. PR segment elevation: This is not a typical finding in hypokalemia. PR segment depression may occur with more severe hypokalemia. E. Absence of P waves: This is not a typical finding in hypokalemia. It is more commonly seen in atrial fibrillation or other atrial arrhythmias. Therefore, based on the patient's symptoms, laboratory tests, and the effects of hypokalemia on the ECG, T-wave flattening or inversion is the most likely ECG finding.

104. The correct answer is C. Administer intravenous calcium gluconate.

The patient's symptoms and laboratory tests are consistent with hyperkalemia, which can disrupt the electrical activity of the heart, leading to characteristic changes on an ECG such as tall peaked T waves. Hyperkalemia can be life-threatening due to the risk of cardiac arrhythmias and cardiac arrest.

The initial management of hyperkalemia involves counteracting the cardiac manifestations of hyperkalemia. Intravenous calcium gluconate is used to stabilize the cardiac membrane and reduce the risk of arrhythmias. It does not lower the potassium level but it helps to counteract the effects of hyperkalemia on the heart.

The other options are less likely: A. Administer sodium polystyrene sulfonate: This medication helps to eliminate potassium from the body and is usually used for chronic management of hyperkalemia, not for initial acute management. B. Start him on a loop diuretic: This can help to eliminate potassium from the body through the urine, but it is not the first-line treatment for acute hyperkalemia. D. Discontinue lisinopril: ACE inhibitors like lisinopril can cause hyperkalemia, so it may be appropriate to discontinue this medication. However, this is not the first-line treatment for acute hyperkalemia. E. Start him on a beta-blocker: Beta-blockers are not used in the management of hyperkalemia. Therefore, based on the patient's symptoms, laboratory tests, and the effects of hyperkalemia on the ECG, the most appropriate initial step in management is to administer intravenous calcium gluconate.

105. The correct answer is A. Prolonged QT interval.

The patient's symptoms, history of thyroidectomy (which can sometimes inadvertently result in removal or damage to the parathyroid glands leading to hypocalcemia), and laboratory tests are consistent with hypocalcemia. Hypocalcemia can disrupt the electrical activity of the heart, leading to characteristic changes on an ECG. The most consistent and characteristic ECG finding in hypocalcemia is a prolonged QT interval, which arises due to delayed ventricular repolarization caused by calcium's role in cell membrane stability. Hypocalcemia, characterized by low blood calcium levels, can leave its mark on your electrocardiogram (ECG). Recognizing these changes is crucial for prompt diagnosis and treatment. Here's a breakdown of the key findings:

The Hallmarks:

- Prolonged QT interval: This is the most consistent and characteristic ECG finding in hypocalcemia. It arises due to delayed ventricular repolarization caused by calcium's role in cell membrane stability.
- Lengthened ST segment: This often accompanies the prolonged QT interval, appearing as a subtle elevation of the baseline between the QRS complex and the T wave.
- Other potential findings:
-
- T-wave changes: T waves may be flattened or slightly inverted, initially in leads II, III, and aVF, and progress to deeper and more widespread inversion with worsening hypocalcemia.
- U waves: Prominent U waves may become evident, sometimes merging with the T wave.
- PR segment depression and QT-interval prolongation: These occur less frequently but can be seen in severe cases.
- QRS widening: In extreme cases, prolonged conduction through the ventricles can lead to widening of the QRS complex.

106. The correct answer is B. Shortened QT interval.

The patient's symptoms and laboratory tests are consistent with hypercalcemia, which is characterized by high blood calcium levels. One of the key ECG findings in hypercalcemia is a shortened QT interval. It arises due to accelerated ventricular repolarization caused by high calcium levels.

The other options are less likely:

A. Prolonged QT interval: This is a characteristic finding in hypocalcemia, not hypercalcemia. C. Prominent U waves: Prominent U waves may be seen in hypokalemia, but they are not a typical finding in hypercalcemia. D. PR segment elevation: PR segment elevation is not a typical finding in hypercalcemia. E. QRS narrowing: QRS widening may occur in extreme cases of hypocalcemia, indicating prolonged conduction through the ventricles, but it is not a typical finding in hypercalcemia. Therefore, based on the patient's symptoms, laboratory tests, and the ECG findings associated with hypercalcemia, the most likely finding on the ECG is a shortened QT interval.

107. The correct answer is C. Inferior ST-elevation myocardial infarction.

The patient's symptoms and ECG findings are consistent with an ST-elevation myocardial infarction (STEMI), a type of heart attack characterized by complete blockage of blood flow to a portion of the heart. The presence of ST elevations in leads III and aVF, which represent the inferior (or bottom) part of the heart, suggests an inferior STEMI. The ST depressions in leads I and aVL are reciprocal changes often seen in inferior STEMI. The ST depressions in leads V2 and V3 may indicate posterior myocardial ischemia, and the T-wave inversions in V4 to V6 could suggest lateral wall ischemia. This patient meets STEMI criteria and requires urgent revascularization.

The other options are less likely:

A. Anterior ST-elevation myocardial infarction: This would typically present with ST elevations in the anterior leads (V1-V4), which is not the case here. B. Pericarditis: This condition typically presents with diffuse ST elevations in multiple leads, not the localized changes seen in this patient. D. Stable angina: This condition does not typically cause ST elevations on ECG. E. Unstable angina: This condition may cause ST depressions or T wave inversions, but not the ST elevations seen in this patient. Therefore, based on the patient's symptoms and ECG findings, the most likely diagnosis is an inferior ST-elevation myocardial infarction.

108. Answer: B. Begin chest compressions and prepare for defibrillation.

This patient's presentation is consistent with ventricular tachycardia (VT) leading to cardiac arrest. The absence of a central pulse indicates that the patient is in a state of hemodynamic compromise, and immediate intervention is required.

The most appropriate initial management in this case is to begin chest compressions and prepare for defibrillation (Option B) as per the Advanced Life Support (ALS) guidelines This is because VT is a shockable rhythm, and immediate defibrillation is the treatment of choice in a pulseless patient.

Option A (Administer intravenous beta-blockers): Beta-blockers are used in the management of stable VT or in cases of long QT syndrome to prevent torsade de pointes . However, in a cardiac arrest situation, immediate life-saving measures like chest compressions and defibrillation are needed. Option C (Administer intravenous amiodarone): Amiodarone is a Class III antiarrhythmic drug that can be used in the management of VT However, it is not the first-line treatment in a cardiac arrest situation. Defibrillation is the priority in this scenario. Option D (Perform immediate DC cardioversion): While DC cardioversion is indeed used in the management of VT, in a cardiac arrest situation, chest compressions should be initiated first. This is because the patient may be in a state of low perfusion, and chest compressions can help to improve perfusion and increase the chances of successful defibrillation. Option E (Administer intravenous fluids): Intravenous fluids are not the first-line treatment in a cardiac arrest situation. They may be used as part of the post-resuscitation care to maintain adequate perfusion, but they are not the immediate priority.

109. Answer: D. Junctional supraventricular tachycardia (SVT); treat with vagal maneuvers and adenosine.

The patient's presentation is consistent with junctional supraventricular tachycardia (SVT), a narrow-complex tachycardia originating from the AV node. This diagnosis is supported by the sudden onset of palpitations, the regular rhythm, the heart rate above 120 beats per minute, and the absence of visible P waves on the ECG. The initial treatment for SVT includes vagal maneuvers followed by adenosine. Vagal maneuvers, such as the Valsalva maneuver or carotid sinus massage, can help slow the heart rate and potentially terminate the tachycardia. If these maneuvers are unsuccessful, adenosine can be administered intravenously to block AV node conduction and terminate the tachycardia.

Option A (Sinus tachycardia; treat with beta-blockers): While sinus tachycardia can be caused by stress and anxiety, it rarely goes above 120 beats per minute. Also, sinus tachycardia typically presents with visible P waves on the ECG, which are not seen in this case. Option B (Atrial flutter; treat with electrical cardioversion): Atrial flutter typically presents with a "sawtooth" pattern on the ECG, which is not described here. Also, the heart rate in atrial flutter is usually closer to 300 beats per minute. Option C (Ventricular tachycardia; treat with defibrillation): Ventricular tachycardia is a wide-complex tachycardia, whereas the question describes a narrow-complex tachycardia. Also, ventricular tachycardia is typically associated with structural heart disease, which the patient does not have. Option E (Atrial fibrillation; treat with anticoagulation): Atrial fibrillation is characterized by an irregularly irregular rhythm, which is not described in this case. Also, anticoagulation is not the initial treatment for a new onset of atrial fibrillation; rate or rhythm control would be the first step. In summary, the most likely diagnosis for this patient is junctional SVT, and the initial treatment should include vagal maneuvers followed by adenosine.

110.Answer: B. Hyperkalemia; treat with calcium gluconate, insulin and dextrose, and urgent dialysis

The patient's presentation and ECG findings are consistent with severe hyperkalemia. The sine wave pattern on the ECG is a classic sign of severe hyperkalemia, which can quickly deteriorate into ventricular fibrillation. Other ECG changes in hyperkalemia can include peaking of the T-waves, a decrease in the height of the P-wave and an increase in the PR interval, and widening of the QRS complex. The immediate treatment for severe hyperkalemia includes administration of calcium gluconate for cardioprotection, insulin and dextrose to drive potassium into the intracellular space, and urgent dialysis to decrease total body potassium. Option A (Hypokalemia; treat with oral potassium supplements): Hypokalemia would present with different ECG changes, such as flattened T waves, prominent U waves, and ST segment depression. Option C (Hypocalcemia; treat with intravenous calcium): Hypocalcemia can cause prolonged QT interval on ECG, which is not described in this case. Option D (Hypercalcemia; treat with intravenous fluids and furosemide): Hypercalcemia can cause a shortened QT interval on ECG, which is not described in this case. Option E (Hyponatremia; treat with hypertonic saline): Hyponatremia does not typically cause specific ECG changes.

111. Answer: C. Wolff-Parkinson-White (WPW) syndrome; treat with catheter ablation.

The patient's presentation and ECG findings are consistent with Wolff-Parkinson-White (WPW) syndrome. This condition is characterized by the presence of an accessory pathway that bypasses the normal electrical conduction system of the heart, leading to a shortened PR interval and a 'delta wave' on the ECG. The initial treatment for WPW syndrome is typically catheter ablation. This procedure involves the use of radiofrequency energy to destroy the accessory pathway, thereby restoring normal electrical conduction in the heart.

Option A (Atrial fibrillation; treat with electrical cardioversion): Atrial fibrillation is characterized by an irregularly irregular rhythm and absence of P waves on the ECG, which is not described in this case.

Option B (Ventricular tachycardia; treat with defibrillation): Ventricular tachycardia is a wide-complex tachycardia, whereas the question describes a narrow-complex tachycardia. Also, ventricular tachycardia is typically associated with structural heart disease, which the patient does not have. Option D (Long QT syndrome; treat with beta-blockers): Long QT syndrome is characterized by a prolonged QT interval on the ECG, which is not described in this case. Option E (Brugada syndrome; treat with an implantable cardioverter-defibrillator (ICD)): Brugada syndrome is characterized by specific ST-segment elevation in the right precordial leads (V1-V3) on the ECG, which is not described in this case.

112. Answer: C. Posterior myocardial infarction; treat with percutaneous coronary intervention (PCI).

The patient's presentation and ECG findings are consistent with an acute posterior myocardial infarction (MI). The 'upside down' ST elevation seen in the anterior leads represents what is happening in the posterior region of the heart. This is a classic sign of a posterior MI. The bradycardia could be due to the involvement of the 'pacemaker' region of the SA node, which is often supplied by the same vessels that supply the posterior region of the heart. The initial treatment for an acute MI, whether it is anterior or posterior, is typically percutaneous coronary intervention (PCI), if it can be performed in a timely manner. This procedure involves the use of a catheter to open up the blocked coronary artery and restore blood flow to the heart muscle.

Option A (Anterior myocardial infarction; treat with PCI): The ECG findings are not consistent with an anterior MI, which would show ST elevation in the anterior leads. Option B (Posterior myocardial infarction; treat with thrombolytic therapy): While thrombolytic therapy can be used in the treatment of an acute MI, PCI is generally the preferred initial treatment if it can be performed in a timely manner. Option D (Anterior myocardial infarction; treat with thrombolytic therapy): Again, the ECG findings are not consistent with an anterior MI. Option E (Pericarditis; treat with NSAIDs): Pericarditis would typically present with diffuse ST elevation and PR depression on the ECG, which is not described in this case.

113. Answer:C. Torsades de pointes; treat with intravenous magnesium

The patient's presentation and ECG findings are consistent with Torsades de pointes, a type of polymorphic ventricular tachycardia. This condition can be precipitated by a number of causes, including medications and electrolyte imbalances, and is often associated with a prolonged QT interval. The initial treatment for Torsades de pointes is typically intravenous magnesium, regardless of the patient's serum magnesium concentration. This can help to stabilize the heart's electrical activity and prevent further episodes of this potentially life-threatening arrhythmia.

Option A (Ventricular fibrillation; treat with defibrillation): Ventricular fibrillation is a life-threatening condition that requires immediate defibrillation. However, the ECG findings described in the question are more consistent with Torsades de pointes. Option B (Atrial fibrillation; treat with electrical cardioversion): Atrial fibrillation is characterized by an irregularly irregular rhythm, which is not described in this case. Option D (Supraventricular tachycardia; treat with adenosine): Supraventricular tachycardia is a narrow-complex tachycardia, whereas the question describes a polymorphic ventricular tachycardia. Option E (Sinus tachycardia; treat with beta-blockers): Sinus tachycardia is a regular tachycardia originating from the sinus node, which is not described in this case.

114. Answer:B. Atrial fibrillation; treat with rate control and anticoagulation

The patient's presentation and ECG findings are consistent with atrial fibrillation (AF). This condition is characterized by an irregularly irregular rhythm and the absence of P waves on the ECG. AF can be triggered by a number of factors, including heavy alcohol consumption, which is often referred to as 'holiday heart' syndrome. The initial treatment for AF typically involves rate control and anticoagulation. Rate control can be achieved with medications such as beta-blockers or calcium channel blockers, while anticoagulation is used to reduce the risk of stroke.

Option A (Sinus tachycardia; treat with beta-blockers): Sinus tachycardia is characterized by a regular rhythm with a rate above 100 beats per minute, which is not described in this case. Option C (Ventricular fibrillation; treat with defibrillation): Ventricular fibrillation is a life-threatening condition that requires immediate defibrillation. However, the ECG findings described in the question are more consistent with AF. Option D (Supraventricular tachycardia; treat with adenosine): Supraventricular tachycardia is a narrow-complex tachycardia with a regular rhythm, which is not described in this case. Option E (Atrial flutter; treat with electrical cardioversion): Atrial flutter is characterized by a regular rhythm with a 'sawtooth' pattern on the ECG, which is not described in this case.

115. Answer:B. Atrial flutter; treat with electrical cardioversion.

The patient's presentation and ECG findings are consistent with atrial flutter. This condition is characterized by a regular rhythm with a rate typically around 150 beats per minute and a 'seesaw' baseline on the ECG. Atrial flutter can be triggered by a number of factors, including heavy alcohol consumption.

The initial treatment for atrial flutter is typically electrical cardioversion. This procedure involves the use of a controlled electric shock to restore the heart's normal rhythm.

Option A (Atrial fibrillation; treat with rate control and anticoagulation): Atrial fibrillation is characterized by an irregularly irregular rhythm, which is not described in this case.

Option C (Ventricular tachycardia; treat with defibrillation): Ventricular tachycardia is a life-threatening condition that requires immediate defibrillation. However, the ECG findings described in the question are more consistent with atrial flutter.

Option D (Supraventricular tachycardia; treat with adenosine): Supraventricular tachycardia is a narrow-complex tachycardia with a regular rhythm, which is not described in this case.

Option E (Sinus tachycardia; treat with beta-blockers): Sinus tachycardia is characterized by a regular rhythm with a rate above 100 beats per minute, which is not described in this case.

116. Answer:C. Mobitz type 2 second-degree AV block; treat with pacemaker implantation.

The patient's presentation and ECG findings are consistent with Mobitz type 2 second-degree AV block. This condition is characterized by a constant PR interval with occasional non-conducted beats. It can lead to episodes of dizziness due to the intermittent drop in heart rate. The initial treatment for Mobitz type 2 second-degree AV block is typically pacemaker implantation. This is because this type of block can unpredictably progress to complete heart block, which can be life-threatening.

Option A (Sinus bradycardia; treat with atropine): Sinus bradycardia is characterized by a regular rhythm with a rate below 60 beats per minute, which is not described in this case. Option B (Mobitz type 1 second-degree AV block; treat with observation): Mobitz type 1 second-degree AV block, also known as Wenckebach block, is characterized by a progressively lengthening PR interval until a beat is dropped. This is not described in this case. Option D (Third-degree AV block; treat with pacemaker implantation): Third-degree AV block, or complete heart block, is characterized by a complete dissociation between the atrial and ventricular rhythms. This is not described in this case. Option E (Supraventricular tachycardia; treat with adenosine): Supraventricular tachycardia is characterized by a regular, rapid rhythm, which is not described in this case.

117. D. Third-degree AV block; treat with pacemaker implantation.

The patient's presentation and ECG findings are consistent with third-degree AV block, also known as complete heart block. This condition is characterized by a complete loss of communication between the atria and the ventricles. The atrial rate continues as normal, but the ventricular rate is slower and not associated with the P waves. The initial treatment for third-degree AV block is typically pacemaker implantation. This is because this type of block can lead to a dangerously slow heart rate, causing symptoms such as dizziness and fatigue. Option A (First-degree AV block; treat with observation): First-degree AV block is characterized by a prolonged PR interval, which is not described in this case. Option B (Mobitz type 1 second-degree AV block; treat with observation): Mobitz type 1 second-degree AV block, also known as Wenckebach block, is characterized by a progressively lengthening PR interval until a beat is dropped. This is not described in this case. Option C (Mobitz type 2 second-degree AV block; treat with pacemaker implantation): Mobitz type 2 second-degree AV block is characterized by a constant PR interval with occasional non-conducted beats. This is not described in this case. Option E (Supraventricular tachycardia; treat with adenosine): Supraventricular tachycardia is characterized by a regular, rapid rhythm, which is not described in this case.

118. Answer:D. Trifascicular block; treat with pacemaker implantation

The patient's presentation and ECG findings are consistent with trifascicular block. This condition is characterized by a block in two fascicles and a delay in the third, which is indicated by a bifascicular block with a prolonged PR interval. Trifascicular block can lead to episodes of dizziness and fainting due to the intermittent drop in heart rate. The initial treatment for trifascicular block is typically pacemaker implantation. This is because this type of block can unpredictably progress to complete heart block, which can be life-threatening.

11

Index

Made in the USA
Monee, IL
28 December 2024